Osteoporosis

Guest Editor

SOL EPSTEIN, MD

ENDOCRINOLOGY AND METABOLISM CLINICS OF NORTH AMERICA

www.endo.theclinics.com

Consulting Editor
DEREK LEROITH, MD, PhD

September 2012 • Volume 41 • Number 3

SAUNDERS an imprint of ELSEVIER, Inc.

W.B. SAUNDERS COMPANY
A Division of Elsevier Inc.

1600 John F. Kennedy Boulevard ● Suite 1800 ● Philadelphia, Pennsylvania 19103-2899

http://www.theclinics.com

ENDOCRINOLOGY AND METABOLISM CLINICS OF NORTH AMERICA Volume 41, Number 3
September 2012 ISSN 0889-8529, ISBN-13: 978-1-4557-4843-3

Editor: Pamela Hetherington

Endocrinology and Metabolism Clinics of North America (ISSN 0889-8529) is published quarterly by Elsevier Inc., 360 Park Avenue South, New York, NY 10010-1710. Months of issue are March, June, September, and December. Periodicals postage paid at New York, NY and additional mailing offices. Subscription prices are USD 313.00 per year for US individuals, USD 536.00 per year for US institutions, USD 158.00 per year for US students and residents, USD 393.00 per year for Canadian individuals, USD 656.00 per year for Canadian institutions, USD 456.00 per year for international individuals, USD 656.00 per year for international institutions, and USD 233.00 per year for international and Canadian and foreign students/residents. To receive student/resident rate, orders must be accompanied by name of affiliated institution, date of term, and the signature of program/ residency coordinator on institution letterhead. Orders will be billed at individual rate until proof of status is received. Foreign air speed delivery is included in all *Clinics* subscription prices. All prices are subject to change without notice. **POSTMASTER:** Send address changes to *Endocrinology and Metabolism Clinics of North America*, Elsevier Health Sciences Division, Subscription Customer Service, 3251 Riverport Lane, Maryland Heights, MO 63043. **Customer Service: Telephone: 1-800-654-2452** (U.S. and Canada); **1-314-447-8871** (outside U.S. and Canada). **Fax: 1-314-447-8029. E-mail: journalscustomerservice-usa@elsevier.com** (for print support); **journalsonlinesupport-usa@elsevier.com** (for online support).

Reprints. For copies of 100 or more, of articles in this publication, please contact the Commercial Rights Department, Elsevier Inc., 360 Park Avenue South, New York, NY 10010-1710; phone: (+1) 212-633-3813; fax: (+1) 212-462-1935; e-mail: reprints@elsevier.com.

Endocrinology and Metabolism Clinics of North America is covered in *MEDLINE/PubMed (Index Medicus), EMBASE/Excerpta Medica, Current Contents/Clinical Medicine, Current Contents/Life Sciences, Science Citation Index, ISI/BIOMED, BIOSIS,* and *Chemical Abstracts.*

Printed and bound by CPI Group (UK) Ltd, Croydon, CR0 4YY

Transferred to Digital Print 2012

Contributors

CONSULTING EDITOR

DEREK LEROITH, MD, PhD
Chief, Division of Endocrinology, Metabolism, and Bone Diseases, Department of Medicine, Mount Sinai School of Medicine, New York, New York

GUEST EDITOR

SOL EPSTEIN, MD, FRCP, FACP
Professor of Medicine and Geriatrics, Mount Sinai School of Medicine, New York, New York; Director of Clinical Research, Doylestown Hospital, Doylestown, Pennsylvania

AUTHORS

LAURA A.G. ARMAS, MD, MS
Assistant Professor of Medicine, Osteoporosis Research Center, Endocrine Division, Department of Internal Medicine, Creighton University Medical Center, Omaha, Nebraska

JOHN P. BILEZIKIAN, MD
Professor, Department of Medicine, College of Physicians and Surgeons, Columbia University, New York, New York

HENRY BONE, MD, FACP, FACE
Director, Michigan Bone and Mineral Clinic, and Head, Section of Endocrinology and Metabolism, St. John Hospital and Medical Center, Detroit, Michigan

NATALIE E. CUSANO, MD
Instructor, Division of Endocrinology, Department of Medicine, College of Physicians and Surgeons, Columbia University, New York, New York

DIMA L. DIAB, MD
Assistant Professor of Clinical Medicine, Division of Endocrinology, Diabetes and Metabolism, Department of Internal Medicine, Cincinnati VA Medical Center, University of Cincinnati, Cincinnati, Ohio

MATTHEW T. DRAKE, MD, PhD
Assistant Professor of Medicine, Department of Medicine, Division of Endocrinology, College of Medicine, Mayo Clinic, Rochester, Minnesota

GREGORY R. EMKEY, MD
Pennsylvania Regional Center for Arthritis & Osteoporosis Research, Wyomissing, Pennsylvania

RONALD D. EMKEY, MD, FACP, FACR
Pennsylvania Regional Center for Arthritis & Osteoporosis Research, Wyomissing, Pennsylvania

CONNY GYSEMANS, PhD
Laboratory for Clinical and Experimental Endocrinology, Catholic University Leuven (KUL), Leuven, Belgium

SUNDEEP KHOSLA, MD
Professor of Medicine and Physiology, Department of Medicine, Division of Endocrinology, College of Medicine, Mayo Clinic, Rochester, Minnesota

BENJAMIN Z. LEDER, MD
Associate Professor of Medicine, Harvard Medical School, Endocrine Unit, Massachusetts General Hospital, Boston, Massachusetts

CHANTAL MATHIEU, MD, PhD
Laboratory for Clinical and Experimental Endocrinology, Catholic University Leuven (KUL), Leuven, Belgium

PAUL D. MILLER, MD
Distinguished Clinical Professor of Medicine, University of Colorado Medical School; Medical Director, Colorado Center for Bone Research, Lakewood, Colorado

ROBERT R. RECKER, MD, MACP, FACE
Professor of Medicine, Director, Osteoporosis Research Center, Endocrine Division, Department of Internal Medicine, Creighton University Medical Center, Omaha, Nebraska

PAULA H. STERN, PhD
Professor and Vice-Chair, Department of Molecular Pharmacology and Biological Chemistry, Northwestern University Feinberg School of Medicine, Chicago, Illinois

ALEXANDER V. UIHLEIN, MD
Fellow in Endocrinology and Metabolism, Endocrine Unit, Massachusetts General Hospital, Boston, Massachusetts

ANNEMIEKE VERSTUYF, PhD
Laboratory for Clinical and Experimental Endocrinology, Catholic University Leuven (KUL), Leuven, Belgium

NELSON B. WATTS, MD
Director, Mercy Health Osteoporosis and Bone Health Services, Cincinnati, Ohio

ROBERT S. WEINSTEIN, MD
Division of Endocrinology and Metabolism, Department of Internal Medicine, Center for Osteoporosis and Metabolic Bone Diseases, The Central Arkansas Veterans Healthcare System, and the University of Arkansas for Medical Sciences, Little Rock, Arkansas

HEIDI WOLDEN-KIRK, MSc
Laboratory for Clinical and Experimental Endocrinology, Catholic University Leuven (KUL), Leuven, Belgium

TOMOHIKO YOSHIDA, MD, PhD
Assistant Professor of Clinical Cell Biology and Medicine, Division of Endocrinology, Diabetes and Metabolism, Chiba University Hospital, Chiba, Japan

Contents

> Understanding of the pathophysiology of osteoporosis has evolved to include compromised bone strength and skeletal fragility caused by several factors: (1) defects in microarchitecture of trabeculae, (2) defective intrinsic material properties of bone tissue, (3) defective repair of microdamage from normal daily activities, and (4) excessive bone remodeling rates. These factors occur in the context of age-related bone loss. Clinical studies of estrogen deprivation, antiresorptives, mechanical loading, and disuse have helped further knowledge of the factors affecting bone quality and the mechanisms that underlie them. This progress has led to several new drug targets in the treatment of osteoporosis.

> Bisphosphonates are widely used in the treatment of osteoporosis to reduce fracture risk. Because of their long retention time in bone and uncommon side effects, questions have been raised about the optimal duration of therapy. Potential side effects appear to be rare and may not be causally related. Although there is no strong science to guide "drug holidays," there appears to be some lingering antifracture benefit when treatment is stopped, so some time off treatment should be offered to most patients on long-term bisphosphonate therapy. For most patients with osteoporosis, the benefits of treatment outweigh the risks.

> As the first FDA-approved anabolic agent for osteoporosis, teriparatide has proven effective for people at highest risk of fracture, despite limitations of expense, route of delivery, and length of treatment. Available data show that combination therapy with teriparatide and antiresorptive agents does not offer a therapeutic advantage. However, treatment with an antiresorptive agent after teriparatide discontinuation is essential to prevent the ensuing bone loss. Although pretreatment with bisphosphonates may somewhat attenuate the anabolic effect of teriparatide, significant gains in bone mineral density are still achieved and prior bisphosphonate use should not dissuade clinicians from using teriparatide in select patients.

Calcium is the most abundant cation in the human body, of which approximately 99% occurs in bone, contributing to its rigidity and strength. Bone also functions as a reservoir of Ca for its role in multiple physiologic and biochemical processes. This article aims to provide a thorough understanding of the absorptive mechanisms and factors affecting these processes to enable one to better appreciate an individual's Ca needs, and to provide a rationale for correcting Ca deficiencies. An overview of Ca requirements and suggested dosing regimens is presented, with discussion of various Ca preparations and potential toxicities of Ca treatment.

Vitamin D is important for the normal development and maintenance of bone. The elucidation of the vitamin D activation pathway and the cloning of the vitamin D receptor have advanced our understanding of the actions of vitamin D on bone. The preponderance of evidence indicates that 1,25(OH)2D3 enhances bone mineralization through its effects to promote calcium and phosphate absorption. Although 1,25(OH)2D3 stimulates bone resorption in vitro, treatment in vivo can prevent bone loss and fracture through several potential mechanisms. The development of vitamin D analogues has provided new therapeutic options for increasing bone mineral density and reducing fractures.

The presence of vitamin D receptors in diverse tissues like immune cells, beta-cells in the pancreas, and cardiac myocytes has prompted research to evaluate the impact of vitamin D deficiency on the occurrence of immune diseases, diabetes, and cardiovascular disease (CVD). The expression of receptors not only in normal cells, but also in cancer cells including breast, prostate, and colon cancer cells has moreover opened the path to therapeutic exploitation of vitamin D or its metabolites and hypocalcemic structural analogues as pharmaceutical tools in the fight against chronic non-communicable diseases like diabetes, CVD, and cancer.

Glucocorticoid administration is the most common cause of secondary osteoporosis and the leading cause of nontraumatic osteonecrosis. In patients receiving long-term therapy, glucocorticoids induce fractures in 30% to 50% and osteonecrosis in 9% to 40%. This article reviews glucocorticoid-induced osteoporosis and osteonecrosis, addressing the risk factors, pathogenesis, evaluation, treatment, and uncertainties in the clinical management of these disorders.

There are a substantial number of secondary causes of osteoporosis that can be identified through appropriate evaluation. Unrecognized celiac disease, Monoclonal gamopathy of undetermined significance (MGUS), impaired renal function, diabetes mellitus, and renal tubular acidosis are just a few of the more common secondary causes of osteoporosis. Through targeted laboratory tests, many secondary causes of osteoporosis can be identified.

Osteoporosis is now recognized as a major threat to health in aging men. Morbidity and mortality, particularly following hip fracture, are substantial. Although trabecular bone loss starts in early adulthood, loss of cortical bone only seems to occur from midlife onwards. Declining bioavailable estradiol levels plays an integral role in male age-associated bone loss. Both pharmacologic and supportive care interventions are important for optimal care in men at an increased fracture risk.

Osteoanabolic agents directly stimulate bone formation to improve bone mass and skeletal microarchitecture. At present, parathyroid hormone (PTH), in the form of the full-length molecule (PTH(1–84)) and its fully active, but truncated amino-terminal fragment, PTH(1–34) (teriparatide), are the only medications that belong to the osteoanabolic class. It is appealing to consider simultaneous combination therapy with antiresorptive and osteoanabolic drugs as potentially more beneficial than monotherapy with either class, given that their mechanisms of action differ. This review focuses on the research that has been conducted on combination therapy with PTH and an antiresorptive drug.

Future directions in osteoporosis treatment will include development of medications with increasingly precise mechanistic targets, including the RANK-ligand pathway, cathepsin K inhibition, and Wnt signaling manipulation. More gains are likely with anabolics and newer antiresorptives that cause little or no suppression of formation. Optimal treatment of osteoporosis may require coordination of anabolic and antiresorptive treatment, following stimulation of bone formation with consolidation and long-term maintenance. Some well-established drugs may be useful in such regimens. We can also anticipate emphasis on cost containment using currently available drugs, especially as they become generic. Effective implementation and treatment continuity will be important themes.

ENDOCRINOLOGY AND METABOLISM CLINICS OF NORTH AMERICA

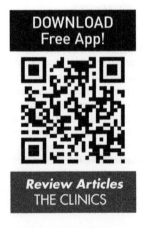

NOW AVAILABLE FOR YOUR iPhone and iPad

Foreword

Osteoporosis has always been an important endocrinologic disorder. In the past decade or so it has grown in clinical importance owing to the newer therapeutic options available to prevent bone loss from either a primary or a secondary standpoint. This has also spurred an interest in basic and clinical research on the topic. In this issue we present articles that include selected topics of the disorder.

While bisphosphonates have proven to be important therapy for the treatment of osteoporosis and prevention of fracture risk, they are not without side effects. These side effects include but perhaps are not limited to osteonecrosis of the jaw, esophageal cancer, and atrial fibrillation. Whether these side effects are off-target effects and specific to one or another of the bisphosphonates is debatable and, despite the side effects, the benefit-to-risk ratio is still strongly in favor of their widespread use. One question that is also debatable and discussed in the article by Drs Diab and Watts is the "holiday" period that has been introduced after a 5-year treatment period. The duration of the holiday period and resumption of treatment and for how long is unclear but should be considered by the practicing physician and the patient. This complex issue was the subject of an FDA report as well as articles in the *New England Journal of Medicine.*

As discussed by Drs Leder and Uilein, anabolic therapy for bone formation to treat osteoporosis has become an important modality. The use of teriparatide is perhaps the first of potentially many anabolic hormones. Its effect when given before the use of bisphosphonates is maximal but it is still effective even following bisphosphonates therapy, although some evidence does point to a blunting of the effect in the spine, the significance of which is clinically unclear. Newer regimens of "add-on" therapy for short periods of time are also being studied. Naturally, there are side effects such as dizziness, cramps, hypercalcemia, and a debatable increase in osteosarcomas. Once again the benefit-to-risk ratio is markedly in favor of teriparatide. Future therapies for use as anabolic hormones affecting bone are currently being studied.

Drs Emkey and Emkey raise the question of how much calcium supplements are needed by individuals. Initially they describe whole body calcium homeostasis and the importance of calcium for bone and focus on calcium absorption from the gastrointestinal tract, an important process involving calcium supplementation, and factors that affect calcium absorption. Most importantly, they discuss the critical issue of supplementation with vitamin D and calcium. This has become an important issue, of late, as some randomized, controlled clinical trials have suggested a link between levels of calcium intake and cardiovascular disorders. Indeed, there have been discussions regarding recommending lower levels of calcium intake for safety reasons.

Vitamin D has received lots of attention over the past decade, not only for its effects on bone but also potentially for its role in many other disorders. While the evidence for vitamin D as preventing cancer, diabetes, and other disorders are experimental and not yet confirmed, its effect on bone are convincing. However, as discussed in the article by Drs Yoshida and Stern, the exact effects of vitamin D on bone are still not fully understood. They discuss the in vitro effects of vitamin D and the clinical effects and conclude that while in vitro and in vivo effects do not always correlate, the end result in humans is enhanced bone formation.

Endocrinol Metab Clin N Am 41 (2012) ix–xi
doi:10.1016/j.ecl.2012.05.007
0889-8529/12/$ – see front matter © 2012 Elsevier Inc. All rights reserved.

endo.theclinics.com

One of the more interesting aspects of vitamin D research involves its extraskeletal effects. Drs Wolden-Kirk, Gysemans, Verstuyf, and Mathieu describe the presence of vitamin D receptors in many cells and tissues other than bone cells and that these findings suggest potential effects on diabetes (both pancreatic as well as insulin-sensitive tissues), cardiovascular disorders, immune disorders, and even cancer. Because epidemiologic studies as specific non-bone effects are being reported in increasing numbers, a true causal link has yet to be defined and thus vitamin D supplementation is primarily essential for bone health.

A major side effect of glucocorticoid use is secondary osteoporosis and avascular osteonecrosis. The induction of osteoporosis is apparently secondary to reduced osteoblasts and osteocytes, whereas in the case of osteoclasts, while their number is reduced, they have a longer half-life. Dr Weinstein in his article also describes the therapeutic options available to reduce this devastating side effect in the chronic use of glucocorticoids. Osteonecrosis most commonly occurs in the hip and may be secondary to glucocorticoid injections. While osteocyte apoptosis has been invoked as being involved in the pathogenesis, this mechanism is also not well established. It has been suggested that avoidance of intra-articular glucocorticoid injections could reduce the incidence.

Glucocorticoid therapy produces secondary osteoporosis; however, there are a number of other secondary causes, as described by Dr Miller in his article. Some of these relate to chronic kidney disease, monoclonal gammopathy and multiple myeloma, mastocytosis, gastrointestinal malabsorption syndromes including the growing procedures of bariatric surgery, diabetes and hyperparathyroidism, and very importantly, drug-induced osteoporosis. Thus physicians are urged not to accept osteoporosis as a primary postmenopausal disorder but to consider all other causes as these have different pathophysiologic mechanisms and potential therapies.

While osteoporosis is commonly seen in postmenopausal women, male osteoporosis is now considered a major issue in relation to the health of the aging man. Epidemiologic and clinical studies have shown us that low bone mass is increased in aging men with the threat of hip fractures increasing accordingly. Drs Drake and Khosla discuss that while it is commonly believed that low testosterone maybe causative, bioavailable estradiol (E2) may correlate better with the reduction in bone mass in aging men, although the causal relations between E2 and bone loss in men are unclear.

Drs Cusano and Bilezikian discuss the combination of anabolic and antiresorptive therapy for osteoporosis. The major anabolic hormone available is parathyroid hormone (1-84), specifically the 1-34 N-terminal fragment (teriparatide), a well-studied therapy now used quite widely. Studies have been performed using a combination with bisphosphonates either simultaneously or sequentially. The evidence to date is that a combination of these two medications has not proven more efficacious than teriparatide alone and thus as suggested it may be more beneficial to consider sequential therapy.

An important topic in these publications is the issue of future directions. Dr Bone has undertaken this task in his interesting article. He discusses the potential of newer calcitonin preparations, a drug that has been used extensively for pain after vertebral fractures, with a good safety record, but in its current form does not have the same fracture efficacy as other available therapies. There is tremendous excitement regarding the future use of Rank ligand inhibitors; one such therapy, Denosunab, a monoclonal antibody, reduces the Rank ligand's effect on osteoclasts and has very impressive fracture reduction at the spine, hip, and nonvertebral sites. In the future, we will hear more about other potential therapies including Cathepsin K inhibitors. Cathepsin K, a cysteine protease, mediates degradation of demineralized bone matrix and inhibition blocks this degradation but seems to allow bone formation to continue. Sclerostin blockade is an exciting new option as an anabolic agent and acts by reducing Wnt signaling, which inhibits bone resorption. In addition, there is growing interest in potential therapies that can affect the osteocytes, as this cell is a major source of sclerostin and other bone regulators. The periosteum will assume greater importance as it is now recognized that drugs that potentially enhance periosteal apposition by increasing the thickness and diameter of bone should enhance the strength of bone.

Undoubtedly, the reader will derive great benefit from this issue with a clearer understanding of the basic pathophysiology of osteoporosis and a more in-depth understanding of how the newer medications work as well as the future directions in research and clinical therapeutics. For this we owe our appreciation to Dr Sol Epstein and his colleagues for their hard work and scholarly approaches to bringing this information to the readers.

Derek LeRoith, MD, PhD
Division of Endocrinology, Metabolism, and Bone Diseases
Department of Medicine
Mount Sinai School of Medicine
One Gustave L. Levy Place
Box 1055, Altran 4-36
New York, NY 10029, USA

E-mail address:
derek.leroith@mssm.edu

Preface

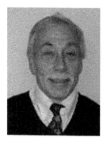

Sol Epstein, MD, FRCP, FACP
Guest Editor

This volume deals with selected topics in osteoporosis that are normally not covered extensively in textbooks, in journals, or on Internet web sites. The decisions for highlighting these topics and the disease state in general are the following. Osteoporosis is a neglected and unrecognized, and even considered an inconsequential, disease in the minds of both physicians and the public. The reason is that it is largely asymptomatic and the consequence of the disease, namely fractures, has been overshadowed by breast cancer, heart disease, and, recently, obesity and diabetes, both diseases which are inseparably linked. This despite the fact that there are 1.5 million fractures per year, that the mortality from a hip fracture can approximate anywhere from 20 to 40% in the first year, and that 50% of patients lose some form of independence after a hip fracture. The cost to the US health system is staggering in terms of billions of dollars annually and this is mirrored in other Western societies. Although the incidence of hip fracture has declined in some parts of the United States and Canada perhaps due to the advent of very effective drugs, it is increasing in almost all other parts of the world, and in China the disease will affect huge numbers of the aging population.

Thus, with this in mind, the articles were designed to provide up-to-date information on hot topics in the field. It was not meant to cover all aspects of the disease as this would have resulted in a very large volume, which would defeat the objective of having a readily accessible, readable, erudite, and informative book. The reader will notice that there are no separate articles on drug therapies such as bisphosphonates or alternatives (with the exception of anabolic and combination therapies, which are not ordinarily discussed in depth) as this has been covered so extensively recently in medical journals, web seminars, and in the lay press publications.

It was my distinct pleasure to serve as guest editor for this volume but in truth my job was made easy by the willingness, enthusiasm, and hard work demonstrated by the contributing authors. I derived a great deal of enjoyment from reading the articles, which added to my knowledge as the subjects covered were topical, academic, but also practical. I therefore would like to thank and congratulate the authors for their splendid contributions.

Endocrinol Metab Clin N Am 41 (2012) xiii–xiv
doi:10.1016/j.ecl.2012.05.006
0889-8529/12/$ – see front matter © 2012 Elsevier Inc. All rights reserved.

endo.theclinics.com

I would also like to express my appreciation to the staff at Elsevier, who supported my efforts in all ways possible.

Please enjoy this volume.

Sol Epstein, MD, FRCP, FACP
One Gustave L. Levy Place
New York, NY 10029-6574, USA

E-mail address:
bonedocsol@aol.com

Pathophysiology of Osteoporosis
New Mechanistic Insights

Laura A.G. Armas, MD, MS[a],*, Robert R. Recker, MD, MACP, FACE[b]

KEYWORDS

- Osteoporosis • Remodeling • Bone quality • Mechanical loading • Microdamage

KEY POINTS

- The definition of osteoporosis includes bone strength and fragility.
- Factors other than bone mineral density contribute to bone strength and resistance to fracture:
  - Defects in the microarchitecture of bone
  - Poor intrinsic material properties of bone
  - Defective repair of microdamage to bone
  - Excessive bone remodeling.

EPIDEMIOLOGY OF OSTEOPOROSIS

Osteoporosis, defined by the World Health Organization (WHO) as a bone mineral density (BMD) T-score less than -2.5 as measured by dual-emission x-ray absorptiometry (DXA) is a common condition affecting 30% of women and 12% of men at some point in their lifetimes. The risk of fracture increases with age, and is increasingly common in the elderly. In the United States, the lifetime risk in white women more than 50 years old is 50%.[1,2] A white man has a 6% risk of hip fracture and 16% to 25% risk of any low-trauma fracture.[3] Fractures lead to significant health care costs ($19 billion in 2005, $25.3 billion by 2025), and impairment of physical function. Hip fractures are particularly risky and are associated with high rates of disability and mortality.

OSTEOPOROSIS DEFINITION

Changing ideas regarding the pathophysiology of osteoporosis are reflected in the changing definitions of osteoporosis as noted in National Institutes of Health

The authors have no conflicts of interest.
[a] Osteoporosis Research Center, Endocrine Division, Department of Internal Medicine, Creighton University Medical Center, 601 North 30th Street, Suite 4820, Omaha, NE 68131, USA; [b] Osteoporosis Research Center, Endocrine Division, Department of Internal Medicine, Creighton University Medical Center, 601 North 30th Street, Suite 5766, Omaha, NE 68131, USA
* Corresponding author.
E-mail address: larmas@creighton.edu

Endocrinol Metab Clin N Am 41 (2012) 475–486
doi:10.1016/j.ecl.2012.04.006
0889-8529/12/$ – see front matter © 2012 Elsevier Inc. All rights reserved.

consensus conferences held in 1984 and again in 2001. In 1984, it was defined as follows: "Primary osteoporosis is an age-related disorder characterized by decreased bone mass and by increased susceptibility to fractures in the absence of other recognizable causes of bone loss."[4] In 2001 it was changed to, "Osteoporosis is defined as a skeletal disorder characterized by compromised bone strength predisposing a person to an increased risk of fracture. Bone strength primarily reflects the integration of bone density and bone quality."[5] The change in 2001 came from review of literature published between 1995 and 1999 (2449 references). Extensive research conducted since then has further emphasized that, although bone mass or density, however measured, remains an important element in the risk of fracture, it reveals only a portion of that risk in postmenopausal osteoporosis or other syndromes of excess skeletal fragility. Thus, the clinical diagnosis of osteoporosis (ie, the definition) now seems to depend on the presence of low-trauma fracture, defined as fracture resulting from trauma equal to, or less than, a fall from a standing height, excluding fractures of face, skull, or digits. In addition, although risk of fracture is inversely related to bone density, and positively related to age, most low-trauma fractures occur in patients in whom bone density is greater than the WHO threshold for a densitometric diagnosis of osteoporosis (ie, a T-score <-2.5 by DXA).[6,7]

For the purposes of this discussion, osteoporosis is defined as the presence of low-trauma fractures in women after menopause or in men of similar age in the absence of a primary diagnosis or condition that weakens the skeleton. These primary diagnoses or conditions include osteomalacia from any cause; disuse; treatment with corticosteroids or other bone-active medications; gastrointestinal diseases that cause nutritional defects or systemic inflammation; chronic kidney, lung, or liver disease; and a host of conditions/diagnoses that damage the skeleton. Although bone loss, changes in bone quality, and resultant propensity to fracture are usually referred to as osteoporosis when occurring in patients with these diagnoses, the osteoporosis occurring with them is regarded as secondary, and is not included in the definition of postmenopausal or idiopathic osteoporosis as discussed herein. This article addresses the clinical effects of increased bone remodeling rates and defects in bone quality that contribute to the development of osteoporosis. To reiterate, features of bone quality that contribute to skeletal fragility and risk of low-trauma fracture, separately or in combination, are defects in microarchitecture of trabeculae, defective intrinsic material properties of bone tissue, and defective repair of microdamage. Defective repair of microdamage results from physiologic loading occurring in normal daily life. These features occur in the context of age-related bone loss, and bone remodeling rates greater than those found in normal premenopausal women.[8–10]

CLINICAL OBSERVATIONS PERTINENT TO THE PATHOPHYSIOLOGY OF OSTEOPOROSIS
Menopause: The Effect of Estrogen Deprivation on Bone

Menopause is the cessation of menstruation, which is preceded by 1 to 2 years of gradual decline in ovarian estrogen production. It occurs in most women at approximately age 51 years.[11] Estrogen inhibits osteoclast activity and estrogen deprivation removes this inhibition and contributes to loss of bone mass. Estrogen deprivation is also associated with decreased intestinal calcium absorption and increasing urinary calcium loss, likely secondary to infusion of calcium into the plasma from the estrogen-deprived bone, and resultant reduction in parathyroid hormone levels.[12] The rapid bone loss associated with menopause is impressive. In the 5 to 7 years surrounding menopause, women lose approximately 12% of their bone mass[13]; the equivalent of 1 T-score measured by DXA. The trabecular bone is especially affected with thinning and loss of trabeculae.[8] Cortical bone also becomes porous and thin[8,14] through endosteal and intracortical resorption. Immobilization or disuse has similar effects on the skeleton, with increased endosteal bone resorption and decreased bone formation,[15,16] which suggests that estrogen deficiency at menopause affects the signaling from normal skeletal loading, and this is elaborated on later in this article. The most pronounced skeletal effect of menopause is a doubling of remodeling early, and tripling 10 to 15 years later, in healthy postmenopausal women in the absence of increased skeletal loading. These increased remodeling rates persist in most patients with fracturing osteoporosis, although 5% have depressed remodeling rates.[17]

Increased Bone Remodeling Rates

Bone remodeling definition

In adults, remodeling, or removing and replacing packets of bone, is the primary mechanism whereby bone is renewed and adapts to changes in load bearing. From an evolutionary standpoint, it is a useful process for decreasing skeleton size in the event of immobilization,[18] and for repairing microdamage or small areas of damage before they become clinically apparent.[19]

Remodeling is triggered by signaling from osteoblasts or their matured form, osteocytes, which in turn activate osteoclasts (**Fig. 1**). Osteoclasts are multinuclear cells derived from the myeloid hematopoietic cell lines and are principally involved in bone resorption. Receptor activator of nuclear factor κB ligand (RANKL), a member of the tumor necrosis factor (TNF) receptor family, is produced by osteoblasts/osteocytes and binds to the RANK receptor on osteoclast precursors. This binding is a key step in the activation of osteoclast precursors to form multinucleated cells that differentiate to form osteoclasts and activate to resorb bone. Osteoclasts attach firmly to the bone surface, sealing them to the bone surface. They then secrete hydrochloric acid to dissolve bone mineral and the enzyme, cathepsin K, to dissolve bone matrix. The osteoclasts work in packs to remove discreet volumes of bone from locations, creating what are called bone structural units. After resorption is complete, the resorbed surface is covered with mononuclear cells that prepare the surface for deposition of the reversal or cement line, a thin layer of matrix. Osteoblasts then lay down layers of bone collagen matrix, which is then mineralized. Some osteoblasts become incorporated into the bone matrix, forming osteocytes that are extensively connected with the surface of the bone and with each other by cytoplasmic processes that course through canaliculi. The osteocytes are important in cell signaling, regulating osteoblast

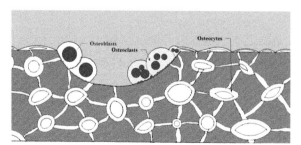

Fig. 1. The osteoclasts remove bone from discrete locations. After resorption is complete, osteoblasts lay down layers of bone collagen matrix that is then mineralized. Some osteoblasts become incorporated into the bone matrix forming osteocytes that are extensively connected with the surface of the bone and with each other by cytoplasmic processes that course through canaliculi. (*Courtesy of* Christopher D. Graeff. Copyright © 2012; used with permission.)

and osteoclast function, and sensing mechanical loading.[20,21] The number of active bone structural units created per unit time at any chosen surface locus is measured histomorphometrically as activation frequency and is a tissue-level measure of the rate of bone remodeling. This sequence of bone resorption followed by bone formation is tightly linked, ensuring that resorption is followed by formation. The net amount of bone formed is termed bone balance. A negative bone balance occurs at menopause when more bone is resorbed than is replaced, resulting in lower bone mass.

The mechanisms controlling remodeling are largely unknown, but mechanical loading has a large effect. Disuse can cause an increase in remodeling and negative bone balance and loss of bone mass, which is observed in immobilized patients and in astronauts in a microgravity environment.[22]

Remodeling Effect on Osteoporosis

Remodeling causes transient weakness at the locus of resorption but is necessary for repairing microdamage. Remodeling is also necessary as a reservoir of calcium to meet the needs of plasma calcium homeostasis. Thus, there are 2 categories of remodeling: (1) targeted remodeling to repair microdamage and preserve the mechanical integrity of the skeleton, and (2) stochastic remodeling that supports plasma calcium homeostasis. The latter, if excessive, can affect overall bone strength. It may weaken through loss of bone mass that occurs because of trabecular penetration. Once a trabecular surface is eliminated, subsequent formation cannot take place at that location. Further, an excess of bone structural units, during excessive activation of resorption and reversal phases, causes an excess of weakened loci in trabeculae and an increase in microdamage that outpaces the ability to repair. Thus, microdamage can accumulate and result in structural failure (ie, fractures). Trabecular connectivity can be lost, and/or trabeculae can grow thinner and fewer.[8,23] This is most evident at menopause when remodeling rates, activation frequency, double 12 months after the last menstrual period, and triple about 13 years later.[17] Patients with postmenopausal osteoporosis continue to maintain these high rates of bone remodeling.[17] A noninvasive assessment of remodeling rates using markers of bone resorption, such as N-terminal telopeptide (NTX) or C-telopeptides of type I collagen (CTX), and markers of bone formation such as osteocalcin, procollagen type I N-terminal propeptide (PINP), or bone-specific alkaline phosphatase (BSAP), shows similar increases in remodeling rates. A large number of studies have shown that increased remodeling activity as measured by these markers predicts fracture risk[24] and that change in remodeling markers correlates with risk, sometimes predicting fracture risk better than BMD.[25] However, this is difficult to apply clinically to the individual patient.

Reducing Excess Remodeling Reduces Fracture Risk

Some of the best evidence that decreasing remodeling rates decreases fracture risk comes from clinical trials of antiresorptives. Antiresorptive treatment of postmenopausal osteoporosis increases BMD but, more importantly, decreases remodeling rates. In a meta-analysis of 12 clinical trials of antiresorptives, Cummings and colleagues[26] found that, based on BMD gain, antiresorptive treatments were predicted to reduce fracture by 20%, but they reduced fracture by as much as 45%. Another example comes from the MORE (Multiple Outcomes of Raloxifene Evaluation) trial. The data showed that raloxifene (a selective estrogen receptor modulator) decreased vertebral fracture risk by ~40% irrespective of change in bone mass. However, 96% of the fracture risk reduction was not related to change in BMD.[27] There is considerable literature showing that change in BMD accounts for some of the antifracture effect of antiresorptive medicines,[26–30] but, although a low BMD is predictive of fracture in an untreated patient, reduction in treated patients' fracture risks has less to do with their BMD response to treatment. This means that change in BMD is not a good marker of clinical response, or lack thereof. Other aspects of bone quality, not measureable clinically, are most likely more important for mechanical integrity of bone and resistance to fracture. Experience gained in recent years suggests that the most important pathogenetic factor for excessive skeletal fragility in osteoporosis is excessive rates of nontargeted remodeling (ie, stochastic remodeling).

BONE QUALITY
Intrinsic Material Properties in Osteoporosis

Intrinsic material properties of bone tissue, an essential part of its resistance to fracture, refer to bone's resistance to bending, elasticity, toughness, and/or strength. The relationships between loads and the resultant deformation can be measured using classic engineering properties in animal models. Most of them cannot be measured clinically. New technology such as nanoindentation is being used to test microhardness in human iliac biopsy specimens, but data in humans are scarce. One abstract reported that bone biopsies taken before and after menopause had a slight decrease in microhardness measured by nanoindentation,[10] whereas nanoindentation in biopsies from men and women with osteoporosis had significantly lower microhardness than those of controls.[31] It is likely that the excessive remodeling in patients with osteoporosis has a negative effect on bone material properties (microhardness), independently of changes in bone mass. Because newly deposited osteoid matrix requires an extended period of time to become fully mineralized,[32] excessive remodeling results in a larger than normal fraction of newly formed bone that would be undermineralized and less resistant to bending. This newly formed bone is shielded from load bearing by the older, stiffer, bone tissue, resulting in increased microdamage of the older bone, and less resistance to failure (fracture).

Microarchitecture is Disrupted in Osteoporosis

The microarchitecture of bone is another essential part of the bone's resistance to fracture. It consists in the amount, size, shape, and connectivity of trabecular bone tissue as well as the amount and shape of cortical bone tissue. Osteoporosis is associated with a decrease in the number and size of trabeculae. The trabeculae also became thinner and rodlike in shape, replacing the stronger platelike morphology that is seen in nonosteoporotic bone.[8] Akhter and colleagues[8] reported a significant decrease in trabecular number and transformation to a more rodlike trabeculae during the years surrounding menopause (**Fig. 2**). The excessive remodeling present in most osteoporotics is likely to be the primary cause of these changes in microarchitecture.

All the features of osteoporosis, from an increase in remodeling to defects in microarchitecture and intrinsic material properties, do not occur in isolation. No single feature shown to be associated with skeletal fragility is responsible for the disorder. They are likely to be interactive and self-perpetuating, although the excess in nontargeted remodeling may be the most important single factor. To date, there is no biological explanation for this excess remodeling. Perhaps the most attractive hypothesis is that estrogen deprivation, and/or some other change, results in reduction of skeletal sensitivity to loading. The gross and microscopic morphology of the skeleton during bone loss at menopause and in patients with osteoporosis resembles that seen in

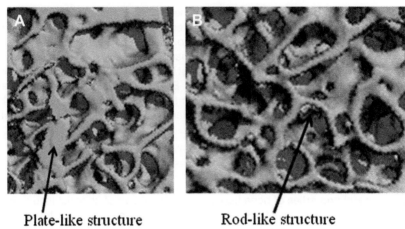

Plate-like structure   Rod-like structure

Fig. 2. As osteoporosis progresses, the trabeculae become thinner and rodlike in shape (*B*) compared with a stronger platelike morphology (*A*) that is seen in nonosteoporotic bone. Akhter and colleagues[8] provided these micro–computed tomography photomicrographs of the transformation of bone from before menopause (*A*) to directly after menopause (*B*) in women. (*Courtesy of* Mohammed P. Akhter. Copyright © 2012; used with permission.)

disuse experiments and in paralysis, which lends support to this hypothesis (discussed later).[18,33,34]

The Role of Cortical Bone in Osteoporosis

Cortical bone forms the outer shell over the skeleton. It is a compact, dense bone that makes up 80% of the weight of the skeleton. Age and menopause both cause loss of cortical bone, which occurs primarily on the endosteal (inner) surface. This bone loss is partially offset by adding bone to the periosteal (outer) surface, which increases the bones' size (diameter) and strength and helps partially compensate for the loss of bone mass.[35,36] This process occurs in both men and women, and in women is a response to estrogen deficiency at menopause.[35]

THE PATHOPHYSIOLOGY OF OSTEOPOROSIS
Mechanical Loading

Mechanical loading of the skeleton, or bearing the weight of the body through daily activity, has an influence on the development of osteoporosis. At one extreme, disuse or lack of loading, which is seen in paralysis or in astronauts in a microgravity environment, leads to profound bone loss with associated increased bone remodeling. During clinical studies of disuse, as much as 10% of bone mass can be lost, especially in the lower extremities.[37] The body is programmed to shed unnecessary unused bone. On the other extreme is overuse of bone, which is seen most commonly in athletes[38,39] or in military recruits.[40] The marked increase in skeletal loading with increased activity over a short period of time can lead to increased skeletal microdamage. In the absence of sufficient recovery time for repair, it can result in clinically apparent stress fractures. The optimal range of mechanical loading exists somewhere in between these extremes. At this level of activity, remodeling is effective in repair of microdamage, and is not excessive. Given time, the skeleton adapts to increased loading by increasing its mass and morphology to accommodate the increase in loading without allowing microdamage to accumulate and result in clinical fractures.

Microdamage

Microdamage occurs in response to repeated submaximal loading. Microdamage can transect lamellae and canaliculi and disrupt the communication of osteocytes **(Fig. 3)**.[41] Osteocytes are the most abundant cells in bone, and seem to be especially important in bones' sensing and signaling involved in adaptation to varying levels of mechanical usage and repair of microdamage. There is an extensive network of cell processes located in the canaliculi, ideally located to sense and signal responses to mechanical loads. Loading causes shifts in fluid flow in the lacunae and canaliculi.[42] When osteocyte communication is disrupted by microcracks transecting canaliculi, osteocyte apoptosis occurs, which causes signaling molecules such as RANKL and other cytokines to be transmitted to bone surfaces.[43] These signal osteoclast precursors to differentiate into osteoclasts that target the microdamage for removal and repair by osteoblasts. Increase in unrepaired microdamage beyond the level that is successfully repaired by targeted remodeling is associated with loss of stiffness and strength. Small cracks may coalesce, forming larger cracks that, if left unrepaired, result in clinically apparent fractures.[19,44] Microdamage increases with age, but does so more quickly in women,[45] leaving them potentially more vulnerable to fracture. Targeting repair of this microdamage is an area that needs more study in humans. In the authors' opinion, the most important translational research needed is investigation into the biological regulation of targeted and stochastic remodeling and the development of clinical biomarkers that accurately measure their rates independently of one another.

Genetics and Osteoporosis

There are both heritable and nonheritable factors that play a role in the development of osteoporosis and the occurrence of fragility fracture. The nonheritable factors include features of the general environment such as smoking, nutrition, other illness, and those factors more immediately related to falls such as visual acuity, neuromuscular function, and soft tissue padding. The heritable factors related to osteoporosis are those genes that determine bone mass, bone size, architecture, microarchitecture, and intrinsic properties. A large number of genes and polymorphisms have been identified as possible candidates for regulating bone mass, including transforming growth factor B1 (TGF-B1), bone morphogenic proteins (BMPs), sclerostin (SOST),

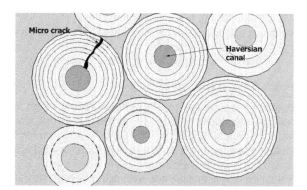

Fig. 3. Microdamage can transect lamellae and canaliculi and disrupt the communication of osteocytes. This process can trigger osteocyte apoptosis, which signals osteoclast precursors to differentiate into osteoclasts that target the microdamage for removal and repair by osteoblasts. (*Courtesy of* Christopher D. Graeff. Copyright © 2012; used with permission.)

transcription factors such as Runx2, cathepsin K, type 1 collagen (TCIRG1), chloride channel 7 (CLCN7), vitamin D receptor (VDR), and estrogen receptor (ER-α). Liu and colleagues[46] in 2003 produced a comprehensive review of candidate genes for osteoporosis. Despite the large number of genes associated with osteoporosis, many have not been replicated, nor have the mechanisms of these candidates been elucidated. The most well studied are those related to bone mass, but, as already discussed, genetic determinants of bone quality are as important as those determining bone mass. As much as 60% to 80% of peak bone mass attained at the end of growth and development is genetically determined.[47,48] Peak bone mass is especially important because it determines the amount of bone a person retains until the end of life. Some authors have aptly called osteoporosis a children's disease because bone is accrued in childhood and puberty.[49]

The genetic predisposition to osteoporosis is the end result of multiple gene polymorphisms and gene-by-environment interactions, each contributing a small amount to BMD variance. There are few instances in which a single gene is responsible for a direct effect on BMD, and most of these genes have resulted in clinically apparent bone disease. Examples include mutations of COLI, the gene for type 1 collagen, which is responsible for osteogenesis imperfecta.[50] TCIRGI, the gene coding for a subunit in the osteoclast-specific proton pump, is mutated in osteopetrosis.[51] Mutations of the SOST gene, the gene coding for sclerostin, are responsible for sclerosing bone dysplasias, van Buchem disease, and sclerosteosis.[52] Although these specific gene mutations are not necessarily related to typical postmenopausal osteoporosis seen in the clinic, polymorphisms of these genes are potential contributors to low bone mass, and may indicate potential targets for drug therapy.[53]

The G171V mutation of LRP5 (low-density lipoprotein receptor–related protein 5) is unique in that it gives rise to very high bone mass without a dysmorphic phenotype.[54] The bones are of normal shape and there is no impingement on neural structures as seen in other diseases with high bone mass. The bone is operating normally, but has higher sensitivity for adaptation to load and bone mass accrual.[55] This discovery in humans led to studies of this gene in transgenic mice and the characterization of its signaling pathway, the Wnt/B catenin system.[56] The main effect of the mutation is to cause an increased sensitivity to mechanical loading. Loading studies of these mice show increased bone formation compared with nontransgenic mice in response to a given load and its corresponding surface strain pattern. However, the bone is not immune from other influences. Ovariectomy and estrogen deprivation produced bone loss similar to that seen in nontransgenic mice.[57] In addition, disuse in transgenic mice leads to loss of bone similar to that in littermates.[58] This discovery has provided an understanding of the signaling pathway for the adaptive response to mechanical loading.

Estrogen Deficiency: Effects at the Cellular Level

Estrogen deficiency at menopause removes its inhibitory effect on osteoclasts. Increased numbers of osteoclasts and increased lifespan of the osteoclasts lead to more and deeper bone remodeling sites.[59,60] There is some compensation by the increase in osteoblastogenesis, but it is offset by early osteoblast apoptosis.[61] Both of these effects lead to trabecular thinning and perforation. However, the mechanism of the inhibitory effect on osteoclasts is not well characterized. As mentioned earlier, the morphology of bone loss at menopause resembles disuse; the increased remodeling is located on trabecular and endocortical surfaces and the inner area of the cortex. The bone loss is also located in these areas. Subperiosteal remodeling is not increased and there is preservation of the total cross-sectional area of the long bones and flat bones. This pattern resembles that seen in disuse experiments in animals and in human studies.[18,34,62] As mentioned earlier, the most attractive hypothesis for explaining the estrogen effect is therefore that it causes skeletal tissue to have optimal sensitivity to loading, and, with estrogen deprivation, that sensitivity is reduced. This loss of sensitivity to loading results in a morphologic pattern of bone loss that closely resembles disuse.

Aging and Oxidative Stress and Osteoporosis

An additional effect of estrogen withdrawal at menopause is the increased production of inflammatory cytokines, which also affect osteoblasts.[63,64] Estrogen deficiency promotes T-cell activation.[65] Activated T-cells can produce cytokines that stimulate osteoclast activity and inhibit osteoblasts. The 2 most common cytokines are TNFs and interleukin 1 (IL-1). They not only stimulate osteoclast activity, they inhibit their apoptosis, thus prolonging their life span.

Aging resulting from intracellular reactive oxidative species (ROS) is not a new concept,[66] but it has recently been proposed as a contributor to osteoporosis, especially in old age.[67] ROS are generated during fatty acid oxidation and in response to inflammatory cytokines. The body can protect itself from some of these effects, but this ability declines with age.[68] Mice studies that manipulated this ability to protect against ROS led to osteoblast and osteocyte apoptosis and decreased bone mass.[67] Estrogens and androgens can also protect against oxidative stress, which has added to understanding of the effect of aging on bone as well as the protective effects of sex steroids on this process.

SUMMARY

Study of osteoporosis has moved away from a single paradigm (bone mass) to explain fragility fractures. The myriad interactions of factors from sex steroids to ROS that have an effect on bone strength and quality and, ultimately, resistance to fracture are complex. This complexity makes the treatment of osteoporosis more complicated, but expands the possibilities for new drug targets. Several articles in this issue address the specifics of various treatment strategies.

REFERENCES

1. Cummings SR, Black DM, Nevitt MC, et al. Bone density at various sites for prediction of hip fractures. The Study of Osteoporotic Fractures Research Group. Lancet 1993;341(8837):72–5.
2. Carmona R. Bone health and osteoporosis. A report of the Surgeon General. Rockville, MD: US Department of Health and Human Services; 2004.
3. Bilezikian JP. Osteoporosis in men. J Clin Endocrinol Metab 1999;84(10):3431–4.
4. Osteoporosis. JAMA 1984;252(6):799–802.
5. NIH Consensus Development Panel on Osteoporosis Prevention, Diagnosis, and Therapy. Osteoporosis prevention, diagnosis, and therapy. JAMA 2001;285(6): 785–95.
6. Muschitz C, Patsch J, Buchinger E, et al. Prevalence of vertebral fracture in elderly men and women with osteopenia. Wien Klin Wochenschr 2009; 121(15–16):528–36.
7. Siris ES, Brenneman SK, Barrett-Connor E, et al. The effect of age and bone mineral density on the absolute, excess, and relative risk of fracture in postmenopausal women aged 50-99: results from the National Osteoporosis Risk Assessment (NORA). Osteoporos Int 2006;17(4):565–74.

8. Akhter MP, Lappe JM, Davies KM, et al. Transmenopausal changes in the trabecular bone structure. Bone 2007;41(1):111–6.

9. Stepan JJ, Burr DB, Pavo I, et al. Low bone mineral density is associated with bone microdamage accumulation in postmenopausal women with osteoporosis. Bone 2007;41(3):378–85.

10. Bala Y, Bare S, Boivin G, et al. Secondary mineralization and the microhardness of bone measured across menopause in women. J Bone Miner Res 2009;24(Suppl 1). Available at http://www.asbmr.org/Meetings/AnnualMeeting/Abstracts09.aspx. Accessed May 16, 2012.

11. McKinlay SM, Bifano NL, McKinlay JB. Smoking and age at menopause in women. Ann Intern Med 1985;103(3):350–6.

12. Heaney RP, Recker RR, Omaha PD. Menopausal changes in calcium balance performance. Nutr Rev 1983;41(3):86–9.

13. Recker R, Lappe J, Davies K, et al. Characterization of perimenopausal bone loss: a prospective study. J Bone Miner Res 2000;15(10):1965–73.

14. Cooper DM, Thomas CD, Clement JG, et al. Age-dependent change in the 3D structure of cortical porosity at the human femoral midshaft. Bone 2007;40(4):957–65.

15. Yeh JK, Liu CC, Aloia JF. Effects of exercise and immobilization on bone formation and resorption in young rats. Am J Physiol Endocrinol Metab 1993;264(2):E182–9.

16. Turner RT, Bell NH. The effects of immobilization on bone histomorphometry in rats. J Bone Miner Res 1986;1(5):399–407.

17. Recker R, Lappe J, Davies KM, et al. Bone remodeling increases substantially in the years after menopause and remains increased in older osteoporosis patients. J Bone Miner Res 2004;19(10):1628–33.

18. Jaworski Z, Liskova-Kiar M, Uhthoff H. Effect of long-term immobilisation on the pattern of bone loss in older dogs. J Bone Joint Surg Br 1980;62(1):104–10.

19. Burr DB, Turner CH, Naick P, et al. Does microdamage accumulation affect the mechanical properties of bone? J Biomech 1998;31(4):337–45.

20. Cardoso L, Herman BC, Verborgt O, et al. Osteocyte apoptosis controls activation of intracortical resorption in response to bone fatigue. J Bone Miner Res 2009;24(4):597–605.

21. Bonewald LF, Johnson ML. Osteocytes, mechanosensing and Wnt signaling. Bone 2008;42(4):606–15.

22. LeBlanc AD, Spector ER, Evans HJ, et al. Skeletal responses to space flight and the bed rest analog: a review. J Musculoskelet Neuronal Interact 2007;7(1):33–47.

23. Parfitt AM, Mathews CH, Villanueva AR, et al. Relationships between surface, volume, and thickness of iliac trabecular bone in aging and in osteoporosis. Implications for the microanatomic and cellular mechanisms of bone loss. J Clin Invest 1983;72(4):1396–409.

24. Garnero P, Sornay-Rendu E, Chapuy M, et al. Increased bone turnover in late postmenopausal women is a major determinant of osteoporosis. J Bone Miner Res 1996;11(3):337–49.

25. Riggs BL, Melton LJ 3rd, O'Fallon WM. Drug therapy for vertebral fractures in osteoporosis: evidence that decreases in bone turnover and increases in bone mass both determine antifracture efficacy. Bone 1996;18(Suppl 3):197S–201S.

26. Cummings SR, Karpf DB, Harris F, et al. Improvement in spine bone density and reduction in risk of vertebral fractures during treatment with antiresorptive drugs. Am J Med 2002;112(4):281–9.

27. Sarkar S, Mitlak BH, Wong M, et al. Relationships between bone mineral density and incident vertebral fracture risk with raloxifene therapy. J Bone Miner Res 2002;17(1):1–10.

28. Watts NB, Geusens P, Barton IP, et al. Relationship between changes in BMD and nonvertebral fracture incidence associated with risedronate: reduction in risk of nonvertebral fracture is not related to change in BMD. J Bone Miner Res 2005; 20(12):2097–104.

29. Watts NB, Cooper C, Lindsay R, et al. Relationship between changes in bone mineral density and vertebral fracture risk associated with risedronate: greater increases in bone mineral density do not relate to greater decreases in fracture risk. J Clin Densitom 2004;7(3):255–61.

30. Austin M, Yang Y, Vittinghoff E, et al. Relationship between bone mineral density changes with denosumab treatment and risk reduction for vertebral and nonvertebral fractures. J Bone Miner Res 2012;27(3):687–93.

31. Boivin G, Bala Y, Doublier A, et al. The role of mineralization and organic matrix in the microhardness of bone tissue from controls and osteoporotic patients. Bone 2008;43(3):532–8.

32. Boivin G, Meunier PJ. The mineralization of bone tissue: a forgotten dimension in osteoporosis research. Osteoporos Int 2003;14(Suppl 3):S19–24.

33. Heaney RP. Is the paradigm shifting? Bone 2003;33(4):457–65.

34. Keshawarz NM, Recker RR. Expansion of the medullary cavity at the expense of cortex in postmenopausal osteoporosis. Metab Bone Dis Relat Res 1984;5(5): 223–8.

35. Heaney RP, Barger-Lux MJ, Davies KM, et al. Bone dimensional change with age: interactions of genetic, hormonal, and body size variables. Osteoporos Int 1997; 7(5):426–31.

36. Ahlborg HG, Johnell O, Turner CH, et al. Bone loss and bone size after menopause. N Engl J Med 2003;349(4):327–34.

37. Leblanc AD, Schneider VS, Evans HJ, et al. Bone mineral loss and recovery after 17 weeks of bed rest. J Bone Miner Res 1990;5(8):843–50.

38. Matheson GO, Clement DB, McKenzie DC, et al. Stress fractures in athletes. A study of 320 cases. Am J Sports Med 1987;15(1):46–58.

39. Khan K, Brown J, Way S, et al. Overuse injuries in classical ballet. Sports Med 1995;19(5):341–57.

40. Milgrom C, Giladi M, Stein M, et al. Stress fractures in military recruits. A prospective study showing an unusually high incidence. J Bone Joint Surg Br 1985;67(5): 732–5.

41. Herman BC, Cardoso L, Majeska RJ, et al. Activation of bone remodeling after fatigue: differential response to linear microcracks and diffuse damage. Bone 2010;47(4):766–72.

42. Bonewald LF. The amazing osteocyte. J Bone Miner Res 2011;26(2):229–38.

43. Mulcahy LE, Taylor D, Lee TC, et al. RANKL and OPG activity is regulated by injury size in networks of osteocyte-like cells. Bone 2011;48(2):182–8.

44. Carter DR, Hayes WC. Compact bone fatigue damage: a microscopic examination. Clin Orthop Relat Res 1977;127(127):265–74.

45. Schaffler MB, Choi K, Milgrom C. Aging and matrix microdamage accumulation in human compact bone. Bone 1995;17(6):521–5.

46. Liu Y, Liu Y, Recker R, et al. Molecular studies of identification of genes for osteoporosis: the 2002 update. J Endocrinol 2003;177(2):147–96.

47. Pocock NA, Eisman JA, Hopper JL, et al. Genetic determinants of bone mass in adults. A twin study. J Clin Invest 1987;80(3):706–10.

48. Tylavsky FA, Bortz AD, Hancock RL, et al. Familial resemblance of radial bone mass between premenopausal mothers and their college-age daughters. Calcif Tissue Int 1989;45(5):265–72.

49. Clinical aspects of metabolic bone disease: Proceedings of the International Symposium on Clinical Aspects of Metabolic Bone Disease, Henry Ford Hospital. Detroit (MI), June 26–29, 1972. Henry Ford Hospital International Symposium. Excerpta Medica, 1973.

50. Efstathiadou Z, Tsatsoulis A, Ioannidis JPA. Association of collagen Iα 1 Sp1 polymorphism with the risk of prevalent fractures: a meta-analysis. J Bone Miner Res 2001;16(9):1586–92.

51. Sobacchi C, Vezzoni P, Reid DM, et al. Association between a polymorphism affecting an AP1 binding site in the promoter of the TCIRG1 gene and bone mass in women. Calcif Tissue Int 2004;74:35–41.

52. Uitterlinden AG, Arp PP, Paeper BW, et al. Polymorphisms in the sclerosteosis/van Buchem disease gene (SOST) region are associated with bone-mineral density in elderly whites. Am J Hum Genet 2004;75(6):1032–45.

53. Silverman SL. Sclerostin. J Osteoporos 2010;2010:941419.

54. Johnson ML, Gong G, Kimberling W, et al. Linkage of a gene causing high bone mass to human chromosome 11 (11q12-13). Am J Hum Genet 1997;60(6):1326–32.

55. Akhter MP, Wells DJ, Short SJ, et al. Bone biomechanical properties in LRP5 mutant mice. Bone 2004;35(1):162–9.

56. Mao J, Wang J, Liu B, et al. Low-density lipoprotein receptor-related protein-5 binds to Axin and regulates the canonical Wnt signaling pathway. Mol Cell 2001;7(4):801–9.

57. Johnson ML. The high bone mass family–the role of Wnt/Lrp5 signaling in the regulation of bone mass. J Musculoskelet Neuronal Interact 2004;4(2):135–8.

58. Akhter MP, Alvarez GK, Cullen DM, et al. Disuse-related decline in trabecular bone structure. Biomech Model Mechanobiol 2011;10(3):423–9.

59. Weitzmann MN, Pacifici R. The role of T lymphocytes in bone metabolism. Immunol Rev 2005;208:154–68.

60. Hughes DE, Dai A, Tiffee JC, et al. Estrogen promotes apoptosis of murine osteoclasts mediated by TGF-beta. Nat Med 1996;2(10):1132–6.

61. Kousteni S, Bellido T, Plotkin LI, et al. Nongenotropic, sex-nonspecific signaling through the estrogen or androgen receptors: dissociation from transcriptional activity. Cell 2001;104(5):719–30.

62. Uhthoff HK, Jaworski ZF. Bone loss in response to long-term immobilisation. J Bone Joint Surg Br 1978;60(3):420–9.

63. Weitzmann MN, Roggia C, Toraldo G, et al. Increased production of IL-7 uncouples bone formation from bone resorption during estrogen deficiency. J Clin Invest 2002;110(11):1643–50.

64. Gilbert L, He X, Farmer P, et al. Inhibition of osteoblast differentiation by tumor necrosis factor-alpha. Endocrinology 2000;141(11):3956–64.

65. Cenci S, Toraldo G, Weitzmann MN, et al. Estrogen deficiency induces bone loss by increasing T cell proliferation and lifespan through IFN-gamma-induced class II transactivator. Proc Natl Acad Sci U S A 2003;100(18):10405–10.

66. Giorgio M, Trinei M, Migliaccio E, et al. Hydrogen peroxide: a metabolic by-product or a common mediator of ageing signals? Nat Rev Mol Cell Biol 2007;8(9):722–8.

67. Manolagas SC. From estrogen-centric to aging and oxidative stress: a revised perspective of the pathogenesis of osteoporosis. Endocr Rev 2010;31(3):266–300.

68. Russell SJ, Kahn CR. Endocrine regulation of ageing. Nat Rev Mol Cell Biol 2007;8(9):681–91.

Bisphosphonates in the Treatment of Osteoporosis

Dima L. Diab, MD[a],*, Nelson B. Watts, MD[b]

KEYWORDS

- Bisphosphonates • Osteoporosis • Long-term safety • Osteonecrosis of the jaw
- Atypical femur fractures • Atrial fibrillation • Esophageal cancer • Drug holidays

KEY POINTS

- Bisphosphonates are popular and effective for the treatment of osteoporosis.
- Since their initial introduction in the United States in 1995, questions have been raised about their association with possible uncommon side effects such as esophageal cancer, atrial fibrillation, musculoskeletal pain, osteonecrosis of the jaw, and atypical fractures.
- Because there seems to be some lingering antifracture benefit when treatment is stopped, "drug holidays" should be offered to most patients on long-term bisphosphonate therapy.
- The duration of treatment and the length of the holiday should be individualized based on fracture risk and the binding affinity of the particular bisphosphonate used.
- The benefits of treatment outweigh the risks for most patients with osteoporosis.

INTRODUCTION

Bisphosphonates are agents that share a common chemical structure, characterized by 2 phosphonic acids joined to a carbon along with 2 side chains designated R^1 and R^2, which influence the binding affinity and antiresorptive potency of the agent (**Fig. 1**).[1] This structure causes these compounds to bind avidly to hydroxyapatite crystals on bone surfaces, particularly at sites of active bone remodeling, which resulted in the use of these agents initially for nuclear bone scintigraphy. In the late 1960s, they began to be used as therapeutic agents for the treatment of a variety of metabolic bone diseases such as heterotopic ossification, fibrous dysplasia, osteogenesis imperfecta, Paget disease of bone, hypercalcemia, bone loss, destructive arthropathy, and skeletal involvement with malignancy.

[a] Division of Endocrinology, Diabetes and Metabolism, Department of Internal Medicine, Cincinnati VA Medical Center, University of Cincinnati, 3125 Eden Avenue, PO Box 670547, Cincinnati, OH 45267, USA; [b] Mercy Health Osteoporosis and Bone Health Services, 4760 E. Galbraith Road, Cincinnati, OH 45236, USA
* Corresponding author.
E-mail address: dima.diab@uc.edu

Endocrinol Metab Clin N Am 41 (2012) 487–506
doi:10.1016/j.ecl.2012.04.007
0889-8529/12/$ – see front matter © 2012 Elsevier Inc. All rights reserved.

endo.theclinics.com

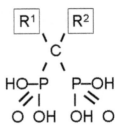

Fig. 1. Structure of pyrophosphate and germinal bisphosphonates. (*From* Watts NB. Bisphosphonate treatment for postmenopausal osteoporosis. In: Avioli L, editor. The osteoporotic syndrome. 4th edition. San Diego: Academic Press; 2000; with permission.)

PHARMACOLOGY, PHARMACOKINETICS, AND MECHANISM OF ACTION

Bisphosphonates can be taken by mouth or given intravenously. These agents are poorly absorbed when taken orally; less than 1% of an orally administered dose is absorbed under ideal conditions, and little or none under less than ideal situations. Therefore, they must be taken after a prolonged fast, with water only, followed by at least 30 minutes with nothing else by mouth to allow for adequate absorption. Atelvia, which is risedronate in a delayed-release formulation, is taken immediately following breakfast. About half of the absorbed dose binds to bone surfaces, mostly avidly at sites of active remodeling, and the other half is rapidly excreted by the kidneys.

The 4 bisphosphonates currently in clinical use for the treatment of osteoporosis are nitrogen-containing and differ in the strength for binding to bone (**Table 1**). The rank order for binding affinity is zoledronate > alendronate > ibandronate > risedronate.[2] Higher-affinity bisphosphonates will bind avidly to the bone surface but will spread through bone more slowly, whereas lower-affinity agents with be distributed more widely through the bone but have a shorter residence time in bone if treatment is stopped.[2]

Bisphosphonates reduce osteoclastic bone resorption by entering the osteoclast and causing loss or resorptive function as well as accelerating apoptosis by interfering with protein prenylation via inhibiting farnesyl pyrophosphate synthase, an enzyme in the HMG-CoA reductase pathway.[2,3] The rank order of potency for inhibiting farnesyl pyrophosphate synthase is zoledronate > risedronate >> ibandronate > alendronate.[2,3] The net result is a rapid and substantial decrease in bone turnover markers that is dose

Table 1 Structures of some of the bisphosphonates in clinical use		
	R¹	R²
Non–Nitrogen-Containing Compounds		
Etidronate	OH	CH_3
Clodronate	Cl	Cl
Tiludronate	H	SC_6H_3Cl
Nitrogen-Containing Compounds		
Pamidronate	OH	$CH_2CH_2NH_2$
Alendronate	OH	$CH_2CH_2CH_2NH_2$
Risedronate	OH	CH_2-3-pyridinyl
Zoledronate	OH	$CH_2C_3N_2H_3$

From Watts NB. Bisphosphonate treatment for postmenopausal osteoporosis. In: Avioli L, editor. The osteoporotic syndrome. 4th edition. San Diego: Academic Press; 2000; with permission.

dependent and compound dependent, with a maximum effect in 3 to 6 months. With continued treatment, this effect is maintained in a new steady state for 10 years and perhaps longer.[4,5] Treatment with bisphosphonates also results in a modest increase in bone mineral density (BMD).

The unique profile of binding affinity and antiresorptive potency for each bisphosphonate most likely results in clinically meaningful differences in the speed of onset and offset of effect, the degree of reduction of bone turnover, uptake in cortical versus trabecular bone, and types of antifracture effect (vertebral versus nonvertebral).

CLINICAL TRIALS AND EXPERIENCE WITH BISPHOSPHONATES

Bisphosphonates are currently approved for prevention of bone loss through aging, estrogen deficiency, and glucocorticoid use, and for prevention of fractures in women with postmenopausal osteoporosis and in women and men with glucocorticoid-induced osteoporosis. The first bisphosphonate approved in the United States for treatment of osteoporosis was alendronate (1995), followed by risedronate (approved for Paget disease in 1998 and for osteoporosis in 2000), zoledronic acid (approved for skeletal complications of malignancy in 2001 and for osteoporosis in 2007), and ibandronate (approved for osteoporosis in 2005). The placebo-controlled trials of these agents that prove antifracture efficacy are summarized in **Table 2**. Of all the agents approved in the United States for use in osteoporosis, only alendronate, risedronate, and zoledronate have evidence for reducing the risk of hip fractures. These same 3 agents have also been shown to reduce the risk of nonvertebral fractures as a composite end point, establishing these compounds as the agents of choice for most patients with osteoporosis. The current indications for these agents and the available dosing forms are shown in **Tables 3** and **4**, respectively.

SIDE EFFECTS AND SAFETY ISSUES
Gastrointestinal Side Effects and Esophageal Cancer

Gastrointestinal side effects, which may irritate the esophagus and cause reflux, esophagitis, or esophageal ulcers, have been the primary concern for patients taking oral bisphosphonates. The incidence of these side effects is low if proper instructions for administration are followed; bisphosphonates should not be given orally to patients who cannot remain upright, who have active upper gastrointestinal symptoms, or have delayed esophageal emptying, such as patients with strictures, achalasia, or severe dysmotility.

Between 1995 and 2009, 34 cases of esophageal cancer among patients using oral bisphosphonates in the United States were reported to the Food and Drug Administration (FDA).[6,7] In addition, 34 cases of esophageal cancer from Europe and Japan were reported in patients after receiving oral bisphosphonate therapy.[6,7] However,

Table 2			
Placebo-controlled studies with bisphosphonates that show antifracture efficacy			
Bisphosphonate	**Vertebral Fractures**	**Hip Fracture**	**Nonvertebral Fracture**
Alendronate	Black, Cummings	Black	Black, Pols
Risedronate	Harris, Reginster	McClung	Harris, McClung
Ibandronate	Chesnut	No effect demonstrated	
Zoledronate	Black[38]	Black[38]	Black[38]

From Watts NB, Diab DL. Long-term use of bisphosphonates in osteoporosis. J Clin Endocrinol Metab 2010;95:1557. Copyright 2010, The Endocrine Society; with permission.

Table 3
FDA-approved indications for nitrogen-containing bisphosphonates

Drug	Postmenopausal Osteoporosis		Glucocorticoid-Induced Osteoporosis		Men
	Prevention	Treatment	Prevention	Treatment	
Alendronate (Fosamax)	√	√	—	√	√
Risedronate (Actonel)	√	√	√	√	√
Risedronate (Atelvia)	—	√	—	—	—
Ibandronate (Boniva)	√	√	—	—	—
Zoledronate (Reclast)	√	√	√	√	√

information regarding risk factors for esophageal cancer in this population and the expected incidence of esophageal cancer in this age group was lacking.[8] Furthermore, the usefulness of these observations is limited by the lack of a control group, which made it impossible to assess the association between esophageal cancer and bisphosphonate use.[9] Lastly, the median time from use to diagnosis was brief (1–2 years), and hence not consistent with a causal relationship.[10,11]

One report using data from European national registries and another from the United States Medicare database have not shown an increased risk of esophageal cancer among individuals who were receiving oral bisphosphonates in comparison with those who were not.[12,13]

In a recent case-control cohort study of more than 40,000 bisphosphonate users in a comparison with a similar number of age-matched and gender-matched controls in the UK General Practice Research Database, there was no difference between the 2 cohorts in the incidence of esophageal cancer after a mean follow-up time of about 4.5 years.[14] All of the bisphosphonate cohort and 9% of the control cohort received at least one prescription for oral bisphosphonates during follow-up. There was also no increased risk of other types of cancer.[15]

Another recent large nested case-control study of more than 15,000 adults with gastrointestinal cancer in a comparison with approximately 78,000 matched controls found a doubling of the risk of esophageal cancer among patients who had 10 or more prescriptions for bisphosphonates or who had taken these drugs over 3 years, compared with patients not prescribed bisphosphonates (about 30% vs 17%).[16] Specifically, of nearly 3000 patients with esophageal cancer, 2864 patients did not receive any bisphosphonate prescription and 90 subjects received at least one. Furthermore, those who received at least one bisphosphonate prescription had an

Table 4
Available dosing forms of nitrogen-containing bisphosphonates in the United States

Drug	Oral Dosing (mg)			Intravenous
	Daily	Weekly	Monthly	
Alendronate (Fosamax)	5 & 10	35 & 70	—	—
Risedronate (Actonel)	5	35	150	—
Risedronate (Atelvia)[a]	—	35	—	—
Ibandronate (Boniva)	2.5	—	150	3 mg every 3 mo
Zoledronate (Reclast)	—	—	—	5 mg/y

[a] Atelvia is risedronate in a delayed-release formulation; it is taken once weekly in the morning immediately following breakfast.

increased risk of esophageal cancer compared with patients who did not receive any (adjusted relative risk 1.30, 95% confidence interval [CI] 1.02–1.66). In this study, the risk of gastric or colorectal cancers was not increased after prescription of bisphosphonates. The mean observation period was 7.5 years. This study estimated that the incidence of esophageal cancer in Europe and North America in people aged 60 to 79 years, which is typically 1 per 1000 population over 5 years in both sexes combined, will increase to about 2 per 1000 with 5 years' use of oral bisphosphonates.

In summary, the data linking the use of bisphosphonates with an increased risk of esophageal cancer are conflicting, which may be due to differences in study design and duration of follow-up. The theoretical rationale for a possible association of esophageal cancer and bisphosphonate use arises from the fact that this class of medications can cause erosive esophagitis, and esophageal biopsies of patients on alendronate have revealed crystalline material similar to this drug as well as persistent mucosal abnormalities consistent with chronic inflammation.[17,18] Although further studies looking at the potential risk for carcinogenicity, particularly the association between esophageal cancer and different types and formulations of bisphosphonates, are clearly needed, the current data do not support a causal association between oral bisphosphonates and esophageal carcinoma. Nevertheless, it may be prudent to avoid prescribing oral bisphosphonates to patients with known esophageal abnormality such as Barrett esophagus. At this time, the FDA's review is ongoing and the agency has not concluded that patients taking oral bisphosphonate drugs have an increased risk of esophageal cancer, which is a rare cancer, especially in women. The FDA believes that the benefits of oral bisphosphonate drugs in reducing the risk of serious fractures in people with osteoporosis continue to outweigh their potential risks.[19]

Acute-Phase Reaction

Intravenous and high-dose oral bisphosphonates are often associated with an acute-phase reaction within 24 to 72 hours of the infusion, characterized by fever, myalgias, and arthralgias.[20–22] Treatment with antipyretic agents generally improves the symptoms, and these rarely recur with subsequent infusions.

Hypocalcemia

Hypocalcemia may occur with bisphosphonate use, but is usually mild and not clinically important except in patients with hypoparathyroidism, calcium deficiency, or vitamin D deficiency.[23] Disturbances of mineral metabolism should be corrected before initiating bisphosphonate therapy.

Ocular Side Effects

Ocular side effects including pain, blurred vision, conjunctivitis, iritis, uveitis, and scleritis have been reported with most bisphosphonates (more with intravenous than oral agents), but these complications are a rare occurrence.[24,25]

Renal Safety

The only route of elimination for bisphosphonates is renal excretion. Little information is available on dosing in patients who have impaired renal function, and renal toxicity may occur with rapid intravenous administration.

Bisphosphonates in the treatment of osteoporosis have not been associated with renal adverse events in patients with creatinine clearance (CCr) above 30 to 35 mL/min, but the FDA product labeling states that it is not recommended to use these medications in patients with CCr below 30 (risedronate, ibandronate) to 35 (alendronate, zoledronate) mL/min, because of the lack of data for this population,[26,27] although it may be safe in some cases.[28,29] In fact, the revised zoledronate label (August 2011) states that zoledronate is contraindicated in patients with creatinine clearance less than 35 mL/min or in patients with evidence of acute renal impairment.

However, 2 post hoc studies of the pivotal risedronate and alendronate registration trials revealed that the approved doses of risedronate and alendronate did not alter renal function in postmenopausal women with CCr as low as 15 mL/min as estimated by the Cockcroft-Gault formula, although none of these patients had intrinsic kidney disease or a CCr less than 15 mL/min.[28,29] Compared with placebo, there was no difference in the incidence of adverse events in the treatment groups regardless of renal function, and therapy was as effective in terms of preservation of BMD and reduction of fractures.

Studies of intravenous (IV) ibandronate and zoledronate showed that these agents are safe in patients with CCr greater than 30 to 35 mL/min if administered correctly.[30–33] Although transient changes in renal function may occur after receiving IV zoledronate, renal function returns to baseline in the long term.[34] Adverse effects on renal function seem to be primarily related to the peak concentration, which is determined by the dose of the agent and the infusion rate. Before each zoledronate infusion, clinicians should measure serum creatinine and make sure that patients are adequately hydrated. IV zoledronate should be infused over a period of at least 15 minutes. Furthermore, IV zoledronate labeling indicates that it should be used with caution in the presence of other nephrotoxic drugs.

In summary, bisphosphonates appear to be safe and effective in individuals with mild or moderate renal impairment, and no dosage adjustment is recommended for these patients. It also appears that the risk of kidney damage in patients receiving IV bisphosphonates is very small, and can be reduced further by adequate hydration and the use of longer infusion times. However, there is a dearth of data on use of bisphosphonates in patients with severe renal impairment and in end-stage renal disease (ESRD).[35] Despite the lack of evidence regarding the use of bisphosphonates in patients with stage 5 chronic kidney disease (CCr <15 mL/min) and ESRD, one approach based on the known pharmacokinetics of bisphosphonates in subjects with normal renal function[36] suggests treating patients suffering fragility fractures with half the usual dose of bisphosphonates for up to 3 years, but only after the diagnosis of osteoporosis is confirmed by a bone biopsy because patients with ESRD may have fractures attributable to other forms of metabolic bone disease, such as osteomalacia or adynamic bone disease, for which bisphosphonate use is contraindicated.[35,37]

Atrial Fibrillation

The Health Outcomes and Reduced Incidence with Zoledronic Acid Once Yearly (HORIZON) Pivotal Fracture Trial (PFT) raised concerns of cardiac safety issues surrounding use of bisphosphonates when it unexpectedly reported that zoledronate increased the risk for atrial fibrillation (AF) reported as a serious adverse event (1.3% of the zoledronic acid group compared with 0.5% of the placebo group).[38] The occurrence of AF did not seem to be associated with the timing of the infusion, the acute-phase reaction following the infusion, or any acute electrolyte imbalance. This surprising observation raised the question of whether this may be related to the medication itself or whether this was a chance finding, which prompted further studies to assess this issue.

In the HORIZON Recurrent Fracture Trial (RFT), a smaller and shorter study in which careful evaluation of AF and its serious adverse events was performed,[30] there was no increase in the rate of AF in the treatment group. Similarly, no increase in the rate of AF was noted in an extension of the HORIZON pivotal trial[39] as well as the oncology trials of zoledronic acid, which used a dose approximately 10 times higher than what is typically used to treat osteoporosis.

A retrospective analysis of the alendronate Fracture Intervention Trial showed a nonsignificant trend toward an increase in AF (1.5% vs 1.0%, relative hazard 1.51, 95% CI 0.97–2.40; $P = .07$).[40] A retrospective analysis of the risedronate Vertebral Efficacy with Risedronate Therapy (VERT) study did not find a difference between the treatment and placebo arms.[41] In a case-control study from the United States, the risk of AF was increased in past, not current, users of alendronate.[42] However, a large population-based case control study that analyzed a medical database in Denmark reported no definite association between use of bisphosphonates and risk of atrial fibrillation.[43] Another Danish register-based cohort study performed to evaluate rates of AF in fracture patients starting oral bisphosphonates showed that there was an increased risk of AF in bisphosphonate users versus nonusers, with the main risk factors for AF being old age and patients who are already at an increased cardiovascular risk.[44] Two other large population studies, one using 2 US databases and the other using a UK database, did not find an association between bisphosphonate use and AF.[45,46]

In a meta-analysis of datasets from 4 randomized trials of bisphosphonate therapy for osteoporosis, bisphosphonate exposure was significantly associated with risk of serious but not all AF adverse events.[47] There was no increase in the risk of stroke or cardiovascular mortality in an analysis of 3 of these trial datasets. On the other hand, in a recent meta-analysis of all Merck-conducted, placebo-controlled clinical trials of alendronate the occurrence of AF was uncommon, with no clear association between overall bisphosphonate exposure and the rate of serious or nonserious AF.[48] A recent retrospective cohort analysis of older Korean women with osteoporosis showed that alendronate had a protective effect against the risk of AF, with a hazard ratio of 0.75 (95% CI 0.58–0.97).[49]

Thus, the data linking the use of bisphosphonates with an increased risk of AF are discordant, and the available information does not reveal a consistent association. At present, the overall evidence still does not support a causal relationship between bisphosphonate exposure and AF. In addition, there is no convincing mechanism to account for this effect, which seems to be independent of the dose and duration of therapy. Osteoporosis and AF are more common in the elderly and share similar risk factors, which may explain some of the reported findings. At present, the US FDA recommends that physicians not alter their prescribing patterns for bisphosphonates while it continues to monitor postmarketing reports of AF in such patients.[50] In the absence of more definitive data, the benefits of fracture prevention should outweigh the risks of therapy in most patients.

Musculoskeletal Pain

The product labeling for all bisphosphonates lists musculoskeletal pain as a potential adverse effect and that treatment should be withheld if such symptoms occur. Between 1995 and 2005, 117 cases of severe musculoskeletal pain (bone, joint, and/or muscle pain) in adults on bisphosphonates were reported to the FDA, as described in a letter to the editor by Wysowski and Chang.[51] In this series of cases, pain was not isolated to a particular anatomic site and may have occurred at any time after starting bisphosphonate therapy. Some patients experienced immediate improvement in their symptoms after discontinuation of the offending drug, although for most patients the improvement was gradual or partial. The frequency and mechanism for this adverse effect are not known; likewise, there is no evidence supporting a causal relationship between this side effect and bisphosphonate use. Because many patients with osteoporosis suffer from background musculoskeletal pain, it would be difficult to assess the incidence of this problem, although it seems to be very uncommon based on data from randomized controlled trials. It is interesting to note that particularly severe musculoskeletal pain associated with intravenous bisphosphonate therapy, which can be alleviated by prior glucocorticoid therapy,[52] has been described in patients with cystic fibrosis.[53] Further studies are needed to evaluate this issue and to learn more about the possible risk factors for this problem. In January of 2008, the FDA issued a communication highlighting this side effect, and recommended instructing patients to alert their physician if such symptoms occur for consideration of stopping the medication temporarily or permanently.[54]

Osteonecrosis of the Jaw

Osteonecrosis of the jaw (ONJ) is defined as exposed necrotic bone in the maxillofacial region, not healing after 8 weeks in patients with no history of craniofacial radiation.[55] It appears as areas of exposed yellow-white hard bone with smooth or ragged borders and is often associated with pain, swelling, paresthesias, suppuration, soft-tissue ulceration, intraoral or extraoral sinus tracks, and loosening of teeth.[56]

ONJ has been described in patients receiving chronic bisphosphonate therapy. It has also been seen in subjects not using bisphosphonates, but the background incidence is not known. It often follows invasive dental procedures, or occurs in patients with poorly fitting dentures or bony exostoses. Other risk factors for developing ONJ include intravenous bisphosphonates, cancer and anticancer therapy, duration of exposure to bisphosphonate therapy, glucocorticoids, smoking, and preexisting dental disease. ONJ may or may not be progressive; healing has been reported, but many lesions heal slowly or do not heal.[57]

The first report linking bisphosphonate use to ONJ appeared in 2003.[58] In this series, all 36 patients were being treated with high doses of intravenous bisphosphonates for skeletal complications of malignancy. Subsequent reports of ONJ included patients receiving lower doses of bisphosphonates for treatment of osteoporosis,[56,59] but the vast majority (more than 90%) of reported cases have been in cancer patients receiving doses of bisphosphonates approximately 10 times higher than that used to treat osteoporosis. None of the clinical trials using bisphosphonates for treatment of osteoporosis or Paget disease, which included more than 60,000 patient-years of exposure, identified ONJ prospectively.[60] In the HORIZON trial with IV zoledronate for osteoporosis, a retrospective review identified 1 case of ONJ in the treatment group and another in the placebo group.[61]

There have been more than 190 million prescriptions in the United States for oral bisphosphonates and more than 6 million patients treated with IV bisphosphonates for cancer worldwide.[62] Based on epidemiologic evidence, the incidence of ONJ in oral bisphosphonate users is estimated to range from 1:10,000 (Australia and Israel), to 1:250,000 (Germany), to 1:160,000 worldwide. It is difficult to obtain accurate estimates because not all cases of ONJ are reported, and not all cases reported are truly ONJ.

A causal link between bisphosphonate use and ONJ appears to be likely, although it has not been established. Despite several potential mechanisms, the pathophysiology of ONJ remains poorly defined. Possible mechanisms include oversuppression of bone turnover leading to failure of osteoclasts to remove diseased necrotic bone, imbalance between osteoblasts and osteoclasts leading to overly dense bone (osteopetrosis), inhibition of angiogenesis, inhibition of T-cell function, bony overgrowth impeding flow through the sublingual artery or vascular canals, and death of the mucous membrane overlying bone because of accumulation of the bisphosphonate compound in the jaw bone. ONJ has also been reported with denosumab, a drug that does not accumulate in bone but does reduce bone remodeling, making oversuppression of bone turnover the leading hypothesis. On the other hand, there is some evidence that bisphosphonates may be beneficial in treating avascular necrosis of long bones,[63,64] and that these may also be helpful for preserving alveolar jaw bone in patients who have periodontal disease.[65,66]

The problem of ONJ received considerable media coverage,[67–69] which led to misconceptions among medical and dental professionals as well as the public regarding the frequency and severity of this condition. As a result, many patients decided to stop bisphosphonate treatment although they were at high risk of fracture and low risk of ONJ.

This topic was extensively addressed by a Task Force of the American Society for Bone and Mineral Research,[55] which performed a comprehensive review and recommended that clinicians discuss the risk of ONJ, the signs and symptoms of ONJ, and the risk factors for developing ONJ in patients initiating or receiving treatment with bisphosphonates.

In patients already receiving oral bisphosphonates, there is concern for those scheduled for invasive dental procedures that involve the jaw, such as extractions or implants. Guidelines for oral surgeons have also been published by the American Association of Oral and Maxillofacial Surgeons,[70] who suggest performing dentoalveolar surgery as usual in patients who have been treated with oral bisphosphonates for less than 3 years, and to discontinue the oral bisphosphonate for 3 months before performing the dental surgery if a patient has been treated for more than 3 years, aiming to restart it when the bone has healed. However, there is no evidence to support that this would lower ONJ risk, especially because bisphosphonates stay in bone for years. In fact, the most recent guidelines from the American Dental Association (ADA) state that the benefit provided by antiresorptive therapy outweighs the low risk of developing ONJ, and that discontinuing bisphosphonate therapy may not lower the risk but may have a negative effect on outcomes of treatment of low bone mass.[71] Useful information for patients is also available on the ADA Web site (http://www.ada.org).[71,72]

In summary, patients who are starting or taking bisphosphonates should be informed that ONJ is one the risks of treatment, but that the likelihood is very low. Although good oral hygiene and regular dental visits are recommended for everyone, a dental visit before beginning oral bisphosphonate therapy is not required, but an oral examination should be conducted. Routine dental cleaning and restorative procedures should be strongly encouraged, and patients with periodontal disease should receive appropriate nonsurgical therapy. Patients considering dentoalveolar surgery while taking bisphosphonates should be advised of the risks and alternatives. Invasive surgical procedures should be avoided if possible, and if dental treatment is necessary it should progress in a stepwise fashion if possible. Patients initiating bisphosphonates who need invasive dental procedures should have these done, with healing complete before starting these agents if circumstances allow. Patients already taking a bisphosphonate may elect to take some time off therapy because it is unlikely that there would be adverse consequences on BMD or facture risk, although there is no evidence that this will improve outcomes.

Atypical Femur Fractures

Although evidence clearly supports the beneficial effect of bisphosphonates on the prevention of osteoporotic fracture, there is theoretical concern that prolonged therapy can lead to oversuppression of bone turnover leading to impaired bone remodeling, accumulation of microdamage in bone, and increased skeletal fragility.[73–76] Several case reports have suggested a link between bisphosphonate use and the development of atypical insufficiency fractures, described as unusual low-energy subtrochanteric femoral fractures and pelvic insufficiency fractures, which exhibited problems with healing in patients on long-term bisphosphonate therapy.[77–84] These fractures, which are frequently bilateral, are typically associated with minimal or no trauma and present with prodromal pain in the region of the fracture. These "chalk-stick" fractures also have characteristic radiographic findings including cortical hypertrophy, a transverse fracture pattern, and medial cortical spiking (**Fig. 2**).[85] Even though iliac crest biopsies in such patients often show severely suppressed bone turnover,[36,37,74] at least one patient with this type of subtrochanteric fracture had a completely normal iliac crest biopsy (Watts NB, personal communication, 2008).

Several retrospective studies have also suggested an association between bisphosphonate use and atypical femur fractures,[86–88] although the results from larger observational studies are discordant. A register-based Danish national cohort study showed that the occurrence of classic to atypical hip fractures was similar in the alendronate-treated subjects versus matched untreated controls.[89] In addition, the risk of both typical and atypical fractures was reduced by adherence to alendronate, suggesting that these atypical fractures were more likely due to osteoporosis rather than to treatment with alendronate. On the other hand, a Canadian case-control study of more than 200,000 older women found that treatment with a bisphosphonate for 5 or more years was associated with a higher incidence of atypical and a lower incidence of typical osteoporotic fractures,[90] although the absolute risk of the atypical fractures was low.

In a 2010 report from an international task force appointed by the American Society of Bone and Mineral Research to review this issue, major and minor criteria for atypical fractures were defined.[91] The incidence of atypical fractures associated with bisphosphonate use was acknowledged to be very low, although there was concern that the risk may increase with prolonged bisphosphonate exposure.[91] Furthermore,

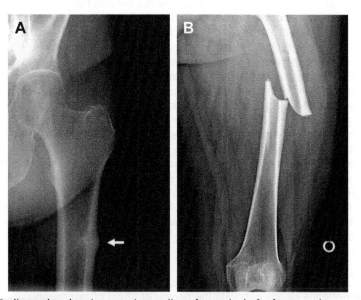

Fig. 2. Radiographs showing an impending femoral shaft fracture (*A, arrow*) and a representative "atypical" diaphyseal femoral fracture (*B*) with thickened cortices and a "beak" or "spike." (*Courtesy of* Drs Joseph Lane and Aasis Unnanuntana, Hospital for Special Surgery, New York, NY; and *From* Watts NB, Diab DL. Long-term use of bisphosphonates in osteoporosis. J Clin Endocrinol Metab 2010;95:1561. Copyright 2010, The Endocrine Society; with permission.)

no definite causal relationship between atypical fractures and bisphosphonate use was demonstrated.

A recent large retrospective United States study found that 70% of subjects with an atypical fracture had no recorded dispensing of bisphosphonates at any time before the fracture event.[92] Individuals with only major features of atypical fractures appeared to be different (older and with lower BMD) from individuals with atypical fractures that had both major and minor features.[92] Another recent study using the French National Database showed that the adjusted risk of having an atypical femur fracture compared with that of having a hip fracture was significantly higher in the context of obesity and dementia, but decreased with age and hypertension.[93] There was no information regarding bisphosphonate use in this study.

The FDA currently recommends that bisphosphonate users with new-onset groin or thigh pain be further evaluated.[94] Conventional radiography is usually the initial imaging procedure of choice, followed by magnetic resonance imaging or bone scintigraphy if clinical suspicion is high and conventional radiography is unrevealing. In patients confirmed to have an atypical fracture, antiresorptive medications should be discontinued and these fractures should be reported. A high index of suspicion for a contralateral fracture should be maintained in patients with such fractures because these are often bilateral, as already mentioned.

In summary, although many studies support an association between duration of bisphosphonate therapy and risk of atypical fractures, a direct causal association has yet to be established. Additional prospective studies are needed to elucidate this issue further and determine the subgroups of long-term users at highest risk for this type of fracture. More definitive data may influence decisions regarding duration of therapy in selected individuals,[95] but concern about oversuppression of bone turnover is not a reason to stop bisphosphonate therapy in the vast majority of postmenopausal women who are at high risk for osteoporotic fracture.[96,97]

POSSIBLE "SIDE BENEFITS" OF BISPHOSPHONATE THERAPY

Recent preclinical and clinical studies indicate that bisphosphonates might also exhibit antitumor activity.[98,99] There is increasing evidence that use of bisphosphonates is associated with a decreased risk of breast cancer.[100–107] In a population-based case control study, the use of bisphosphonates for longer than 1 year was associated with a significant reduction in the relative risk of breast cancer after adjusting for several factors including age, fruit and vegetable intake, physical activity, family history of breast cancer, body mass index, use of hormone replacement therapy, pregnancies, and breast-feeding (odds ratio 0.72, 95% CI 0.57–0.90).[106] Likewise, there are data to suggest that bisphosphonate use is associated with a decreased risk of colorectal cancer. A similar study showed that the use of oral bisphosphonates for more than 1 year was associated with a significant reduction in the relative risk of colorectal cancer after adjusting for vegetable intake, physical activity, family history of colorectal cancer, body mass index, and use of aspirin, statins, vitamin D, and postmenopausal hormone therapy (relative risk 0.41, 95% CI 0.25–0.67).[108]

A growing body of evidence also suggests that bisphosphonate use is associated with a decreased risk of stroke and improved survival. A recent large population cohort study revealed that patients who received bisphosphonate therapy were less likely to suffer a stroke than comparison patients during a 2-year follow-up period after adjusting for demographic variables and medical comorbidities (hazard ratio 0.79, 95% CI 0.66–0.99).[109] Nevertheless, other studies suggest that this association depends on the agent and dosing regimen used.[110,111] In one study of female patients with chronic kidney disease, treatment with bisphosphonates was associated with a lower risk of death (adjusted hazard ratio 0.78, 95% CI 0.67–0.91; $P =$ .003), but not cardiovascular events.[112] A large prospective study from Australia revealed that bisphosphonate therapy appeared to reduce mortality risk in women and possibly men.[113] In another study of 2005 institutionalized older people, use of oral bisphosphonates was associated with a 27% reduction in risk of death in comparison with nonusers over 5 years of follow-up after adjusting for potential confounders.[114] In a randomized, double-blind, placebo-controlled trial of patients who received an infusion of zoledronic acid within 90 days after surgical repair of a low-trauma hip fracture, 101 of 1054 patients in the zoledronic acid group (9.6%) and 141 of 1057 patients in the placebo group (13.3%) died, a reduction of 28% in deaths from any cause in the zoledronic acid group ($P =$ .01).[30] Similarly, a study using prospectively collected long-term data from a randomized trial of osteoporosis quality improvement for hip fracture showed that oral bisphosphonate exposure led to about a 60% reduction in mortality per year of use.[115]

DURATION OF THERAPY AND DRUG HOLIDAYS

Approval of bisphosphonates in the United States was mostly based on studies of 3 to 4 years' duration. Some of these studies have been extended, with alendronate[4,5] and risedronate[116,117] demonstrating efficacy for up to 10 and 7 years, respectively.

The extension of the alendronate Fracture Intervention Trial (FLEX) enrolled subjects who had approximately 5 years of alendronate treatment in the Fracture Intervention Trial into a second 5-year study where subjects were randomized to either continue alendronate or start placebo. At the end of the FLEX study, 5-year fracture rates for new clinical vertebral fractures were reduced by 55% in the subjects who had 10 years of treatment compared with those who were changed to placebo. Although the published report suggested no differences in radiographic vertebral fractures or nonvertebral fractures, a subsequent analysis indicated that, among subjects with T-scores of −2.5 or less at the femoral neck at the time of beginning the second 5 years of treatment, nonvertebral fracture risk was reduced by 50%.[118]

The extension of the risedronate VERT-NA study was a 1-year follow-up of subjects who completed 3 years of blinded therapy with risedronate 5 mg daily or placebo, then stopped their study medications. In the year off treatment, BMD decreased in the former risedronate users (but remained higher than baseline and higher than in the former placebo subjects), and bone turnover markers increased (and were no different from the former placebo subjects). Despite the apparent resolution of treatment effect on these intermediate markers, the risk of new vertebral fractures was reduced by 46% in the former risedronate users compared with the former placebo subjects.[116] Similarly, a recent study looking at the effect of discontinuing risedronate for 1 year after 2 or 7 years also showed decreasing BMD in the total hip and trochanter regions as well as increasing bone turnover markers.[119]

A recently published 3-year extension of the zoledronate HORIZON PFT showed that there were small differences in bone density and bone turnover markers in those who continued versus those who stopped treatment, suggesting residual effects. However, there were significantly fewer morphometric vertebral fractures in the group that continued treatment compared with the placebo group (14 vs 30), suggesting that patients at high fracture risk may benefit by continued treatment.[39]

With respect to long-term safety, no specific issues were identified in the aforementioned studies despite recent evidence that supports an association between prolonged bisphosphonate exposure and the 2 rare but serious conditions, ONJ and atypical fractures. As mentioned previously, only 1 case of ONJ was reported in the treatment group and another in the placebo group in a retrospective review of the HORIZON trial with IV zoledronate for osteoporosis,[61] and no atypical fractures were seen in any of these studies. Although some have expressed concern about possible oversuppression of bone turnover, iliac crest biopsies after up to 10 years of treatment have not shown oversuppression. Nevertheless, these quite uncommon but possibly time-related adverse effects have led to considerable debate about how long to treat with bisphosphonates, and currently no consensus is available.

A "drug holiday" is a period of time when treatment is stopped after continuous bisphosphonate therapy. The rationale for considering a drug holiday stems from the unique pharmacokinetics of bisphosphonates that accumulate in the skeleton, leading to a reservoir that continues to be released for months or years after treatment is stopped.[120] The skeletal binding sites for bisphosphonates are virtually unsaturable, so a considerable amount could accumulate. When treatment is stopped, their long retention time in bone may lead to some lingering antifracture effect. However, the term "holiday" implies that treatment will be restarted after some time off.

On September 9, 2011, the FDA reviewed the long-term safety and efficacy of bisphosphonates including alendronate, risedronate, ibandronate, and zoledronate.[121] The majority of the advisory committee (17 to 6) voted that labeling for these drugs should further clarify the duration of use for bisphosphonates, but could not agree on language for this. This resolution may result in limiting the duration of bisphosphonate therapy if implemented. The American Association of Clinical Endocrinologists responded to the FDA hearing by recommending to maintain current practice until the FDA publishes its final ruling.[122]

At present, the data suggest that although there is some residual benefit in terms of fracture reduction for some time after a 3- to 5-year course of bisphosphonate therapy, continuing treatment for 10 years is better for high-risk patients regardless of the differences between individual bisphosphonates. Even though the risks of bisphosphonate therapy for osteoporosis are small, the risk/benefit ratio may be negative for low-risk patients. For patients who were candidates for treatment, treatment may be stopped for a drug holiday after a course of some years. At present, it is difficult to find evidence to support the need for a drug holiday or to establish the effectiveness of treatment after restarting therapy. Similarly, there is no strong evidence to provide guidance in terms of how long to treat, how long the holiday should be, and when the holiday should be stopped. Nevertheless, the authors believe there is logic to support the following clinical scenarios, as shown in **Table 5**:

1. Low risk of fracture: Treatment is not needed. If a bisphosphonate has been prescribed, it should be discontinued and not restarted unless/until the patient meets treatment guidelines.
2. Mild risk of fracture: Treat with bisphosphonate for 3 to 5 years, then stop. The drug holiday can be continued until there is significant loss of BMD (ie, more than the least significant change as determined by the testing center) or the patient has a fracture, whichever comes first.
3. Moderate risk of fracture: Treat with bisphosphonate for 5 to 10 years, offer a drug holiday of 3 to 5 years or until there is significant loss of BMD or the patient has a fracture, whichever comes first.
4. High risk of fracture: Treat with bisphosphonate for 10 years, offer a drug holiday of 1 to 2 years or until there is significant loss of BMD or the patient has a fracture, whichever comes first. A nonbisphosphonate treatment (eg, raloxifene, teriparatide) may be offered during the holiday from the bisphosphonate.

Table 5
Suggested duration of bisphosphonate treatment and drug holidays

Patient's Fracture Risk	Suggested Duration of Treatment	Suggested Duration of Drug Holiday[a]
Low	Treatment rarely indicated	Not applicable
Mildly increased	Treat for approximately 5 y	Stay off bisphosphonate until BMD decreases significantly or fracture occurs
Moderately increased	Treat for 5–10 y	Stay off bisphosphonate for 2–3 y (or less if BMD decreases or fracture occurs)
High	Treat for 10 y	Stay off bisphosphonate for 1–2 y (or less if BMD decreases or fracture occurs); alternative medication (eg, raloxifene, teriparatide) may be given during the holiday from bisphosphonates

This table is based largely on personal opinion.

[a] Longer holidays might be appropriate for patients treated with bisphosphonates that bind most strongly to bone (ie, zoledronic acid, alendronate), whereas shorter holidays might be considered for patients treated with compounds that bind less strongly (ie, risedronate, ibandronate).

From Watts NB, Diab DL. Long-term use of bisphosphonates in osteoporosis. J Clin Endocrinol Metab 2010;95:1562. Copyright 2010, The Endocrine Society; with permission.

If a drug holiday is advised, reassessment of risk should occur after 1 year for risedronate, 1 to 2 years for alendronate, and 2 to 3 years for zoledronate.[123] Although it has been suggested that a decrease in BMD or an increase in bone turnover marker (BTM) might be used to decide when to end a drug holiday, the risedronate study showed that fracture risk remained reduced despite what appeared to be unfavorable changes in these parameters.[116] Conversely, there is no evidence that fracture risk is reduced if BMD is stable or BTM is low off treatment. All things considered, the strength of the evidence for fracture reduction in high-risk individuals and the rarity of long-term adverse effects indicate that the benefits of continued treatment outweigh the risks in individuals at high risk of fracture.

SUMMARY

Bisphosphonates are popular and effective for the treatment of osteoporosis and for reducing the risk of fracture, with evidence for broad-spectrum (ie, spine, hip, and nonvertebral) reduction of fracture risk. These agents can be administered orally or intravenously. Since their initial introduction in the United States in 1995, questions have been raised about their association with possible side effects (such as esophageal cancer, AF, musculoskeletal pain, ONJ, and atypical fractures), but these appear to be rare. Moreover, no causal relationship has been established between prolonged bisphosphonate exposure and any of these adverse effects.

Because bisphosphonates accumulate in bone and provide some residual antifracture benefit after therapy is stopped, it is reasonable to consider drug holidays (time off bisphosphonate therapy but possibly on another agent) and then resumption of therapy. Although there is no strong evidence for guidance, the authors recommend a drug holiday after 3 to 10 years of bisphosphonate treatment. The duration of treatment and the length of the holiday should be individualized based on fracture risk and the binding affinity of the particular bisphosphonate used. High-risk patients should be treated for 10 years and have a short holiday of 1 to 2 years, as opposed to patients at mild risk of fracture who may stop treatment after 3 to 5 years and continue off treatment as long as bone density is stable and no fractures occur.

REFERENCES

1. Watts NB. Bisphosphonate treatment for osteoporosis. In: Avioli LV, editor. The osteoporotic syndrome. San Diego: Academic Press; 2000. p. 121–32.
2. Russell RG, Watts NB, Ebetino FH, et al. Mechanisms of action of bisphosphonates: similarities and differences and their potential influence on clinical efficacy. Osteoporos Int 2008;(733):759.
3. Rogers MJ, Frith JC, Luckman SP, et al. Molecular mechanisms of action of bisphosphonates. Bone 1999;24(5):73S–9S.
4. Bone HG, Hosking D, Devogelaer JP, et al. Ten years' experience with alendronate for osteoporosis in postmenopausal women. N Engl J Med 2004;350:1189–99.
5. Black DM, Schwartz AV, Ensrud KE, et al. Effects of continuing or stopping alendronate after 5 years of treatment. The Fracture Intervention Trial long-term extension (FLEX): a randomized trial. JAMA 2006;296:2927–38.
6. Wysowski DK. Reports of esophageal cancer with oral bisphosphonate use. N Engl J Med 2009;360:89.
7. Wysowski DK. Oral bisphosphonates and oesophageal cancer. BMJ 2010;341: c4506.
8. Siris ES, Oster MW, Bilezikian JP. More on reports of esophageal cancer with oral bisphosphonate use. N Engl J Med 2009;360:1791 [author reply: 1791].
9. Shaheen NJ. More on reports of esophageal cancer with oral bisphosphonate use. N Engl J Med 2009;360:1790.
10. Hofbauer LC, Miehlke S. More on reports of esophageal cancer with oral bisphosphonate use. N Engl J Med 2009;360:1790 [author reply: 1791].
11. Robins HI, Holen KD. More on reports of esophageal cancer with oral bisphosphonate use. N Engl J Med 2009;360:1790 [author reply: 1791].
12. Abrahamsen B, Eiken P, Eastell R. More on reports of esophageal cancer with oral bisphosphonate use. N Engl J Med 2009;360:1789 [author reply: 1791].
13. Solomon DH, Patrick A, Brookhart MA. More on reports of esophageal cancer with oral bisphosphonate use. N Engl J Med 2009;360:1789.
14. Cardwell CR, Abnet CC, Cantwell MM, et al. Exposure to oral bisphosphonates and risk of esophageal cancer. JAMA 2010;304:657.
15. Cardwell CR, Abnet CC, Veal P, et al. Exposure to oral bisphosphonates and risk of cancer. Int J Cancer 2011. [Epub ahead of print].
16. Green J, Czanner G, Reeves G, et al. Oral bisphosphonates and risk of cancer of oesophagus, stomach, and colorectum: case-control analysis within a UK primary care cohort. BMJ 2010;341:c4444.
17. Ribeiro A, DeVault KR, Wolfe JT 3rd, et al. Alendronate-associated esophagitis: endoscopic and pathologic features. Gastrointest Endosc 1998;47:525.
18. Abraham SC, Cruz-Correa M, Lee LA, et al. Alendronate-associated esophageal injury: pathologic and endoscopic features. Mod Pathol 1999;12:1152.
19. Available at: http://www.fda.gov/Drugs/DrugSafety/ucm263320.htm. Accessed January 2012.
20. Adami S, Bhalla AK, Dorizzi R, et al. The acute phase response after bisphosphonate administration. Calcif Tissue Int 1987;41:326–31.
21. Gallacher SJ, Ralston SH, Patel U, et al. Side-effects of pamidronate. Lancet 1989;2:42–3.
22. Zojer N, Keck AV, Pecherstorfer M. Comparative tolerability of drug therapies for hypercalcaemia of malignancy. Drug Saf 1999;21(5):389–406.
23. Maalouf NM, Heller HJ, Odvina CV, et al. Bisphosphonate-induced hypocalcemia: report of 3 cases and review of literature. Endocr Pract 2006;12:48–53.

24. Fraunfelder FW, Fraunfelder FT. Bisphosphonates and ocular inflammation. N Engl J Med 2003;348:1187.
25. Lewiecki EM. Safety of long-term bisphosphonate therapy for the management of osteoporosis. Drugs 2011;71:791.
26. Recker RR, Lewiecki EM, Miller PD, et al. Safety of bisphosphonates in the treatment of osteoporosis. Am J Med 2009;122:S22.
27. Miller PD. Treatment of osteoporosis in chronic kidney disease and end-stage renal disease. Curr Osteoporos Rep 2005;3:5.
28. Miller PD, Roux C, Boonen S, et al. Safety and efficacy of risedronate in patients with age-related reduced renal function as estimated by the Cockcroft and Gault method: a pooled analysis of nine clinical trials. J Bone Miner Res 2005;20:2105.
29. Jamal SA, Bauer DC, Ensrud KE, et al. Alendronate treatment in women with normal to severely impaired renal function: an analysis of the Fracture Intervention Trial. J Bone Miner Res 2007;22:503.
30. Lyles KW, Colon-Emeric CS, Magaziner JS, et al. Zoledronic acid and clinical fractures and mortality after hip fracture. N Engl J Med 2007;357:1799.
31. Lewiecki EM, Miller PD. Renal safety of intravenous bisphosphonates in the treatment of osteoporosis. Expert Opin Drug Saf 2007;6:663.
32. Eisman JA, Civitelli R, Adami S, et al. Efficacy and tolerability of intravenous ibandronate injections in postmenopausal osteoporosis: 2-year results from the DIVA study. J Rheumatol 2008;35:488.
33. Miller PD, Ward P, Pfister T, et al. Renal tolerability of intermittent intravenous ibandronate treatment for patients with postmenopausal osteoporosis: a review. Clin Exp Rheumatol 2008;26:1125.
34. Boonen S, Sellmeyer DE, Lippuner K, et al. Renal safety of annual zoledronic acid infusions in osteoporotic postmenopausal women. Kidney Int 2008;74:641.
35. Miller PD. Diagnosis and treatment of osteoporosis in chronic renal disease. Semin Nephrol 2009;29:144.
36. Miller PD. Is there a role for bisphosphonates in chronic kidney disease? Semin Dial 2007;20:186.
37. Miller PD. The role of bone biopsy in patients with chronic renal failure. Clin J Am Soc Nephrol 2008;3(Suppl 3):S140.
38. Black DM, Delmas PD, Eastell R, et al. Once-yearly zoledronic acid for treatment of postmenopausal osteoporosis. N Engl J Med 2007;356:1809.
39. Black DM, Reid IR, Boonen S, et al. The effect of 3 versus 6 years of zoledronic acid treatment of osteoporosis: a randomized extension to the HORIZON-Pivotal Fracture Trial (PFT). J Bone Miner Res 2012;27(2):243.
40. Cummings SR, Schwartz AV, Black DM. Alendronate and atrial fibrillation. N Engl J Med 2007;356:1895.
41. Karam R, Camm J, McClung M. Yearly zoledronic acid in postmenopausal osteoporosis. N Engl J Med 2007;357:712.
42. Heckbert SR, Li G, Cummings SR, et al. Use of alendronate and risk of incident atrial fibrillation in women. Arch Intern Med 2008;168:826.
43. Sorensen HT, Christensen S, Mehnert F, et al. Use of bisphosphonates among women and risk of atrial fibrillation and flutter: population based case-control study. BMJ 2008;336:813.
44. Abrahamsen B, Eiken P, Brixen K. Atrial fibrillation in fracture patients treated with oral bisphosphonates. J Intern Med 2009;265:581.
45. Bunch TJ, Anderson JL, May HT, et al. Relation of bisphosphonate therapies and risk of developing atrial fibrillation. Am J Cardiol 2009;103:824.

46. Grosso A, Douglas I, Hingorani A, et al. Oral bisphosphonates and risk of atrial fibrillation and flutter in women: a self-controlled case-series safety analysis. PLoS One 2009;4:e4720.
47. Loke YK, Jeevanantham V, Singh S. Bisphosphonates and atrial fibrillation: systematic review and meta-analysis. Drug Saf 2009;32:219.
48. Barrett-Connor E, Swern AS, Hustad CM, et al. Alendronate and atrial fibrillation: a meta-analysis of randomized placebo-controlled clinical trials. Osteoporos Int 2012;23:233.
49. Rhee CW, Lee J, Oh S, et al. Use of bisphosphonate and risk of atrial fibrillation in older women with osteoporosis. Osteoporos Int 2012;23:247.
50. Available at: http://www.fda.gov/Drugs/DrugSafety/PostmarketDrugSafety InformationforPatientsandProviders/DrugSafetyInformationforHeathcare Professionals/ucm136201.htm. Accessed January 2012.
51. Wysowski DK, Chang JT. Alendronate and risedronate: reports of severe bone, joint, and muscle pain. Arch Intern Med 2005;165:346.
52. Haworth CS, Selby PL, Webb AK, et al. Oral corticosteroids and bone pain after pamidronate in adults with cystic fibrosis. Lancet 1999;353:1886.
53. Haworth CS, Selby PL, Webb AK, et al. Severe bone pain after intravenous pamidronate in adult patients with cystic fibrosis. Lancet 1998;352:1753.
54. Available at: http://www.fda.gov/drugs/drugsafety/postmarketdrugsafetyinformation forpatientsandproviders/ucm124165.htm. Accessed January 2012.
55. Khosla S, Burr D, Cauley J, et al. Bisphosphonate-associated osteonecrosis of the jaw: report of a task force of the American Society for Bone and Mineral Research. J Bone Miner Res 2007;22:1479.
56. Woo SB, Hellstein JW, Kalmar JR. Systematic review: bisphosphonates and osteonecrosis of the jaws. Ann Intern Med 2006;206(144):753–61.
57. Triester N, Woo S-B. Bisphosphonate-associated osteonecrosis of the jaw. N Engl J Med 2006;335:2348.
58. Marx RE. Pamidronate (Aredia) and zoledronate (Zometa) induced avascular necrosis of the jaws: a growing epidemic [letter]. J Oral Maxillofac Surg 2003; 61:1115–7.
59. Ruggiero SL, Mehrotra B, Rosenberg TJ, et al. Osteonecrosis of the jaws associated with the use of bisphosphonates: a review of 63 cases. J Oral Maxillofac Surg 2004;62:527–34.
60. Bilezikian JP. Osteonecrosis of the jaw: do bisphosphonates pose a risk? N Engl J Med 2006;355:2278–82.
61. Black DM, Boonen S, Cauley J, et al. Effect of once-yearly infusion of zoledronic acid 5 mg on spine and hip fracture reduction in postmenopausal women with osteoporosis: the HORIZON pivotal fracture trial [abstract]. J Bone Miner Res 2006;21(Suppl 1):S16.
62. IMS HEALTH. NPA Plus May 2006.
63. Agarwala S, Sule A, Pai BU, et al. Alendronate in the treatment of avascular necrosis of the hip. Rheumatology 2002;41(3):346–7.
64. Desai MM, Sonone S, Bhasme V. Efficacy of alendronate in the treatment of avascular necrosis of the hip. Rheumatology 2005;44(10):1331–2.
65. Jeffcoat MK. Safety of oral bisphosphonates: controlled studies on alveolar bone. Int J Oral Maxillofac Surg 2006;21:349–53.
66. Palomo L, Bissada NF, Liu J. Periodontal assessment of postmenopausal women receiving risedronate. Menopause 2005;12:685–90.
67. Kolata G. Drug for bones is newly linked to jaw disease. New York Times 2006.
68. Rubin R. Drug linked to death of jawbone. USA Today 2005.

69. Knox R. Side effects noted with bone-loss drugs. National Public Radio, broadcast 2006. Available at: http://www.npr.org/templates/story/story.php?storyId=5358285.

70. Advisory Task Force on Bisphosphonate-Related Osteonecrosis of the Jaws, American Association of Oral and Maxillofacial Surgeons. American Association of Oral and Maxillofacial Surgeons position paper on bisphosphonate-related osteonecrosis of the jaws. J Oral Maxillofac Surg 2007;65:369–76.

71. Hellstein JW, Adler RA, Edwards B, et al. Managing the care of patients receiving antiresorptive therapy for prevention and treatment of osteoporosis: executive summary of recommendations from the American Dental Association Council on Scientific Affairs. J Am Dent Assoc 2011;142:1243.

72. Osteoporosis medications and your dental health. J Am Dent Assoc 2011;142:1320.

73. Visekruna M, Wilson D, McKiernan FE. Severely suppressed bone turnover and atypical skeletal fragility. J Clin Endocrinol Metab 2008;93:2948.

74. Mashiba T, Hirano T, Turner CH, et al. Suppressed bone turnover by bisphosphonates increases microdamage accumulation and reduces some biomechanical properties in dog rib. J Bone Miner Res 2000;15(4):613–20.

75. Odvina CV, Zerwekh JE, Rao DS, et al. Severely suppressed bone turnover: A potential complication of alendronate therapy. J Clin Endocrinol Metab 2005;90(3):1294–301.

76. Armamento-Villareal R, Napoli N, Diemer K, et al. Bone turnover in bone biopsies of patients with low-energy cortical fractures receiving bisphosphonates: a case series. Calcif Tissue Int 2009;85:37–44.

77. Imai K, Yamamoto S, Anamizu Y, et al. Pelvic insufficiency fracture associated with severe suppression of bone turnover by alendronate therapy. J Bone Miner Metab 2007;25:333.

78. Kwek EB, Goh SK, Koh JS, et al. An emerging pattern of subtrochanteric stress fractures: a long-term complication of alendronate therapy? Injury 2008;39:224.

79. Lee P, Seibel MJ. More on atypical fractures of the femoral diaphysis. N Engl J Med 2008;359:317 [author reply: 317].

80. Lee P, van der Wall H, Seibel MJ. Looking beyond low bone mineral density: multiple insufficiency fractures in a woman with post-menopausal osteoporosis on alendronate therapy. J Endocrinol Invest 2007;30:590.

81. Lenart BA, Lorich DG, Lane JM. Atypical fractures of the femoral diaphysis in postmenopausal women taking alendronate. N Engl J Med 2008;358:1304.

82. Odvina CV, Levy S, Rao S, et al. Unusual mid-shaft fractures during long term bisphosphonate therapy. Clin Endocrinol (Oxf) 2010;72(2):161–8.

83. Schneider JP. Should bisphosphonates be continued indefinitely? An unusual fracture in a healthy woman on long-term alendronate. Geriatrics 2009;61:31–3.

84. Armamento-Villareal R, Napoli N, Panwar V, et al. Suppressed bone turnover during alendronate therapy for high-turnover osteoporosis. N Engl J Med 2009;355:2048–50.

85. Capeci CM, Tejwani NC. Bilateral low-energy simultaneous or sequential femoral fractures in patients on long-term alendronate therapy. J Bone Joint Surg Am 2009;91:2556.

86. Goh SK, Yang KY, Koh JS, et al. Subtrochanteric insufficiency fractures in patients on alendronate therapy: a caution. J Bone Joint Surg Br 2007;89:349.

87. Lenart BA, Neviaser AS, Lyman S, et al. Association of low-energy femoral fractures with prolonged bisphosphonate use: a case control study. Osteoporos Int 2009;20:1353.

88. Neviaser AS, Lane JM, Lenart BA, et al. Low-energy femoral shaft fractures associated with alendronate use. J Orthop Trauma 2008;22:346.

89. Abrahamsen B, Eiken P, Eastell R. Subtrochanteric and diaphyseal femur fractures in patients treated with alendronate: a register-based national cohort study. J Bone Miner Res 2009;24:1095.

90. Park-Wyllie LY, Mamdani MM, Juurlink DN, et al. Bisphosphonate use and the risk of subtrochanteric or femoral shaft fractures in older women. JAMA 2011; 305:783.

91. Shane E, Burr D, Ebeling PR, et al. Atypical subtrochanteric and diaphyseal femoral fractures: report of a task force of the American Society for Bone and Mineral Research. J Bone Miner Res 2010;25:2267.

92. Feldstein A, Black D, Perrin N, et al. Incidence and demography of femur fractures with and without atypical features. J Bone Miner Res 2012;27:977–86.

93. Maravic M, Ostertag A, Cohen-Solal M. Subtrochanteric/femoral shaft versus hip fractures: Incidences and identification of risk factors. J Bone Miner Res 2011. [Epub ahead of print].

94. Available at: http://www.fda.gov/drugs/drugsafety/ucm229009.htm. Accessed January 2012.

95. Kuehn BM. Long-term risks of bisphosphonates probed. JAMA 2009;301:710.

96. Solomon DH, Rekedal L, Cadarette SM. Osteoporosis treatments and adverse events. Curr Opin Rheumatol 2009;21:363.

97. Kennel KA, Drake MT. Adverse effects of bisphosphonates: implications for osteoporosis management. Mayo Clin Proc 2009;84:632–7.

98. Clezardin P. Bisphosphonates' antitumor activity: an unravelled side of a multifaceted drug class. Bone 2011;48:71.

99. Daniele G, Giordano P, De Luca A, et al. Anticancer effect of bisphosphonates: new insights from clinical trials and preclinical evidence. Expert Rev Anticancer Ther 2011;11:299.

100. Chlebowski RT. Bisphosphonates and breast cancer incidence and recurrence. Breast Dis 2011;33(2):93–101.

101. Chlebowski RT, Chen Z, Cauley JA, et al. Oral bisphosphonate use and breast cancer incidence in postmenopausal women. J Clin Oncol 2010;28: 3582.

102. Chlebowski RT, Col N. Bisphosphonates and breast cancer prevention. Anticancer Agents Med Chem 2012;12:144.

103. Dreyfuss JH. Oral bisphosphonate use associated with a decreased risk of breast cancer. CA Cancer J Clin 2010;60:343.

104. Gnant M. Can oral bisphosphonates really reduce the risk of breast cancer in healthy women? J Clin Oncol 2010;28:3548.

105. Newcomb PA, Trentham-Dietz A, Hampton JM. Bisphosphonates for osteoporosis treatment are associated with reduced breast cancer risk. Br J Cancer 2010;102:799.

106. Rennert G, Pinchev M, Rennert HS. Use of bisphosphonates and risk of postmenopausal breast cancer. J Clin Oncol 2010;28:3577.

107. Vestergaard P, Fischer L, Mele M, et al. Use of bisphosphonates and risk of breast cancer. Calcif Tissue Int 2011;88:255.

108. Rennert G, Pinchev M, Rennert HS, et al. Use of bisphosphonates and reduced risk of colorectal cancer. J Clin Oncol 2011;29:1146.

109. Kang JH, Keller JJ, Lin HC. A population-based 2-year follow-up study on the relationship between bisphosphonates and the risk of stroke. Osteoporos Int 2012. [Epub ahead of print].

110. Lu PY, Hsieh CF, Tsai YW, et al. Alendronate and raloxifene use related to cardio-vascular diseases: differentiation by different dosing regimens of alendronate. Clin Ther 2011;33:1173.

111. Vestergaard P, Schwartz K, Pinholt EM, et al. Stroke in relation to use of raloxi-fene and other drugs against osteoporosis. Osteoporos Int 2011;22:1037.

112. Hartle JE, Tang X, Kirchner HL, et al. Bisphosphonate therapy, death, and cardiovascular events among female patients with CKD: a retrospective cohort study. Am J Kidney Dis 2012;59(5):636–44.

113. Center JR, Bliuc D, Nguyen ND, et al. Osteoporosis medication and reduced mortality risk in elderly women and men. J Clin Endocrinol Metab 2011;96:1006.

114. Sambrook PN, Cameron ID, Chen JS, et al. Oral bisphosphonates are associ-ated with reduced mortality in frail older people: a prospective five-year study. Osteoporos Int 2011;22:2551.

115. Beaupre LA, Morrish DW, Hanley DA, et al. Oral bisphosphonates are associ-ated with reduced mortality after hip fracture. Osteoporos Int 2011;22:983.

116. Watts NB, Chines A, Olszynski WP, et al. Fracture risk remains reduced one year after discontinuation of risedronate. Osteoporos Int 2008;19:365–72.

117. Mellström DD, Sörensen OH, Goemaere S, et al. Seven years of treatment with risedronate in women with postmenopausal osteoporosis. Calcif Tissue Int 2004; 75(6):462–8.

118. Schwartz AV, Bauer DC, Cauley JA, et al. Efficacy of continued alendronate for fractures in women without prevalent vertebral fracture: the FLEX trial (abstract). J Bone Miner Res 2007;22(Suppl 1):S16–7.

119. Eastell R, Hannon RA, Wenderoth D, et al. Effect of stopping risedronate after long-term treatment on bone turnover. J Clin Endocrinol Metab 2011;96:3367.

120. Papapoulos SE, Cremers SC. Prolonged bisphosphonate release after treat-ment in children. N Engl J Med 2007;356:1075–6.

121. Available at: http://www.fda.gov/AdvisoryCommittees/Calendar/ucm262477.htm. Accessed January 2012.

122. Available at: http://media.aace.com/press-release/aace-responds-fda-hearing-bisphosphonates. Accessed January 2012.

123. Compston JE, Bilezikian JP. Bisphosphonate therapy for osteoporosis: the long and short of it. J Bone Miner Res 2012;27:240.

Anabolic Therapies for Osteoporosis

Alexander V. Uihlein, MD, Benjamin Z. Leder, MD*

KEYWORDS

- Teriparatide • Osteoporosis • Bone mineral density • Parathyroid hormone
- Anabolic therapy

KEY POINTS

- Teriparatide (parathyroid hormone 1–34) is the only currently approved anabolic therapy for osteoporosis in the United States. It is approved for use in postmenopausal women, men with idiopathic or hypogonadal osteoporosis, and men and women with glucocorticoid-induced osteoporosis.
- Teriparatide significantly increases areal spine bone mineral density (BMD) and trabecular volumetric BMD at multiple anatomic sites, and reduces vertebral and nonvertebral fractures in postmenopausal women with osteoporosis.
- Treatment with an antiresorptive agent after completion of teriparatide therapy is essential to prevent the significant bone loss that is seen after teriparatide discontinuation.
- Currently available evidence does not generally support the simultaneous use of teriparatide and antiresorptive agents.
- The risk of osteosarcoma at the approved dose and duration of therapy with teriparatide is likely small or absent. Nonetheless, care should be taken to avoid prescribing it to patients whose baseline risk of osteosarcoma may be elevated.
- Several promising new anabolic agents are currently being developed for osteoporosis.

INTRODUCTION

As the population ages and lifespan is extended, osteoporosis will become an increasingly urgent public health concern. Although the arrival of potent antiresorptive medications was a major step forward in the ability to prevent fractures, they do not reverse the bone loss that has already occurred, and fractures are still common in people at highest risk. Medications that stimulate new bone formation (anabolic agents) have the potential to restore skeletal integrity, even in patients who have lost significant bone mass and whose skeletal microarchitecture is severely compromised.

Endocrine Unit, Massachusetts General Hospital, 50 Blossom Street, Thier 1051, Boston, MA 02114, USA
* Corresponding author.
E-mail address: bzleder@partners.org

Endocrinol Metab Clin N Am 41 (2012) 507–525
doi:10.1016/j.ecl.2012.05.002
0889-8529/12/$ – see front matter © 2012 Elsevier Inc. All rights reserved.

Sodium fluoride was one of the first anabolic agents investigated as a treatment for osteoporosis. Although it is a potent stimulator of trabecular bone formation, its propensity to increase appendicular skeletal fractures renders it an inappropriate agent for therapeutic use.[1] In 2002, teriparatide (parathyroid hormone [PTH] 1–34) became the first anabolic agent approved by the U.S. Food and Drug Administration (FDA) for the treatment of postmenopausal osteoporosis, and was subsequently approved for male osteoporosis and glucocorticoid-induced osteoporosis. In the coming decade, the hope is that additional anabolic agents will make their way into clinical use. Moreover, as the limitations of antiresorptive agents become better defined, it is becoming increasingly clear that anabolic agents will have the greatest potential to reduce the individual and systemic health burden of osteoporosis. This article focuses primarily on data supporting the current use of PTH and its analogs in treating osteoporosis in men and women. Additionally, the use of PTH-derived therapies in sequence or in combination with antiresorptive agents is explored in detail.

HISTORICAL PERSPECTIVE

PTH, the major hormonal regulator of calcium homeostasis, is secreted by the chief cells of the parathyroid gland as a polypeptide containing 84 amino acids. Bauer and colleagues first discovered the anabolic effect of PTH in rats in 1929.[2] In these series of experiments, daily injection of PTH in growing rats was shown to have an anabolic effect in trabecular bone. Largely because of the known proresorptive effects of PTH excess in other settings, this finding was set aside for the next half century.

After the purification of PTH in the 1970s, enthusiasm again developed for investigating exogenously administered PTH analogs as potential treatments for osteoporosis. In these early studies, administration of the first 34 amino acids of PTH (PTH 1–34, teriparatide) was shown to stimulate bone formation to a greater degree than the concomitant increase in bone resorption, resulting in net increases in trabecular bone mass.[3–9] These studies and others clearly showed that although continuous activation of the PTH receptor has a predominately proresorptive effect on skeletal metabolism, intermittent administration of PTH could act as a net anabolic agent, particularly at anatomic sites rich in trabecular bone.[4,10]

In 2001, a multinational clinical trial showed for the first time that teriparatide administration could reduce the incidence of vertebral and nonvertebral fractures.[11] This study led to FDA approval of teriparatide as the first available anabolic agent. Although PTH (1–84) has been approved in Europe to treat postmenopausal osteoporosis, it is not available in the United States. Nevertheless, many clinical trials have been performed with PTH (1–84) and both molecules are discussed in detail.

MECHANISM OF ACTION

Although the mechanisms through which PTH analogs exert their anabolic effects are incompletely understood, evidence suggests that multiple pathways are involved. On a cellular level, the PTH-induced increase in osteoblast number has been shown to be related to both reduced osteoblast apoptosis[12,13] and transformation of bone-lining cells to osteoblasts.[14] On a molecular level, current evidence suggests that PTH may decrease the production of osteocyte-derived sclerostin, an endogenous inhibitor of Wnt signaling.[15,16] Through decreasing sclerostin expression, PTH may remove the inhibition of the Wnt signaling cascade, which is the final common pathway leading to osteoblast differentiation and activation.[17] Another suggested mechanism of PTH's anabolic action is the direct stimulation of local production of insulin-like growth factor I or other bone-stimulating growth factors that are known to be necessary for PTH to exert its anabolic effect.[18–20] Furthermore, evidence shows that through stimulating receptor activator of nuclear factor κβ (RANK) ligand–mediated bone resorption, PTH promotes the release of preformed growth factors that are adsorbed to the bone matrix, contributing to skeletal anabolism.[20]

EFFECT OF PTH ON BONE TURNOVER

Intermittent PTH administration stimulates both bone resorption and formation, and thus its effects on bone turnover markers differ significantly from those seen with antiresorptive treatments for osteoporosis. Serum bone formation markers (eg, pro-collagen type 1 amino-terminal propeptide [P1NP], osteocalcin, alkaline phosphatase) increase significantly within days of initiation of either teriparatide or PTH (1–84).[21] Although bone resorption markers also rise early in the course of therapy, the rate and relative magnitude of their rise are considerably smaller than those of formation markers (**Fig. 1**).[22–24] This observation has led to the hypothesis that an anabolic window exists in the first several months of PTH analog therapy, during which its effect is purely anabolic. As discussed below, several clinical trials have been designed to extend this period of increased formation without increased resorption. In addition, the dramatic stimulation of bone formation seen with PTH therapy peaks at 6 to 12 months of therapy, after which bone formation markers generally revert toward base-line levels (see **Fig. 1**).[24] This waning of osteoblast stimulation may be one of the limiting factors in the clinical use of teriparatide and PTH (1–84), although the mechanisms underlying this effect remain unknown.

EFFECTS OF PTH ON BONE MINERAL DENSITY

Teriparatide and PTH (1–84) induce the most significant increases in bone mineral density (BMD) at the spine, an anatomic site rich in trabecular bone. In the teriparatide fracture prevention study, 1637 postmenopausal women received either placebo, 20 mcg/d of teriparatide, or 40 mcg/d of teriparatide through subcutaneous injection for a mean treatment period of 18 months. Posteroanterior spine BMD as assessed with dual-energy x-ray absorptiometry (DXA) increased by 9.7% in the 20-mcg group and by 13.7% in the 40-mcg group (**Fig. 2**).[11] Although changes in trabecular volumetric BMD (via quantitative CT [QCT]) were not assessed in this study, a smaller

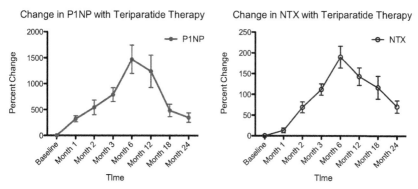

Fig. 1. Change in P1NP and type I collagen N-telopeptide in 31 postmenopausal osteoporotic women treated for 24 months with 40 mcg/d of teriparatide. (*Data from* Finkelstein JS, Wyland JJ, Lee H, et al. Effects of teriparatide, alendronate, or both in women with postmenopausal osteoporosis. J Clin Endocrinol Metab 2010;95(4):1838–45.)

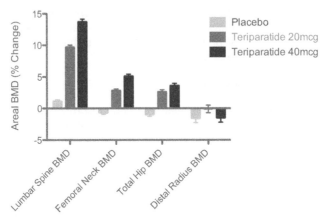

Fig. 2. BMD changes in 1637 postmenopausal women receiving placebo, 20 mcg/d of teriparatide, or 40 mcg/d of teriparatide after a mean of 18 months of treatment and median follow-up of 21 months. (*Data from* Neer RM, Arnaud CD, Zanchetta JR, et al. Effect of parathyroid hormone (1–34) on fractures and bone mineral density in postmenopausal women with osteoporosis. N Engl J Med 2001;344:1434–41.)

study showed that QCT-derived spinal trabecular volumetric BMD increased by 61% in postmenopausal women treated with 40 mcg/d of teriparatide for 24 months.[24]

Another trial randomized 2532 postmenopausal women to receive either placebo or 100 mcg of PTH (1–84) for 18 months. DXA-derived BMD of the posteroanterior spine increased by 6.9% and QCT-derived trabecular volumetric bone mineral density increased by 37% in the PTH (1–84) group.[23]

Several studies have also directly compared the BMD response to PTH analogs and bisphosphonates. In one trial, after 12 months of treatment with 100 mcg/d of PTH (1–84) or 10 mg/d of alendronate, spine BMD increased by 6.3% and 4.6%, respectively, a difference that did not reach statistical significance.[25] In a 12-month trial comparing 20 mcg/d of teriparatide with a single infusion of 5 mg of zoledronic acid, spine BMD increased by 7.0% and 4.4%, respectively (a statistically significant difference).[26]

Changes in total hip and femoral neck DXA-derived BMD are often negligible in the first year of therapy with teriparatide or PTH (1–84) but then increase more substantially thereafter. In the teriparatide fracture prevention study, femoral neck and total hip BMD decreased by 0.7% and 1.0%, respectively, in subjects receiving 20 mcg/d of teriparatide (the FDA-approved dose). In the 40-mcg group, femoral neck BMD increased by 5.1%, whereas total hip BMD increased by 3.6%.[11] PTH (1–84) showed similar effects at the hip in postmenopausal women, with total hip BMD increasing by 2.1% and femoral neck increasing by 2.5% after 18 months of treatment.[23] In a comparison of teriparatide with a parenteral bisphosphonate, BMD at the total hip increased by 2.2% in patients receiving a single 5-mg infusion of zoledronic acid versus 1.1% in subjects receiving 12 months of teriparatide therapy (20 mcg daily), a statistically significant difference.[26] When treatment courses greater than 12 months are administered, head-to-head comparisons of teriparatide or PTH (1–84) and bisphosphonates generally report similar changes in total hip and femoral neck BMD.[22,27] In contrast, 24 months of teriparatide at 40 mcg/d increased areal BMD at the femoral neck and total hip significantly more than 30 months of alendronate at 10 mg/d in postmenopausal women.[24] When QCT is used to assess changes in trabecular volumetric BMD of the hip, PTH (1–84) clearly shows positive effects as early as 12 months.[25]

At the one-third distal radius (a site composed of predominantly cortical bone), teriparatide and PTH (1–84) generally produce an apparent decrease in BMD. In the teriparatide fracture study, distal radius BMD decreased by 1.6% in the placebo group, was unchanged in the 20-mcg group, and decreased by 1.5% in the 40-mcg group (comparisons of treatment groups with placebo did not reach statistical significance). In the subset of patients in the PTH (1–84) fracture trial who underwent one-third distal radius BMD assessment, BMD declined by 5.0%.[23] Whether this decrease in cortical BMD represents true bone loss or subtle changes in bone size and mineralization is unclear.

EFFECTS ON SKELETAL METABOLISM, MICROARCHITECTURE, AND ESTIMATED STRENGTH

The effects of teriparatide on trabecular architecture, cortical parameters, and bone formation rates have been investigated primarily via bone biopsy of the iliac crest. In these studies, teriparatide significantly increased trabecular bone volume,[4,28] trabecular connectivity, and cortical thickness.[28,29] In addition, cancellous, endocortical, and periosteal bone formation rates were increased in bone biopsy specimens from patients who had undergone short-term treatment with teriparatide.[30,31] Although the increase in periosteal bone formation suggests that PTH may have the ability to increase bone size, this remains a very controversial concept and has not been confirmed in all studies. For example, in a study assessing bone biopsy specimens from postmenopausal osteoporotic women who received 100 mcg of PTH (1–84) for 18 or 24 months, no effect on cortical thickness or endocortical and periosteal bone formation rates was observed.[32]

Using finite element analysis of QCT data, estimated vertebral bone strength was compared in subjects who had received 18 months of therapy with either 20 mcg/d of teriparatide or 10 mg/d of alendronate. Estimated strength increased in both groups; however, it increased more in the teriparatide group, primarily because of increased trabecular strength parameters.[33] QCT-derived finite element analysis of the hip was also performed on a subset of subjects participating in a trial that compared treatment with either alendronate, PTH (1–84), or both for 1 year. In this study, estimated bone strength increased equally in both the PTH and alendronate groups.[34]

In a study using high-resolution peripheral quantitative CT, changes in bone microarchitecture and estimated strength at the distal radius and tibia were assessed in 11 osteoporotic postmenopausal women treated with 20 mcg/d of teriparatide. After 18 months of treatment, cortical BMD decreased significantly at both anatomic sites and a trend was seen toward increased cortical porosity, although estimated bone strength did not change.[35]

ANTIFRACTURE EFFICACY

In the teriparatide fracture prevention trial, 1637 postmenopausal women with a history of one moderate or two mild vertebral fractures (women with fewer than two moderate fractures were also required to have a hip or lumbar spine T score of –1 or below) were randomized to receive placebo, 20 mcg/d of teriparatide, or 40 mcg/d of teriparatide. Median treatment duration was 18 months, and median follow-up was 21 months. Teriparatide reduced the risk of a new vertebral fracture by 65% and 69% in the 20-mcg/d and 40-mcg/d groups, respectively (**Fig. 3**). Nonvertebral fragility fractures were reduced by 53% and 54% in the 20-mcg/d and 40-mcg/d groups, respectively.

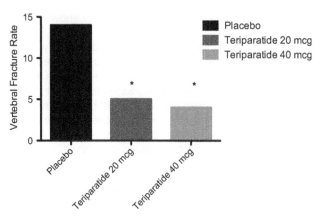

Fig. 3. Vertebral fracture rate in 1637 postmenopausal women treated with placebo, 20 mcg/d of teriparatide, or 40 mcg/d of teriparatide for a median follow-up of 21 months. Asterisk indicates between group statistical significance compared with placebo. (*Data from* Neer RM, Arnaud CD, Zanchetta JR, et al. Effect of parathyroid hormone (1–34) on fractures and bone mineral density in postmenopausal women with osteoporosis. N Engl J Med 2001;344:1434–41.)

The study was not powered to detect a difference in hip fractures. In addition, the study was stopped early because of the discovery of an increased risk of osteosarcoma in animal models. Although DXA-derived BMD increased more at the spine and hip with the 40-mcg dose, a greater incidence of hypercalcemia and other minor side effects, in addition to the lack of a difference in fracture reduction, led to the marketing approval of the 20-mcg dose.[11]

A study of PTH (1–84) was also powered to assess fracture outcomes but included a lower-risk population of postmenopausal women, many of whom had no history of vertebral fracture.[23] The study randomized 2532 osteoporotic postmenopausal women with a mean age of 64 years to either placebo injections or 100 mcg/d of PTH (1–84) for 18 months. The relative risk of new or worsened vertebral fracture decreased by 58% in the PTH group (2% absolute risk reduction). This study had a high adverse event–associated withdrawal rate, with 98 subjects in the placebo group and 172 subjects in the PTH group discontinuing treatment (a statistically significant difference that is likely related, at least partly, to the inclusion of subjects with mild hypercalcemia at baseline).

GLUCOCORTICOID-INDUCED OSTEOPOROSIS

Glucocorticoid-induced osteoporosis is the most common secondary cause of osteoporosis and, unlike postmenopausal osteoporosis, decreased osteoblast number and function play the largest role in its pathogenesis.[36] Although bisphosphonates are effective in treating glucocorticoid-induced osteoporosis, it was hypothesized that an osteoblast-targeted therapy would provide even greater efficacy. This hypothesis was confirmed in an 18-month comparative efficacy trial in which 428 women and men (age 22–89 years) with glucocorticoid-induced osteoporosis were randomized to receive 10 mg/d of alendronate or 20 mcg/d of teriparatide.[37] The mean prednisone-equivalent daily dose of corticosteroids was 7.8 mg in the alendronate group and 7.5 mg in the teriparatide group, whereas the mean glucocorticoid treatment duration was 1.2 and 1.5 years in the alendronate and teriparatide groups, respectively. Lumbar spine BMD increased 7.2% in the teriparatide group and 3.4% in the alendronate group, whereas total hip BMD increased by 3.8% in the teriparatide group and 2.4% in the alendronate group. The rate of new vertebral fractures in the teriparatide group was 0.6% compared with 6.1% in the alendronate group (**Fig. 4**). No difference was seen in nonvertebral fractures between the groups.

In an earlier trial, 51 postmenopausal women aged 50 to 82 years who were taking corticosteroids for rheumatologic disease were randomized to either teriparatide and continued estrogen therapy or continued estrogen therapy alone. Subjects were eligible for the study if they had been taking the equivalent of 5 to 20 mg/d of prednisone for 12 months and were expected to continue on corticosteroids for 12 months or more. DXA and QCT showed that combination therapy with teriparatide and continued estrogen was more effective at increasing lumbar spine BMD than continued estrogen therapy alone.[38]

EFFECTS IN MEN

The effects of teriparatide in men were investigated in a multicenter trial that randomized 437 men with hypogonadal or idiopathic osteoporosis to placebo, teriparatide at 20 mcg/d, or teriparatide at 40 mcg/d for a median treatment duration of 11 months. Spine DXA-derived BMD increased by 5.9% and 9.0% in the 20-mcg and 40-mcg groups, respectively.[39] These changes in BMD were similar to those seen in the parallel trial performed in postmenopausal women.[11] In an observational follow-up study, these men were monitored for an additional 30 months. Although many subjects from the placebo group had been started on an antiresorptive agent, a significant 83% relative risk reduction for moderate or severe vertebral fractures was seen in the combined teriparatide groups.[40] Several additional studies have confirmed the anabolic effects of PTH in men.[41,42]

EXPLORATION OF ALTERNATIVE DOSING REGIMENS

Although the FDA-approved dose of teriparatide is 20 mcg/d, several studies have addressed whether changing the dosing frequency or magnitude would render

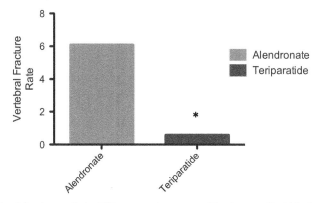

Fig. 4. Vertebral fracture rate in 428 men and women with glucocorticoid-induced osteoporosis after 18 months of treatment with 10 mg/d of alendronate or 20 mcg/d of teriparatide. Asterisk indicates group statistical significance between teriparatide and alendronate groups. (*Data from* Saag KG, Shane E, Boonen S, et al. Teriparatide or alendronate in glucocorticoid-induced osteoporosis. N Engl J Med 2007;357:2028–39.)

a greater increase in bone density. In one study, 80 postmenopausal women were randomized to either constant-dose or escalating-dose teriparatide therapy. The escalating-dose regimen involved administration of 20 mcg/d from baseline to month 6; 30 mcg/d from month 6 to 12; and 40 mcg/d for months 12 to 18. Those in the constant-dose group received 30 mcg/d for 18 months, so the cumulative drug exposure in both groups was equivalent. Although bone turnover markers in the escalating-dose group did not decline during months 12 through 18 as they did in the constant-dose group, changes in BMD did not differ between groups.[43]

Another study designed to determine the efficacy of less-frequent dosing of PTH randomized 50 osteopenic postmenopausal women to treatment with either PTH (1–84) at 100 mcg/d for 1 month followed by 100 mcg weekly for 11 months, or placebo injections with the same schedule. Spine BMD (DXA) increased modestly in the treatment group (2.1% vs placebo), whereas femoral neck and total hip BMD did not change significantly.[44]

The effect of cyclic teriparatide (3 months of daily therapy followed by 3 months without) has also been compared with daily teriparatide therapy among women also receiving alendronate. At 15 months, spine BMD increased by 6.1% in the daily teriparatide group and 5.4% in the cyclic teriparatide group, a difference that was not statistically significant.[45]

The anabolic effects of PTH wane after 6 to 12 months of therapy. In an attempt to overcome this obstacle, 23 osteoporotic men and women were initially treated with 40 mcg of teriparatide for 24 months, maintained off-treatment for 12 months, and then re-treated with 40 mcg/d of teriparatide for an additional 12 months. Although BMD increased during the re-treatment phase, the effects on BMD were approximately 50% less than those seen during the initial 12 months of therapy. Moreover, the increases in biochemical markers of bone formation were significantly attenuated compared with the initial therapeutic period.[46] In another re-treatment trial, increases in spine BMD were similar during an initial and second course of teriparatide treatment, but these subjects were receiving concomitant alendronate, and thus the independent effects of teriparatide cannot be assessed.[47]

NOVEL DELIVERY METHODS

Several alternative teriparatide delivery methods have been investigated, because patient resistance to daily self-injection has been one of several factors limiting its widespread use. In one study, 165 postmenopausal osteoporotic women were randomized to 6 months of therapy with a transdermal teriparatide patch at doses of 20, 30, or 40 mcg/d; a placebo patch; or injections with 20 mcg/d of teriparatide. All three doses of the patch increased lumbar spine BMD to approximately the same degree as the 20-mcg injections. Subjects who received the 40-mcg patch experienced a significantly larger increase in total hip BMD compared with the other treatment groups.[48] In an uncontrolled pilot study of 90 osteoporotic women and men seeking to determine the feasibility of PTH (1–34) nasal spray, 3 months of daily nasal spray therapy (1000 mcg/d) increased lumbar spine BMD by 2.4% and significantly increased bone formation markers.[49]

COMBINATION THERAPY

Over the past decade, investigators have explored the use of antiresorptive agents in combination with teriparatide or PTH (1–84), with the hope that combined therapy would suppress PTH-induced resorption but leave PTH-induced bone formation unaltered. The generally positive response observed in women treated with the combination of estrogen replacement therapy or raloxifene and PTH supported this hypothesis.[50–53] Unfortunately, the results of the randomized trials combining potent oral and intravenous bisphosphonates with teriparatide or PTH (1–84) have generally been disappointing.

In one study, 238 postmenopausal women aged 55 to 85 years with increased fracture risk were randomly assigned to PTH (1–84) at 100 mcg/d, alendronate at 10 mg/d, or the combination of both for 1 year. DXA-derived lumbar spine BMD increased by 4.6%, 6.3%, and 6.1% in the alendronate, PTH, and combination groups, respectively (increases in the PTH and combination groups were significantly greater than those in the alendronate group, although no significant difference was seen between the combination and PTH-alone groups). BMD remained essentially unchanged at the femoral neck and total hip in the PTH group, whereas total hip BMD increased by 1.9% in the combination group. Trabecular BMD of the spine (QCT) increased significantly in all groups, although the increase in the PTH group was approximately double that seen in the combination and alendronate groups (25.5%, 12.9%, and 10.5%, respectively). Trabecular volumetric BMD at the hip (QCT) showed a similar pattern to that seen in the spine, but the differences between groups were not statistically significant. Cortical volumetric BMD of the hip (QCT) decreased significantly in the PTH group, was unchanged in the combination group, and increased in the alendronate group.[25]

In another study, 93 postmenopausal women were randomly assigned to 10 mg/d of alendronate, 40 mcg/d of teriparatide (double the FDA-approved dose), or both medications. Alendronate was started 6 months before teriparatide was added in the combination group. After 24 months of teriparatide therapy, DXA-derived lumbar spine BMD increased by 17.8% in the teriparatide group, 11.9% in the combination group, and 6.8% in the alendronate group (a significant difference among all groups). Total hip and femoral neck BMD also increased more in the teriparatide alone group than in both the combination and alendronate-alone groups (**Fig. 5**). Strikingly, spinal trabecular BMD measured with QCT increased by 61% in the teriparatide group, 24%

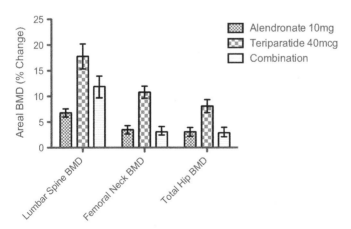

Fig. 5. Change in DXA-derived bone mineral density in 93 postmenopausal women after 30 months of treatment with 10 mg/d of alendronate, 24 months of treatment with 40 mcg/d of teriparatide, or combination therapy with 30 months of 10 mg/d of alendronate and 24 months of 40 mcg/d of teriparatide. Teriparatide was initiated at the 6-month visit in the teriparatide-alone group and the combination therapy group. (*Data from* Finkelstein JS, Wyland JJ, Lee H, et al. Effects of teriparatide, alendronate, or both in women with postmenopausal osteoporosis. J Clin Endocrinol Metab 2010;95(4):1838–45.)

in the combination group, and 1% in the alendronate group (**Fig. 6**). The large increase in biochemical markers of bone formation induced by teriparatide were significantly blunted in the combination therapy group.[24] A study in osteoporotic men using the same protocol as the preceding trial reported similar findings.[41,54]

Another study compared adding 20 mcg/d of teriparatide to preexisting antiresorptive treatment versus switching from antiresorptive therapy to teriparatide monotherapy for 18 months. In this study, 193 postmenopausal women who had previously taken either alendronate or raloxifene for at least 18 months were stratified based on prior antiresorptive treatment and then randomized to either continue the antiresorptive medication and start teriparatide or discontinue the antiresorptive and start teriparatide. Switching from antiresorptive therapy to teriparatide caused a greater increase in bone turnover markers in both raloxifene and alendronate strata. Conversely, adding teriparatide to existing therapy increased BMD slightly more than switching to teriparatide.[55]

Finally, a 12-month randomized controlled trial randomized 412 postmenopausal women with osteoporosis to a single infusion of 5 mg of zoledronic acid, 20 mcg/d of teriparatide, or a combination. DXA-derived lumbar spine BMD increased similarly in the combination group and the teriparatide monotherapy group, and these increases were larger than those observed in the zoledronic acid monotherapy group. Conversely, total hip and femoral neck BMD increased similarly in the combination group and the zoledronic acid monotherapy group, and these increases were larger than those in the teriparatide monotherapy group.[26] Because this study was limited to 12 months, and the positive DXA-derived BMD effects of teriparatide at the total hip and femoral neck are primarily seen in the 12- to 24-month period, the clinical relevance of the between-group difference at hip sites are unclear.

Together these studies suggest that coadministration of bisphosphonates with teriparatide blunts the teriparatide-associated stimulation of bone formation, particularly in predominately trabecular sites, such as the lumbar spine. Although studies

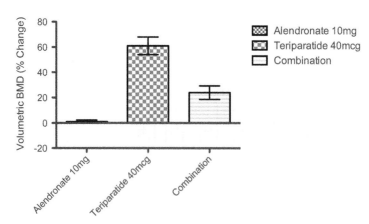

Fig. 6. Change in QCT-derived spinal volumetric bone mineral density in 93 postmenopausal women after 30 months of treatment with 10 mg/d of alendronate, 24 months of treatment with 40 mcg/d of teriparatide, or combination therapy with 30 months of 10 mg/d of alendronate and 24 months of 40 mcg/d of teriparatide. Teriparatide was initiated at the 6-month visit in the teriparatide-alone group and the combination therapy group. (*Data from* Finkelstein JS, Wyland JJ, Lee H, et al. Effects of teriparatide, alendronate, or both in women with postmenopausal osteoporosis. J Clin Endocrinol Metab 2010;95(4):1838–45.)

addressing fracture risk reduction have not been performed, the current data do not support simultaneous therapy with teriparatide and a bisphosphonate.

PRETREATMENT WITH ANTIRESORPTIVE AGENTS

Many patients previously treated with antiresorptive agents will be switched to teriparatide because of suboptimal treatment effect or continued fractures. Thus, it is important to determine the effect of prior exposure to antiresorptive agents on subsequent response to teriparatide therapy. Several trials have addressed this question, although their lack of randomization makes the findings difficult to interpret and may explain their inconsistent results.

Hormone Replacement Therapy

Several studies have examined the effects of adding teriparatide to the treatment of women undergoing estrogen-containing hormone replacement therapy (HRT). Although no direct comparisons were made to teriparatide alone, combination teriparatide and HRT in women pretreated with HRT increased BMD to approximately the same extent seen in the major clinical trials of teriparatide.[50–52] In the largest of these trials, 247 postmenopausal women, 50% of whom had been on HRT for at least 12 months before enrolling in the study, were randomized to either HRT and placebo or HRT and 40 mcg/d of teriparatide for a mean treatment duration of 13.8 months. In the combination group, DXA-derived BMD increased by 14.0%, 5.2%, and 5.2% at the spine, total hip, and femoral neck, respectively, whereas BMD increased by 3.0%, 1.6%, and 2.0%, respectively, in the group receiving HRT alone.[52]

Raloxifene

In a study comparing pretreatment with raloxifene and alendronate, daily teriparatide was administered to 59 postmenopausal women who had previously received one of these antiresorptive agents for 18 months. In the subjects previously treated with raloxifene, lumbar spine BMD increased by 10.2% at 18 months, whereas in alendronate-pretreated subjects, BMD increased significantly less (4.1%). Furthermore, in the raloxifene-pretreated subjects, teriparatide stimulation of bone turnover was similar to that in treatment-naïve subjects.[56]

Bisphosphonates

In addition to the study described earlier, several studies have addressed the issue of prior bisphosphonate treatment on the subsequent response to PTH analogs. In one large trial, a subgroup of 503 postmenopausal women assigned to receive teriparatide for 24 months were prospectively grouped into those who were antiresorptive treatment–naïve and those who had received antiresorptive medications (90% bisphosphonates). Although lumbar spine and hip BMD increased significantly in all groups, spine BMD increased by 13.1% in the treatment-naïve subjects but significantly less (10.2%) in the subjects previously treated with antiresorptive agents.[57] In addition, the increase in bone formation markers at 1 month was diminished in those pretreated with antiresorptive agents compared with treatment-naïve subjects, although levels equalized by 6 months.[58]

In a nonrandomized study that directly compared the effect of pretreatment with two bisphosphonate medications, 324 women previously treated with either alendronate or risedronate for at least 24 months had their bisphosphonate discontinued and were started on 20 mcg/d of teriparatide. Lumbar spine areal BMD and trabecular spine volumetric BMD (by QCT) increased significantly more in women previously treated with risedronate than in those previously treated with alendronate.[59] Whether these findings relate to inherent differences between the antiresorptive agents or to other factors is unclear.

Taken together, these data suggest that prior bisphosphonate use may slightly blunt the anabolic effect of PTH treatment, although the clinical consequences are not clear.

ANTIRESORPTIVES AFTER PTH THERAPY

The use of antiresorptive medications after a course of teriparatide therapy has become the standard of care, because multiple studies have shown that PTH-induced gains in BMD are quickly lost after discontinuation of therapy.[42,50,60–62] In one of the largest of these studies, subjects who had received PTH (1–84) alone for 1 year were randomized to either alendronate or placebo for an additional year. DXA-derived BMD of the spine decreased by approximately 2% in subjects randomized to the placebo arm, and QCT-derived trabecular volumetric BMD of the spine decreased approximately 10%. In contrast, BMD increased in subjects switching from PTH (1–84) to alendronate at most anatomic sites.[62]

TERIPARATIDE INDICATIONS, LIMITATIONS, SIDE EFFECTS, AND SAFETY CONCERNS

Teriparatide is approved for use in postmenopausal women with osteoporosis who are at high risk for fracture, men with primary or hypogonadal osteoporosis at high risk for fracture, and men and women with glucocorticoid-induced osteoporosis. The increased incidence of osteosarcoma in rats receiving high doses of PTH led to an FDA warning that teriparatide should not be prescribed to patients who have an increased baseline risk for osteosarcoma (the risk of osteosarcoma is discussed in detail later). Labeled use of teriparatide is also limited to 2 years partly because of these animal studies and the resultant shortened duration of the teriparatide fracture efficacy study.[11] Aside from concerns over safety, the cost of teriparatide (approximately $12,000 per year) and the requirement for daily subcutaneous delivery have also substantially limited its use to the most severely affected and motivated patients.

The most common side effects of teriparatide at the currently approved dose (20 mcg) are dizziness, leg cramps, hypercalcemia, and hypercalciuria. In trials of PTH (1–84), hypercalcemia, hypercalciuria, nausea, and vomiting were all significantly more common in the treatment group than in the placebo group.[11,23]

In the teriparatide fracture prevention trial, hypercalcemia (defined as a calcium level of 10.6–11.2 mg/dL) occurred in 11% of those treated with the 20-mcg dose and 28% of those with the 40-mcg dose. Hypercalciuria occurred rarely in this trial. Though the incidence of hypercalciuria was higher in the fracture prevention trial of PTH (1–84), this may have been because of the inclusion of more subjects with mild hypercalcemia at baseline. Increased rates of nephrolithiasis, nephrocalcinosis, or worsening renal function have not been observed with teriparatide or PTH (1–84) treatment.

OSTEOSARCOMA RISK

Toxicology studies investigating the effect of PTH (1–34) on young rats showed dose-dependent osteosclerosis, extramedullary hematopoiesis, and increased risk of osteosarcoma.[63–66] PTH (1–84) has also been shown to cause osteosarcoma in rodent models.[66] These toxicology studies were performed in young animals that were administered PTH (1–34) at 6 to 8 weeks of age and continued receiving daily injections between 5 and 75 mg/kg for greater than 12 months. The applicability of the

---

Box 1
Conditions associated with increased risk of osteosarcoma

- Active Paget's Disease
- Unexplained elevations of alkaline phosphatase
- Children or young adults with open epiphyses
- Skeletal metastases
- Skeletal malignant conditions
- History of irradiation to the skeleton

---

results to humans is difficult to assess because of the higher-than-human treatment doses used, initiation of therapy at a young age, continuation of therapy for more than half the life of the animal, and induction of osteosclerosis. Primate models have not shown an increased risk of osteosarcoma,[67] and although three cases of osteosarcoma have been reported in the literature among patients exposed to teriparatide, this is similar to the background rate in the general population.[68,69] In summary, although the risk of precipitating osteosarcoma in humans with the approved dose and duration of teriparatide therapy is likely either absent or small, care should be taken to avoid prescribing PTH to those who may be at increased risk for developing osteosarcoma (see **Box 1**).

EMERGING THERAPIES

Teriparatide is the only currently approved anabolic therapy in the United States for osteoporosis although several promising therapies are on the horizon. Several of these therapies involve the canonical Wnt-β-catenin pathway. Wnt signaling allows accumulation of β-catenin in the nucleus, which results in osteoblastic differentiation and bone formation.[70] Many modulators of the pathway exist; however, an endogenous inhibitor of the pathway, sclerostin, was identified early as a potential drug target because of its tissue specificity.[70]

Sclerostin is an osteocyte-secreted glycoprotein product of the *SOST* gene that competitively binds to LRP5/LRP6 and inhibits Wnt signaling.[71] Its role was discovered as a result of the description of sclerosteosis and van Buchem syndrome, similar human disorders resulting from deletion or abnormal regulation of the *SOST* gene. Both disorders are characterized by larger bones, increased levels of bone formation markers, and complete absence of fractures.[71] *SOST* knockout mice show a greater than 50% increase in BMD at the spine and leg, significant increases in bone volume by micro-CT, and increased histomorphometric bone formation rate.[72]

Preclinical studies have shown significant increases in bone formation, bone density, and bone strength with administration of antisclerostin antibody.[73-76] In a phase I trial, a single dose of an antibody to human sclerostin was given to 72 healthy postmenopausal women. In these patients, biochemical markers of bone formation increased in a dose-responsive fashion while bone resorption markers decreased. Moreover, in less than 3 months postdose, lumbar spine BMD increased by 5.3%.[77]

Dickkopf-1 (Dkk-1) is another tissue-specific inhibitor of the Wnt pathway that has been explored as a potential therapeutic target for osteoporosis. Deletion of a single allele of Dkk-1 in mice significantly increased bone mass, and knockdown of Dkk-1 in rats prevented ovariectomy-induced bone loss.[78,79] An anti–Dkk-1 antibody is currently in development for treatment of osteoporosis.[80]

Finally, PTH-related protein (PTHrP), which shares a receptor with PTH, has also been investigated for therapeutic use in osteoporosis. Although its structure is similar to that of PTH, evidence shows that PTHrP (1–36) may be less calcemic and have less-significant effects on bone resorption than PTH analogs. In a 3-month, double-blind, placebo-controlled trial, 16 postmenopausal women with osteoporosis were randomized to either placebo or 400 mcg/d of PTHrP (1–36). The PTHrP group showed a 4.7% increase in lumbar spine bone mineral density after 3 months of treatment. In addition, although osteocalcin increased significantly, serum concentration of type I collagen N-telopeptide and blood calcium levels did not rise during the treatment period.[81]

SUMMARY

As the first FDA-approved anabolic agent for osteoporosis, teriparatide has proven effective for people at highest risk of fracture, despite limitations of expense, route of delivery, and length of treatment. Based on available data, combination therapy with teriparatide and antiresorptive agents does not seem to offer a therapeutic advantage. However, treatment with an antiresorptive agent after completion of teriparatide therapy is essential to prevent the ensuing bone loss. Although pretreatment with bisphosphonates may somewhat attenuate the anabolic effect of teriparatide, significant gains in BMD are still achieved and prior bisphosphonate use should not dissuade clinicians from using teriparatide in select patients. Although teriparatide is the only anabolic agent available today, the next decade will likely see the arrival of even more potent anabolic agents to reduce the significant morbidity and mortality that result from fragility fractures.

ACKNOWLEDGMENTS

The authors would like to thank Dr Robert Neer for his thoughtful comments during the preparation of this manuscript.

REFERENCES

1. Riggs BL, Hodgson SF, O'Fallon WM, et al. Effect of fluoride treatment on the fracture rate in postmenopausal women with osteoporosis. N Engl J Med 1990;322: 802–9.
2. Bauer W, Aub JC, Albright F. Studies of calcium and phosphorus metabolism: V. A study of the bone trabeculae as a readily available reserve supply of calcium. J Exp Med 1929;49:145–62.
3. Reeve J, Hesp R, Williams D, et al. Anabolic effect of low doses of a fragment of human parathyroid hormone on the skeleton in postmenopausal osteoporosis. Lancet 1976;1:1035–8.
4. Reeve J, Meunier PJ, Parsons JA, et al. Anabolic effect of human parathyroid hormone fragment on trabecular bone in involutional osteoporosis: a multicentre trial. Br Med J 1980;280:1340–4.
5. Slovik DM, Rosenthal DI, Doppelt SH, et al. Restoration of spinal bone in osteoporotic men by treatment with human parathyroid hormone (1-34) and 1,25-dihydroxyvitamin D. J Bone Miner Res 1986;1:377–81.
6. Reeve J, Davies UM, Hesp R, et al. Treatment of osteoporosis with human parathyroid peptide and observations on effect of sodium fluoride. BMJ 1990;301: 314–8.

7. Hesch RD, Busch U, Prokop M, et al. Increase of vertebral density by combination therapy with pulsatile 1-38hPTH and sequential addition of calcitonin nasal spray in osteoporotic patients. Calcif Tissue Int 1989;44:176–80.

8. Finkelstein JS, Klibanski A, Schaefer EH, et al. Parathyroid hormone for the prevention of bone loss induced by estrogen deficiency. N Engl J Med 1994; 331:1618–23.

9. Hodsman AB, Fraher LJ, Ostbye T, et al. An evaluation of several biochemical markers for bone formation and resorption in a protocol utilizing cyclical parathyroid hormone and calcitonin therapy for osteoporosis. J Clin Invest 1993;91:1138–48.

10. Tam CS, Heersche JN, Murray TM, et al. Parathyroid hormone stimulates the bone apposition rate independently of its resorptive action: differential effects of intermittent and continuous administration. Endocrinology 1982;110:506–12.

11. Neer RM, Arnaud CD, Zanchetta JR, et al. Effect of parathyroid hormone (1-34) on fractures and bone mineral density in postmenopausal women with osteoporosis. N Engl J Med 2001;344:1434–41.

12. Jilka RL, Weinstein RS, Bellido T, et al. Increased bone formation by prevention of osteoblast apoptosis with parathyroid hormone. J Clin Invest 1999;104:439–46.

13. Jilka RL, O'Brien CA, Ali AA, et al. Intermittent PTH stimulates periosteal bone formation by actions on post-mitotic preosteoblasts. Bone 2009;44:275–86.

14. Dobnig H, Turner RT. Evidence that intermittent treatment with parathyroid hormone increases bone formation in adult rats by activation of bone lining cells. Endocrinology 1995;136:3632–8.

15. Bellido T, Ali AA, Gubrij I, et al. Chronic elevation of parathyroid hormone in mice reduces expression of sclerostin by osteocytes: a novel mechanism for hormonal control of osteoblastogenesis. Endocrinology 2005;146:4577–83.

16. Drake MT, Srinivasan B, Modder UI, et al. Effects of parathyroid hormone treatment on circulating sclerostin levels in postmenopausal women. J Clin Endocrinol Metab 2010;95:5056–62.

17. Monroe DG, McGee-Lawrence ME, Oursler MJ, et al. Update on Wnt signaling in bone cell biology and bone disease. Gene 2012;492:1–18.

18. Bikle DD, Sakata T, Leary C, et al. Insulin-like growth factor I is required for the anabolic actions of parathyroid hormone on mouse bone. J Bone Miner Res 2002;17:1570–8.

19. McCarthy TL, Centrella M, Canalis E. Parathyroid hormone enhances the transcript and polypeptide levels of insulin-like growth factor I in osteoblast-enriched cultures from fetal rat bone. Endocrinology 1989;124:1247–53.

20. Oreffo RO, Mundy GR, Seyedin SM, et al. Activation of the bone-derived latent TGF beta complex by isolated osteoclasts. Biochem Biophys Res Commun 1989;158:817–23.

21. Glover SJ, Eastell R, McCloskey EV, et al. Rapid and robust response of biochemical markers of bone formation to teriparatide therapy. Bone 2009;45:1053–8.

22. McClung MR, San Martin J, Miller PD, et al. Opposite bone remodeling effects of teriparatide and alendronate in increasing bone mass. Arch Intern Med 2005;165: 1762–8.

23. Greenspan SL, Bone HG, Ettinger MP, et al. Effect of recombinant human parathyroid hormone (1-84) on vertebral fracture and bone mineral density in postmenopausal women with osteoporosis: a randomized trial. Ann Intern Med 2007;146:326–39.

24. Finkelstein JS, Wyland JJ, Lee H, et al. Effects of teriparatide, alendronate, or both in women with postmenopausal osteoporosis. J Clin Endocrinol Metab 2010;95:1838–45.

25. Black DM, Greenspan SL, Ensrud KE, et al. The effects of parathyroid hormone and alendronate alone or in combination in postmenopausal osteoporosis. N Engl J Med 2003;349:1207–15.
26. Cosman F, Eriksen EF, Recknor C, et al. Effects of intravenous zoledronic acid plus subcutaneous teriparatide [rhPTH(1-34)] in postmenopausal osteoporosis. J Bone Miner Res 2011;26:503–11.
27. Body JJ, Gaich GA, Scheele WH, et al. A randomized double-blind trial to compare the efficacy of teriparatide [recombinant human parathyroid hormone (1-34)] with alendronate in postmenopausal women with osteoporosis. J Clin Endocrinol Metab 2002;87:4528–35.
28. Jiang Y, Zhao JJ, Mitlak BH, et al. Recombinant human parathyroid hormone (1-34) [teriparatide] improves both cortical and cancellous bone structure. J Bone Miner Res 2003;18:1932–41.
29. Dempster DW, Cosman F, Kurland ES, et al. Effects of daily treatment with parathyroid hormone on bone microarchitecture and turnover in patients with osteoporosis: a paired biopsy study. J Bone Miner Res 2001;16:1846–53.
30. Lindsay R, Zhou H, Cosman F, et al. Effects of a one-month treatment with PTH(1-34) on bone formation on cancellous, endocortical, and periosteal surfaces of the human ilium. J Bone Miner Res 2007;22:495–502.
31. Lindsay R, Cosman F, Zhou H, et al. A novel tetracycline labeling schedule for longitudinal evaluation of the short-term effects of anabolic therapy with a single iliac crest bone biopsy: early actions of teriparatide. J Bone Miner Res 2006;21:366–73.
32. Recker RR, Bare SP, Smith SY, et al. Cancellous and cortical bone architecture and turnover at the iliac crest of postmenopausal osteoporotic women treated with parathyroid hormone 1-84. Bone 2009;44:113–9.
33. Keaveny TM, Donley DW, Hoffmann PF, et al. Effects of teriparatide and alendronate on vertebral strength as assessed by finite element modeling of QCT scans in women with osteoporosis. J Bone Miner Res 2007;22:149–57.
34. Keaveny TM, Hoffmann PF, Singh M, et al. Femoral bone strength and its relation to cortical and trabecular changes after treatment with PTH, alendronate, and their combination as assessed by finite element analysis of quantitative CT scans. J Bone Miner Res 2008;23:1974–82.
35. Macdonald HM, Nishiyama KK, Hanley DA, et al. Changes in trabecular and cortical bone microarchitecture at peripheral sites associated with 18 months of teriparatide therapy in postmenopausal women with osteoporosis. Osteoporos Int 2011;22:357–62.
36. Weinstein RS. Clinical practice. Glucocorticoid-induced bone disease. N Engl J Med 2011;365:62–70.
37. Saag KG, Shane E, Boonen S, et al. Teriparatide or alendronate in glucocorticoid-induced osteoporosis. N Engl J Med 2007;357:2028–39.
38. Lane NE, Sanchez S, Modin GW, et al. Parathyroid hormone treatment can reverse corticosteroid-induced osteoporosis. Results of a randomized controlled clinical trial. J Clin Invest 1998;102:1627–33.
39. Orwoll ES, Scheele WH, Paul S, et al. The effect of teriparatide [human parathyroid hormone (1-34)] therapy on bone density in men with osteoporosis. J Bone Miner Res 2003;18:9–17.
40. Kaufman JM, Orwoll E, Goemaere S, et al. Teriparatide effects on vertebral fractures and bone mineral density in men with osteoporosis: treatment and discontinuation of therapy. Osteoporos Int 2005;16:510–6.
41. Finkelstein JS, Hayes A, Hunzelman JL, et al. The effects of parathyroid hormone, alendronate, or both in men with osteoporosis. N Engl J Med 2003;349:1216–26.

42. Kurland ES, Cosman F, McMahon DJ, et al. Parathyroid hormone as a therapy for idiopathic osteoporosis in men: effects on bone mineral density and bone markers. J Clin Endocrinol Metab 2000;85:3069–76.

43. Yu EW, Neer RM, Lee H, et al. Time-dependent changes in skeletal response to teriparatide: escalating vs. constant dose teriparatide (PTH 1-34) in osteoporotic women. Bone 2011;48:713–9.

44. Black DM, Bouxsein ML, Palermo L, et al. Randomized trial of once-weekly para-thyroid hormone (1-84) on bone mineral density and remodeling. J Clin Endocrinol Metab 2008;93:2166–72.

45. Cosman F, Nieves J, Zion M, et al. Daily and cyclic parathyroid hormone in women receiving alendronate. N Engl J Med 2005;353:566–75.

46. Finkelstein JS, Wyland JJ, Leder BZ, et al. Effects of teriparatide retreatment in osteoporotic men and women. J Clin Endocrinol Metab 2009;94:2495–501.

47. Cosman F, Nieves JW, Zion M, et al. Retreatment with teriparatide one year after the first teriparatide course in patients on continued long-term alendronate. J Bone Miner Res 2009;24:1110–5.

48. Cosman F, Lane NE, Bolognese MA, et al. Effect of transdermal teriparatide administration on bone mineral density in postmenopausal women. J Clin Endocrinol Metab 2010;95:151–8.

49. Matsumoto T, Shiraki M, Hagino H, et al. Daily nasal spray of hPTH(1-34) for 3 months increases bone mass in osteoporotic subjects: a pilot study. Osteoporos Int 2006;17:1532–8.

50. Lindsay R, Nieves J, Formica C, et al. Randomised controlled study of effect of parathyroid hormone on vertebral-bone mass and fracture incidence among postmenopausal women on oestrogen with osteoporosis. Lancet 1997;350: 550–5.

51. Cosman F, Nieves J, Woelfert L, et al. Parathyroid hormone added to established hormone therapy: effects on vertebral fracture and maintenance of bone mass after parathyroid hormone withdrawal. J Bone Miner Res 2001;16:925–31.

52. Ste-Marie LG, Schwartz SL, Hossain A, et al. Effect of teriparatide [rhPTH(1-34)] on BMD when given to postmenopausal women receiving hormone replacement therapy. J Bone Miner Res 2006;21:283–91.

53. Deal C, Omizo M, Schwartz EN, et al. Combination teriparatide and raloxifene therapy for postmenopausal osteoporosis: results from a 6-month double-blind placebo-controlled trial. J Bone Miner Res 2005;20:1905–11.

54. Finkelstein JS, Leder BZ, Burnett SM, et al. Effects of teriparatide, alendronate, or both on bone turnover in osteoporotic men. J Clin Endocrinol Metab 2006;91: 2882–7.

55. Cosman F, Wermers RA, Recknor C, et al. Effects of teriparatide in postmeno-pausal women with osteoporosis on prior alendronate or raloxifene: differences between stopping and continuing the antiresorptive agent. J Clin Endocrinol Metab 2009;94:3772–80.

56. Ettinger B, San Martin J, Crans G, et al. Differential effects of teriparatide on BMD after treatment with raloxifene or alendronate. J Bone Miner Res 2004;19:745–51.

57. Obermayer-Pietsch B, Marin F, McCloskey EV, et al. Effects of two years of daily teriparatide treatment on BMD in postmenopausal women with severe osteopo-rosis with and without prior antiresorptive treatment. J Bone Miner Res 2008;23: 1591–600.

58. Blumsohn A, Marin F, Nickelsen T, et al. Early changes in biochemical markers of bone turnover and their relationship with bone mineral density changes after 24 months of treatment with teriparatide. Osteoporos Int 2011;22:1935–46.

59. Miller PD, Delmas PD, Lindsay R, et al. Early responsiveness of women with osteoporosis to teriparatide after therapy with alendronate or risedronate. J Clin Endocrinol Metab 2008;93:3785–93.

60. Rittmaster RS, Bolognese M, Ettinger MP, et al. Enhancement of bone mass in osteoporotic women with parathyroid hormone followed by alendronate. J Clin Endocrinol Metab 2000;85:2129–34.

61. Lindsay R, Scheele WH, Neer R, et al. Sustained vertebral fracture risk reduction after withdrawal of teriparatide in postmenopausal women with osteoporosis. Arch Intern Med 2004;164:2024–30.

62. Black DM, Bilezikian JP, Ensrud KE, et al. One year of alendronate after one year of parathyroid hormone (1-84) for osteoporosis. N Engl J Med 2005;353:555–65.

63. Vahle JL, Sato M, Long GG, et al. Skeletal changes in rats given daily subcutaneous injections of recombinant human parathyroid hormone (1-34) for 2 years and relevance to human safety. Toxicol Pathol 2002;30:312–21.

64. Sato M, Vahle J, Schmidt A, et al. Abnormal bone architecture and biomechanical properties with near-lifetime treatment of rats with PTH. Endocrinology 2002;143: 3230–42.

65. Vahle JL, Long GG, Sandusky G, et al. Bone neoplasms in F344 rats given teriparatide [rhPTH(1-34)] are dependent on duration of treatment and dose. Toxicol Pathol 2004;32:426–38.

66. Jolette J, Wilker CE, Smith SY, et al. Defining a noncarcinogenic dose of recombinant human parathyroid hormone 1-84 in a 2-year study in Fischer 344 rats. Toxicol Pathol 2006;34:929–40.

67. Vahle JL, Zuehlke U, Schmidt A, et al. Lack of bone neoplasms and persistence of bone efficacy in cynomolgus macaques after long-term treatment with teriparatide [rhPTH(1-34)]. J Bone Miner Res 2008;23:2033–9.

68. Harper KD, Krege JH, Marcus R, et al. Osteosarcoma and teriparatide? J Bone Miner Res 2007;22:334.

69. Subbiah V, Madsen VS, Raymond AK, et al. Of mice and men: divergent risks of teriparatide-induced osteosarcoma. Osteoporos Int 2010;21:1041–5.

70. Khosla S, Westendorf JJ, Oursler MJ. Building bone to reverse osteoporosis and repair fractures. J Clin Invest 2008;118:421–8.

71. Costa AG, Bilezikian JP. Sclerostin: therapeutic horizons based upon its actions. Curr Osteoporos Rep 2012;10:64–72.

72. Li X, Ominsky MS, Niu QT, et al. Targeted deletion of the sclerostin gene in mice results in increased bone formation and bone strength. J Bone Miner Res 2008; 23:860–9.

73. Li X, Ominsky MS, Warmington KS, et al. Sclerostin antibody treatment increases bone formation, bone mass, and bone strength in a rat model of postmenopausal osteoporosis. J Bone Miner Res 2009;24:578–88.

74. Ominsky MS, Vlasseros F, Jolette J, et al. Two doses of sclerostin antibody in cynomolgus monkeys increases bone formation, bone mineral density, and bone strength. J Bone Miner Res 2010;25:948–59.

75. Ominsky MS, Li C, Li X, et al. Inhibition of sclerostin by monoclonal antibody enhances bone healing and improves bone density and strength of nonfractured bones. J Bone Miner Res 2010;26:1012–21.

76. Li X, Ominsky MS, Warmington KS, et al. Increased bone formation and bone mass induced by sclerostin antibody is not affected by pretreatment or cotreatment with alendronate in osteopenic, ovariectomized rats. Endocrinology 2011;152:3312–22.

77. Padhi D, Jang G, Stouch B, et al. Single-dose, placebo-controlled, randomized study of AMG 785, a sclerostin monoclonal antibody. J Bone Miner Res 2011;26:19–26.

78. Morvan F, Boulukos K, Clement-Lacroix P, et al. Deletion of a single allele of the Dkk1 gene leads to an increase in bone formation and bone mass. J Bone Miner Res 2006;21:934–45.
79. Wang FS, Ko JY, Lin CL, et al. Knocking down dickkopf-1 alleviates estrogen deficiency induction of bone loss. A histomorphological study in ovariectomized rats. Bone 2007;40:485–92.
80. Betts AM, Clark TH, Yang J, et al. The application of target information and preclinical pharmacokinetic/pharmacodynamic modeling in predicting clinical doses of a Dickkopf-1 antibody for osteoporosis. J Pharmacol Exp Ther 2010; 333:2–13.
81. Horwitz MJ, Tedesco MB, Gundberg C, et al. Short-term, high-dose parathyroid hormone-related protein as a skeletal anabolic agent for the treatment of postmenopausal osteoporosis. J Clin Endocrinol Metab 2003;88:569–75.

Calcium Metabolism and Correcting Calcium Deficiencies

Ronald D. Emkey, MD*, Gregory R. Emkey, MD

KEYWORDS

- Calcium metabolism • Calcium absorption • Vitamin D • Osteoporosis
- Calcium requirements

KEY POINTS

- Calcium is the most abundant cation in the human body.
- Calcium contributes to the strength and rigidity of bone.
- Calcium absorption occurs through a process both active and passive, influenced by many factors.
- Large meta-analyses demonstrate a reduction in hip fractures with higher calcium and vitamin D ingestion, most consistently in a higher-risk population.
- It is difficult to separate out the individual contributions of calcium and vitamin D in these studies.
- The importance of concomitant protein and phosphorus ingestion may be underestimated.
- Dietary calcium may be the most reasonable approach to satisfy the body's calcium needs.

INTRODUCTION AND HISTORICAL PERSPECTIVE

Currently accepted tenets of biological theory suggest that current human dietary requirements have evolved over 200 million years, during the first 150 million years of which our ancestors were largely insectivorous and thus consumed a diet higher in calcium content than that of modern man. The average insect calcium content is 124 mg per 100 g portion, and thus much higher than wild game at 14.2 mg per 100 g. Approximately 50 million years ago, our ancestors were omnivorous and consumed a large amount of wild plants (133 mg calcium/100 g portion) in addition to wild game. During this late Paleolithic period, dietary calcium content has been calculated as 1798.9 mg/d.[1] Dietary calcium consumption during the Mesolithic and Neolithic periods decreased substantially to approximately 30% to 50% of the stone-age diet, despite there having been very little change in the genetic makeup

The authors have no disclosures to report.

Pennsylvania Regional Center for Arthritis & Osteoporosis Research, 1200 Broadcasting Road, Suite 200, Wyomissing, PA 19610, USA

* Corresponding author.

E-mail address: bonedocron@yahoo.com

Endocrinol Metab Clin N Am 41 (2012) 527–556

doi:10.1016/j.ecl.2012.04.019

of humans during this time period.[2] Human skeletal remains from the Mesolithic period revealed cortical thickness to be on average 17% greater than those of current whites and blacks.[3] Whether this was due to the increased calcium intake, more physical activity, and/or other dietary changes (more protein, micronutrients, and fiber with less sodium and fat) during the Mesolithic period compared with today is not clear.[1]

Because calcium is a threshold nutrient, would achieving a given threshold for each person be a reasonable goal, and should that level consider the higher calcium intake of our evolutionary ancestors? There is no consensus as to whether exceeding a "threshold" intake may be helpful or harmful to bone or other cellular systems in which calcium plays a significant role. Because fewer than 100 generations have elapsed since the time of calcium surfeit to the present, it is unlikely that adaptive mechanisms for the conservation of calcium would have evolved, thus generating an even more complex dilemma.[4] Modern man is living longer and reproducing successfully, suggesting some evolutionary success. Conversely, our longer life span (and longer postmenopausal interval) may play a major role in the apparent increase in osteoporosis we now see, rather than attributing it anthropologically to a lower calcium intake.

Without doubt we have come a long way in our understanding of the mechanisms of calcium absorption and its effects on bone. Despite this knowledge, a clear demonstration of its therapeutic efficacy in fracture prevention, independent of vitamin D, is lacking. Current evidence warns of the potential toxicity of excess calcium supplementation; however, well-designed clinical trials are necessary to validate these observations and also to define appropriate calcium dosing.[5–7]

DISTRIBUTION

Calcium is the most abundant cation in the human body, approximately 1000 g, of which 99% exists in the mineral phase of bone as hydroxyapatite crystals. One percent of the remaining calcium is contained in the extracellular fluid, blood, and soft tissues. The deposition of calcium into the organic matrix of bone contributes to the rigidity and strength of bone. Bone also functions as a reservoir of calcium, which is readily available for its roles in multiple physiologic and biochemical processes including neuromuscular functioning, coagulation, cell permeability, enzyme activation, hormone secretion and functioning.[8] The calcium required for the latter nonosseous functions is satisfied largely by intracellular stores of the mineral. Because only 5 g of bone contains more calcium than the entire extracellular fluid space of an adult, it would be inconceivable for the requirement of all of the body's cellular functions to ever deplete the bone's calcium reservoir.[4] Nonetheless, protracted periods of inadequate calcium intake require enhanced resorption of bone to satisfy rapidly changing extracellular calcium needs, likely resulting in the loss of key structural elements that could weaken bone. Although nutritional calcium intake may contribute to the mass of the remaining structural elements, there are no data suggesting the lost elements can be replaced.

ABSORPTION
Overview

The ingestion of calcium is the only route by which humans can acquire this important ion needed to serve our cellular functions. Calcium absorption is a multifaceted process, influenced by a large number of factors (**Table 1**) including age, genetics, dietary intake, disease states, race, and medications. Seasonal variations have also been

Table 1
Factors influencing calcium absorption

Increased Calcium Absorption	Decreased Calcium Absorption
Protein	Aging
Fat	Menopause
Carbohydrates	Vitamin D deficiency
1,25(OH)$_2$D	Glucocorticoid excess
Food	Hypoparathyroidism
Lactose	Celiac disease
Lysine	Malabsorptive bariatric surgery
Sarcoidosis	Hyperthyroidism
B-cell lymphoma	Weight loss
Obesity	Caffeine
Primary hyperparathyroidism	Phytate
Pregnancy	Oxalate
Lactation	Cigarette smoking (nicotine)
Growth	Chronic alcoholism
Prebiotics, Probiotics	
Estrogen	

reported,[9,10] as have been nocturnal increases in calcium absorption and bone resorption.

There are 2 major mechanisms of calcium absorption: an active, saturable, transcellular process and a nonsaturable, paracellular process (**Fig. 1**).[11] These mechanisms have largely been elucidated in animal models. The transcellular movement takes place largely in the duodenum and to some extent the jejunum, whereas the paracellular movement occurs throughout the entire small intestine and to a much lesser degree in the colon (**Fig. 2**). A third, relatively minor mechanism called solvent drag also accounts for some degree of calcium absorption in most diets.

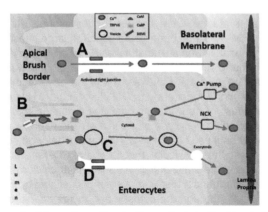

Fig. 1. An overview of calcium absorption in the gastrointestinal tract. Different pathways including (A) paracellular transport, (B) transcellular absorption, (C) vesicular transport, and (D) steady-state tight junction are depicted. CaM, calmodulin; CaBP, calcium-binding protein; BBMI, brush-border myosin.

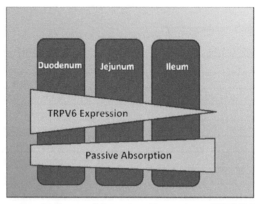

Fig. 2. Calcium absorption in the small intestine. Expression of TRPV6 is more abundant in the duodenum and jejunum, where the bulk of the transcellular absorption of calcium occurs. Paracellular absorption occurs throughout the small intestine, and is maximal in the ileum.

Transcellular Absorption

Transcellular calcium transport is a 3-step, sequential process of which step 1 involves transfer of luminal calcium across the brush-border membrane into the enterocyte[12] using a combination of genomic and nongenomic mechanisms. This step is non–energy dependent, having a favorable electrochemical gradient. It is a cell-mediated process largely regulated by 1,25-dihydroxyvitamin D, involving changes in the lipid content of the brush-border membrane and the presence of an epithelial-specific calcium channel, TRPV6 (also known as CaT1 and ECaC2).[13–16] The membrane changes include an increase in linoleic and arachidonic composition as well as an increase in the phosphatidylcholine:phosphatidylethanolamine ratio, resulting in enhanced membrane fluidity and increased calcium flux. These lipid changes occur within hours and are not blocked by pretreatment with cycloheximide, suggesting a nongenomic effect.[17]

The genomic mechanism involves the expression of TRPV6, which exists in the highest concentrations in the duodenum, with descending amounts in the jejunum and ileum, although earlier studies were unable to demonstrate its presence in the ileum.[18–20] TRPV6 mRNA has also been detected in the large intestine. Production of TRPV6 has been enhanced in human intestinal cell lines and vitamin D–deficient mice by 1,25(OH)$_2$D treatment, although a study of human duodenum by Barley and colleagues[21–24] found no correlation between TRPV6 concentrations and 1,25(OH)$_2$D levels, suggesting vitamin D–independent TRPV6 formation. However, later studies by Walter and colleagues[25,26] suggested a positive correlation with 1,25(OH)$_2$D levels in a vitamin D receptor (VDR) genotype group in men and younger women, but not in older women, possibly because of lower VDR levels in older women. Studies on VDR knockout mice suggest the possibility that in vitamin D–resistant individuals, the TRPV6 channel may be a rate-limiting step in transcellular calcium absorption.[27]

Step 2 is an intracellular transcytosolic movement of calcium from its apical point of entry into the enterocyte, through the cytosol, and to the basolateral membrane for extrusion from the cell. This process is facilitated by calcium-binding proteins calmodulin and calbindins, which are vitamin D–induced, higher-affinity, calcium-binding proteins (CaBP).[28,29] Calbindin, in fact, was the first protein discovered to be induced by Vitamin D.[30] Calmodulin (CaM) is primarily located in the microvillus portion of the cell and, as such, is the major calcium-binding protein in this region (see **Fig. 1**).[28] There is no evidence that 1,25 vitamin D affects the synthesis of calmodulin, but it may cause a redistribution of CaM in the intestinal cell at the brush-border complex, with the highest concentrations being in the villus cells, which have the highest capacity for calcium transport.[31–33] Glenney and Glenney[28] had suggested that calcium transport may flow from CaM in the microvillus to calbindin in the cytosol, which then plays a major role in accelerating the transport of calcium to the basolateral membrane.

Calbindins also seem to have an effect on the control of pore-size properties of the microvillar calcium channels, inactivating expressed TRPV6 protein with high calcium concentrations and activating it with decreased intracellular concentrations, thus suggesting a feedback control mechanism as offered by Hoenderop and colleagues and Peng and colleagues[23,34,35] These mechanisms enhance the availability of calcium at the basolateral membrane for extrusion[36,37] into the extracellular space. Wasserman and colleagues[22,38] discuss data which suggest that calbindins may also stimulate the activity of the basolateral calcium pump. These proposed mechanisms of calbindin function allow it to act as a cytosolic Ca^{2+} buffer in maintaining nontoxic intracellular Ca^{2+} levels during changes in transcellular Ca transport.[37]

Another proposed pathway for transcellular migration of calcium is the vesicular model, in which absorptive cells use lysosomes to sequester Ca ions bound to calmodulin in the vesicles and are transported by microtubules to the basolateral membrane. The role of calbindins in this pathway is unclear, despite their association with lysosomes.[35]

The third step is an extrusion of Ca^{2+} from the basolateral membrane to the capillary bed of the lamina propria against a considerable electrochemical gradient, similar to the gradient that favored calcium entry at the brush-border membrane.[39] There are 2 major energy-requiring mechanisms used to extrude Ca^{2+} against this gradient. The dominant pathway is the adenosine triphosphate–dependent Ca^{2+} pump, a member of the plasma membrane calcium-pumping (PMCA) family, a major isoform of which is PMCA1b in the intestine.[40,41] This pump is induced by $1,25(OH)_2D$, and is activated by CaM and possibly the CaBP.[38] The second pathway to extrude Ca across the basolateral membrane is the sodium/calcium exchanger (NCX), which is essentially linked to downhill movement of extracellular Na into the cell. The NCX is estimated to account for only 20% of the Ca extrusion capacity of the basolateral membrane in the rat intestine.[42] The calcium transported by vesicular mechanism is released from the enterocyte by exocytosis at the basolateral membrane (see **Fig. 1**).[43]

Paracellular Absorption

The second form of Ca absorption is the paracellular route, a nonsaturable, passive, diffusional mode in which calcium is absorbed between adjacent cells on the enterocyte membrane, driven by transepithelial electrochemical gradients. The passive diffusion increases linearly with luminal calcium concentrations independent of vitamin D. These intercellular spaces are very narrow and consist of tight junctions near the apices of the polarized epithelial cells, which are regulated to remain selectively permeable to small molecules and ions.[44] The tight junctions are structures consisting of linear arrays of membrane proteins including claudin-2, claudin-12, and cadherin-17, which are regulated by $1,25(OH)_2D$.[45,46] $1,25(OH)_2D$ can also activate protein kinase C (PKC), which has been shown to increase paracellular permeability of Caco-2 cell monolayers.[47] The extent of the effect of $1,25(OH)_2D$ on paracellular calcium transport, however, is still being debated. Other possible factors that may play a role in this process have been studied, including the L-type calcium-channel isoform Cav1.3, which is found in highest concentrations in the jejunum and ileum, and the 1,25(OH)$_2$D-induced calcium-binding protein sorcin.[48,49] Sorcin has been found to bind and modulate O-type calcium channels, and is also present in high concentrations in the jejunum and ileum (Ajibade and Christakos).[50,51] Paracellular diffusion occurs throughout the entire intestinal tract, and on a normal or high calcium diet accounts for most of the daily calcium absorption (see **Fig. 1**). Additional studies may enable researchers to further elucidate other potential mechanisms involved in these and other pathways to provide an understanding of the more complete role played by vitamin D in intestinal calcium absorption.

Solvent Drag

Of lesser magnitude is solvent drag, a mechanism whereby ingestion of a hyperosmolar concentration of a substance (such as lactose, glucose, NaCl, or zylitol) is accompanied by a 2- to 3-fold increase in calcium transfer in intestinal loops. Concomitant with the lactose ingestion, active calcium transport and intestinal CaBP content are reduced.[52,53] Increases in tight and gap junction spaces between the cells have been postulated as an explanation of the increased calcium absorption.[54]

Absorption Fraction

Whereas total calcium absorption increases with an increase in calcium intake, the absorption fraction is inversely correlated with the amount of calcium ingested. Heaney and colleagues[55] studied calcium absorption in healthy middle-aged women, focusing on its relationships to calcium intake, estrogen status, and age. The data revealed very broad ranges of absorptive performance at all intake levels. The mean absorption fraction declined from a value of 0.45 at very low intakes (about 200 mg Ca/d) to approximately 0.15 at intakes above 2000 mg/d.

Animal data reveal fluctuations in calcium channels, especially TRPV6, in response to dietary calcium-driven variations in 1,25(OH)$_2$D levels.[56] In these studies there is an upregulation with a low calcium diet and downregulation with a high calcium diet. In another study Heaney demonstrated that the calcium intake/absorption slope is nonlinear. The change in slope at an intake of 500 mg/d may reflect the saturation point of the active transport mechanism, considered to be the major method of calcium absorption at low levels of intake.[57] In a study of women aged 22 to 70 years on a calcium-restricted diet (300 mg/d), Dawson-Hughes found a slight reduction in serum ionized calcium and 24-hour urine calcium, and an increase in intact parathyroid hormone (PTH) secretion, 1,25(OH)$_2$D production, and calcium absorption by active transport.[58]

At higher levels of calcium intake the bulk of calcium absorption occurs via the passive diffusion process, which is essentially dependent on the luminal calcium concentration and has no defined upper limit. This process is accompanied by a suppression of the active transcellular transport. The majority of Ca absorption on a normal (adequate or high Ca intake) diet occurs in the ileum because of its slow transit time and the greater luminal calcium content, which often exceeds the blood ionized Ca concentration (1.25 mM), thus providing a favorable electrochemical gradient.[59] The transit time of chyme in the duodenum is brief (minutes) whereas in the distal small bowel the residence time is more than 2 hours, allowing for prolonged mucosal contact and greater calcium absorption.[11,36] In the large intestine calcium absorption undergoes both an active and passive process, though probably accounting for less than 10% of the total absorption at high or low calcium intakes. Thus, at the more usual intakes of calcium, the suggestion of Barger-Lux and colleagues[60] is that the absorptive efficiency varies directly with the mouth-to-cecum transit time. As noted earlier,

1,25(OH)$_2$D is the essential signal driving the active component and appears also to have some role in the passive paracellular component of absorption.

FACTORS INFLUENCING CALCIUM ABSORPTION

Many factors, including various disease states and medications, can affect calcium absorption. A partial list of the conditions known to affect Ca absorption is shown in **Table 1**.[61] It is critically important to keep these in mind when approaching calcium therapy in different populations.

Age

There is considerable evidence that intestinal calcium absorption decreases with increasing age.[55] The combination of a gradual aging effect and one-time estrogen loss resulted in a 20% to 25% decline in absorptive function from age 40 to 60 years. Although declining absorptive capacity with aging has been attributed, in part, to lower 1,25(OH)$_2$D levels, the effect of aging on serum 1,25(OH)$_2$D concentration is controversial. Studies have yielded inconsistent results in terms of changes in 1,25(OH)$_2$D levels over time in both women and men.[62–65] A decrease in serum 1,25(OH)$_2$D levels has been found in elderly men with decreased renal function[63,66] as opposed to those with normal renal function,[67] thus suggesting a correlation between lower concentrations of 1,25(OH)$_2$D in many elderly populations and reductions in glomerular filtration rate. Although renal function tends to decline with age in humans, many individuals maintain good glomerular filtration rates into their eighties.[68,69] In addition, some data suggest that an intestinal resistance to the action of 1,25(OH)$_2$D with age may account for a substantial portion of the reduction in calcium absorption.[55,70–72] The mechanism(s) of this proposed 1,25(OH)$_2$D resistance have not been elucidated. Ebeling and colleagues[72] and Horst and colleagues[73] demonstrated an age-related decline in the 1,25(OH)2D receptor concentration in human duodenal mucosal biopsy specimens, postulated to be one of the mechanisms of 1,25(OH)$_2$D resistance. More recent animal studies reveal decreases in TRPV6 and TRPV5 in the duodenum and kidney, respectively, with aging, and in women there was a significant reduction of both TRPV6 and VDR transcripts in older ages.[26,74]

Menopause

Menopause is accompanied by a reduction in intestinal Ca absorption and increased urinary calcium excretion, each of similar magnitude, leading to negative calcium balance and subsequent bone loss.[75] The intestinal and renal changes are reversible with the administration of 17β-estradiol. Estrogen receptors are present in the intestinal mucosal cells and kidney.[76,77] Estrogen and 1,25(OH)$_2$D independently induce expression of the epithelial calcium channel TRPV6, resulting in enhanced calcium transport.[78] Others report a strong correlation of 1,25(OH)$_2$D levels and the increase in Ca absorption following estrogen administration.[79] Lower levels of total 1,25(OH)$_2$D, but not of free concentrations, have been reported during the menopause, suggesting that the main effect may be on the vitamin D–binding protein.[80] Menopausal PTH concentrations have been inconsistent in many studies, precluding the ability to specifically define its role. Elevated PTH levels were noted in 29% to 35% of postmenopausal patients, in association with low calcium intakes, and tended to be more common in the older subjects and those with lower vitamin D concentrations.[81,82]

Glucocorticoids

Glucocorticoid therapy has been associated with diminished Ca absorption and bone mass without significant effects on circulating vitamin D metabolites.[83,84] In mouse models, glucocorticoids have been shown to reduce intestinal calcium absorption through an inhibition of the expression of active calcium transporters TRPV6 and CaBP-9K in the duodenum.[85,86] These changes occurred during prednisolone treatment[85] and were independent of 1,25(OH)$_2$D and calcium levels, both of which remained unchanged. Lee and colleagues[86] used dexamethasone treatment to demonstrate a reduction in CaBP-9K.

Pregnancy and Lactation

Calcium absorption doubles during pregnancy, beginning as early as the 12th week of gestation, and falls to nonpregnancy levels within days of parturition, corresponding to a rise and decline in both free and bound 1,25(OH)$_2$D levels. In rats, however, the increase in intestinal calcium absorption occurs well before the increase in 1,25(OH)$_2$D levels and may be in part related to prolactin, placental lactogen, estradiol, and other factors.[87–90] A 1,25(OH)$_2$D-mediated increase in intestinal calbindin-9kD is likely responsible for the most of the increase in calcium absorption. PTH-related protein (PTHrP) levels are increased in the last trimester, but its functions are not clearly elucidated. The source includes many maternal and fetal tissues. It is known to stimulate 1α-hydroxylase production, but is weaker than PTH in that capacity. Thus its role in the increased levels of 1,25(OH)2D is in doubt. Consider that PTHrP is a prohormone that produces many peptides with varying physiologic actions and specificities that have not been worked out. For example, a carboxyl-terminal form of PTHrP has been shown in vitro to inhibit osteoclastic bone resorption, thus engendering the idea that PTHrP may protect against bone loss of pregnancy. During lactation the rate of calcium absorption falls to the nonpregnant level, corresponding to the normalization of 1,25(OH)$_2$D levels. After weaning there is again an increase in Ca absorption, which may help restore Ca to the maternal skeleton.[91] In addition, during lactation PTHrP levels are increased and estrogen levels decreased, the effects of which combine to markedly upregulate bone resorption, reduce renal Ca losses, and raise blood Ca levels; however, much of this Ca is released into the breast milk. The major source of PTHrP during lactation appears to be the breast.

Sarcoidosis

Sarcoidosis, as well as many other granulomatous diseases, is associated with an increased intestinal absorption of Ca caused by a dysregulated production of 1,25(OH)$_2$D by activated macrophages.[92,93] Macrophages in sarcoidosis express 1α-hydroxylase, which leads to the production of 1,25(OH)$_2$D. However, unlike the renal expression of 1α-hydroxylase, macrophage-produced 1α-hydroxylase is not suppressed by hypercalcemia or elevated 1,25(OH)$_2$D levels, but is upregulated by various immune stimuli including interferon-γ, via C/EBPβ, an interferon-γ–inducible gene.[94,95] PTH levels are suppressed in sarcoidosis as a result of the hypercalcemia and high levels of calcitriol.[96]

Race

Racial differences in Ca absorption have been reported, with greater rates of absorption noted in adolescent black girls than in corresponding age-matched white girls.[97,98] Bryant and colleagues[97] have demonstrated in adolescent girls that on a calcium intake of 1100 to 1300 mg/d, there was a 70% greater calcium absorption efficiency and a 46% lower urinary calcium excretion in black girls than in white girls. The same group also reported an increase in calcium absorption and reduction in excretion in black girls when compared with white girls over a wide range of calcium intakes (760–2195 mg/d).[99] This study further demonstrated a linear relationship between calcium intake and skeletal retention. Although the slopes for both the black and white girls were parallel, the average calcium retention was greater in black girls. More recent data reveal unusually high levels of single-nucleotide polymorphisms of TRPV6 and, to a lesser extent, TRPV5 in African populations, which likely contribute to the Ca conservation mechanisms in this population.[96] TRPV6 is expressed largely in the intestine as well as in many other tissues, but TRPV5 is located primarily in the apical membrane of the distal convoluted tubule and connecting tubule of the kidney.

Obesity

Obesity has been associated with an increase in both Ca absorption and bone mass in adult women.[100,101] Multiple factors have been implicated in the increased Ca absorption in the obese, including higher intakes of macronutrients such as protein and fat, both of which have a positive effect on absorption. Higher levels of PTH and estradiol in the obese[101-103] also contribute to enhanced Ca absorption.[101-103] Shapses and colleagues[101] studied true fractional Ca absorption (TFCA) in 229 adult women with a mean age of 54 ± 11 years, with the goal of assessing the effect of hormonal and dietary factors in predicting TFCA and whether the TFCA differs with body weight.[101] The groups were divided into tertiles based on body mass index. The results suggest that TFCA is greater in the obese and that dietary fat, estradiol, and $1,25(OH)_2D$ are the most significant positive predictors of TFCA in adult women. Of importance is that the 25(OH)D level was lower in the obese subjects, but did not influence the data significantly. This finding may be due to the fact that 25(OH)D levels are only an indirect marker for $1,25(OH)2D$ and do not always show a positive relationship with TFCA in adults. Also important is the conclusion that dietary fat is the most significant positive predictor of TFCA in the entire study population and that the effect appeared to be greater in the nonobese, which may have implications for dietary management of leaner women who are more likely to have lower Ca absorption and greater risk of fracture.[101,104]

Vitamin D Receptor

Attempts to explain variations in intestinal calcium absorption on a genomic basis led to the study of the VDR, which was first cloned by Baker and colleagues.[105] Miyamoto and colleagues[106] clarified the genomic structure of the VDR gene, of which only a few polymorphisms have been studied to date. Morrison and colleagues[107] reported alleles of the VDR associated with bone mineral density (BMD) in twins and postmenopausal women. Several studies have demonstrated a relationship of calcium absorption and VDR genotypes.[108-110] One study showed the Fok1 polymorphism was significantly associated with BMD and Ca absorption in children. The subjects who were FF homozygotes had a mean Ca absorption that was 17% greater than Ff heterozygotes and 41.5% greater than the ff homozygotes.[111] However, some studies did not find a relationship between the VDR genotype and calcium absorption.[112-114] Although this is a fertile area for ongoing study, the complexities involved with the delineation of functional effects of the individual VDR polymorphisms, as well as the associational analyses for various phenotypic end points, create a daunting task.

Other Factors

Seasonal variations in calcium absorption were noted by Krall and Dawson-Hughes[9] in temperate climates, where absorption was lower in winter than in summer, possibly because of changing 25(OH)D levels. A recent meta-analysis by Hagenau and colleagues[115] of 394 studies consisting of more than 32,000 subjects found no relationship of latitude on 25(OH)D levels. This finding tends to diminish the likelihood that geographic location is a significant variable in the absorption of calcium. A decrease in the absorption of calcium has been described in hyperthyroidism, proposed mechanisms of which include a decrease in intestinal transport, hypovitaminosis D $(1,25(OH)_2D)$, and rapid intestinal transit time.[116–119] Malabsorption of calcium is reported in celiac disease, which can be corrected by a gluten-free diet and compensated for by increasing calcium intake and correcting vitamin D deficiency.[120,121] Bariatric surgeries, either malabsorptive or combined malabsorptive and restrictive, are associated with multiple nutrient deficiencies including protein and vitamin D deficiency, which contribute to an underlying, anatomic Ca malabsorption.[122]

NUTRITION AND CALCIUM ABSORPTION

Heaney and colleagues[123] have studied the effects of meals on the absorption of calcium from various sources, both dietary and supplemental. These investigators reported that there was a significant increase in Ca absorption when calcium was taken with a light meal, even in the presence of achlorhydria as demonstrated by Recker.[124] In general, the direct effects of dietary lipids on Ca absorption are not clear.[125] Experiments on human intestinal-like Caco-2 cells have demonstrated increased paracellular and, subsequently, transepithelial and transcellular Ca^{2+} transport in the presence of conjugated linoleic acid.[126,127] A high-fat diet has been shown to increase adipose tissue production of estrone and dehydroepiandrosterone, and low-fat diets lower serum estradiol levels in women, factors that may contribute to Ca absorption.[128,129] Fat ingestion may hinder the intestinal transit time and thus allow more time for contact with the absorptive surfaces, thus possibly contributing to intestinal Ca absorption.[130]

Carbohydrates have been shown to enhance Ca absorption, particularly the lactose in dairy food.[125] The addition of lactose has not been demonstrated to enhance Ca absorption in lactose-tolerant healthy adults.[131] The carbohydrate effect may be due in part to the "meal effect" as mentioned by Heaney and colleagues,[123] and thus related to other nutrients coingested with the carbohydrate meal. Lactosucrose has been shown to increase Ca absorption in young women, presumably by decreasing the intestinal pH and thus increasing the solubility of Ca^{2+} salts.[132] More recent data suggest that prebiotics and probiotics can increase Ca absorption, but are in need of further investigation.[133] The mechanism has been proposed to be the production of short-chain fatty acids by bacteria.[134]

The effect of dietary fiber on Ca absorption is generally small, but may be significant if calcium intake is quite small and fiber intake is large. Phytates, oxalates, and tannins form insoluble complexes with Ca^{2+} and thus reduce cation absorption. This reduction is most problematic with wheat bran, which can reduce the absorption of coingested calcium because it is a phytate concentrated product.[135] It has been predicted that if an individual with a baseline intake of 0 to 1 g of bran fiber per day increases to 30 g per day, a decrease in absorbability of 20% to 30% can be anticipated, which is not negligible if that person's calcium intake is low.[136] The effect of fiber in various foods is variable. For example, the calcium in beans is about half as available as the calcium in milk, whereas the calcium in spinach and rhubarb is virtually unavailable.[137,138] For beans, phytate is responsible for half of the interference and oxalate the other half. In spinach and rhubarb, oxalate is responsible for most of the absorptive inhibition. However, the interferences in beans, spinach, and rhubarb, for example, tend to only involve the absorption of the calcium contained in the same food and not the coingested calcium from foods such as milk.

The relationship of caffeine to Ca absorption is such that for every 6-ounce serving of brewed coffee, there is a negative calcium balance of 4.6 mg/d.[139] This discrepancy can be balanced by adding 1 to 2 tablespoons of milk to each serving.[139,140] A minimal, acute increase in urinary calcium excretion has been noted. Chronic alcoholism can lead to liver disease and ultimately disturbances in vitamin D metabolism, thus possibly contributing to reduced calcium absorption.[141] Cigarette smoking is associated with a reduction in Ca absorption, possibly related to the decreased PTH, calcitriol, and $25(OH)_2D$ levels as reported by Need and colleagues[142] and Jorde and colleagues.[143] Another contributory factor to be considered is the decreased production and increased degradation of circulating estrogen that has been demonstrated to reduce Ca absorption.[144,145] Nicotine has been shown to inhibit aromatase activity and the conversion of androstenedione to estrogen in a dose-dependent fashion.[144]

EFFECTS OF CALCIUM ON BONE

The driving force behind calcium movement to and from cells is the maintenance of extracellular fluid (ECF) calcium (Ca^{2+}) levels. A decrease in the $ECF(Ca^{2+})$ levels prompts a rapid (within minutes) increase in PTH production, which results in an increase in the $ECF(Ca^{2+})$ levels and, via a negative feedback loop, subsequent reduction in PTH secretion. The involved PTH mechanisms are: (1) an increase in renal phosphate clearance, which results in a lower serum phosphate level, thus leading to an increase in the $ECF(Ca^{2+})$; (2) inactivation of the calcium receptor (CaR) in the parathyroid glands to increase PTH secretion, which acts on the PTH receptor in the kidney to increase tubular calcium reabsorption; and (3) in bone to initiate new bone resorption loci and augment osteoclastic activity at the sites of resorption. The increased PTH also enhances the formation and secretion of $1,25(OH)_2D$ via stimulation of the 1α-hydroxylase enzyme. High levels of $1,25(OH)_2D$ modulate the adaptive changes in intestinal Ca absorption and to some extent renal Ca reabsorption. The latter occurs apparently through vitamin D–mediated transcriptional activation; however, the precise mechanism of the effect of vitamin D in the kidney needs to be elucidated.[146]

The importance of calcium intake on bone mass has been demonstrated in an animal study by Jowsey and Gershon-Cohen,[147] in which calcium deprivation in cats resulted in osteoporosis, followed by recovery of bone mass with restitution of dietary calcium. Jowsey and Raisz[148] subsequently demonstrated that in the absence of PTH, bone loss with calcium deprivation is prevented, but at the same time incurring significant hypocalcemia. This finding tends to emphasize the role of bone as a calcium reserve and of PTH in releasing Ca from bone to maintain $ECF(Ca^{2+})$.

Calcium intake has been demonstrated to have an effect on mineral acquisition in children, with maximal bone turnover occurring during infancy (100%/y) and the adolescent growth spurt during which young boys and girls accrue approximately 37% of their total body mass. Most bone mass is accumulated by age 18 years.[149] Adolescence (9–17 years) is an intensely anabolic period, obviously with greater Ca needs than either childhood or young adulthood. At the very least, a threshold Ca intake would be necessary to attain peak bone mass and help prevent the development of osteoporosis later in life. Although a precise threshold Ca intake level has not been defined, a study by Johnston and colleagues,[150] comparing pairs of monozygotic twins aged 6 to 14 years randomly assigned to placebo or 1000 mg/d of calcium citrate malate, demonstrated a significant increase in BMD of the Ca-treated prepubertal siblings, with no significant changes in the peripubertal or postpubertal children. The baseline Ca intake was 874 mg/d in the girls and 990 mg/d in the boys. However, Nowson and colleagues[151] and Lloyd and colleagues[152] have demonstrated significant increases in BMD in peripubertal and postpubertal girls. In the Lloyd study calcium citrate malate was also used, but at a lower dose (500 mg/d) than that used by Johnston and colleagues,[150,152] yet still demonstrated benefits in sexually maturing children.

Several studies have related adult bone mass to dietary calcium ingestion during adolescence and likely lifetime dietary habits.[153–156] A more recent study using data from the National Health and Nutrition Examination Survey evaluated 3251 non-Hispanic white women, and concluded that those with a low milk intake during childhood and adolescence have lower bone mass in adulthood and a greater risk of fracture.[157] Although most randomized trials during periods of growth show greater BMD gains with increased intakes of Ca, these changes have largely been transient and tend to disappear when Ca supplementation ceases.[158] Intuitively one would expect that attaining a higher peak bone mass by early adulthood could only be helpful in reducing future fracture risk. Matkovic and Ilitch[159] calculate that variations in Ca nutrition early in life could account for as much as a 5% to 10% difference in peak adult bone mass, which could contribute to more than a 50% difference in rate of hip fracture later in life. Whether extrapolations from these types of data are justified may never be proven in a long-term randomized controlled study, but may be supported from components of data in adults with known childhood calcium intakes.

The effect of Ca intake on bone in adults, as well as in children, is intricately tied to vitamin D and, as a result, the end points of various studies, whether randomized controlled trials (RCTs) or observational trials, generally involve components of both factors accompanied by confounding dietary variation. Precisely separating the effects of Ca and vitamin D is generally not possible. However, in trials where both control and calcium-treated individuals were given vitamin D, reductions in fracture rates were demonstrated in the calcium-supplemented individuals.[160,161] In addition, Peacock and colleagues[162] demonstrated that Ca supplementation (750 mg/d) was able to more effectively prevent bone loss than vitamin D alone in the elderly. Bischoff-Ferrari and colleagues[163] performed a meta-analysis demonstrating a dose-dependent reduction of vitamin D in hip fractures. Boonen and colleagues[164] extended the meta-analysis to show that this reduction in hip fractures occurred only when vitamin D was given with calcium supplementation. A meta-analysis of prospective cohort studies and RCTs involving both men and women showed that calcium intake is not significantly associated with risk of hip fracture and may even increase the risk.[165] These conclusions are incongruent with multiple large meta-analyses demonstrating fracture reductions with increased Ca and or Ca/vitamin D supplementation.[164,166–168] In addition, only one of the clinical trials in the meta-analysis by Bischoff-Ferrari and colleagues[165] contained baseline vitamin D levels, and in the meta-analysis by Tang and colleagues[168] the vitamin D status was not always evident in the Ca-alone studies. This finding emphasizes only one of the deficiencies involved in assessing the effect of either Ca or vitamin D on bone parameters.

Another confounding factor is the background intake of calcium by study subjects as reported in the study by Jackson and colleagues,[169] in which the participants had a relatively high intake of calcium (average 1150 mg/d). Subjects were provided 1000 mg Ca and 400 IU vitamin D per day, thus bringing their total Ca intake to approximately 2150 mg/d, much higher than in most other studies. While there was a slight, but significant preservation of total hip BMD in the Ca/vitamin D group, there was a nonsignificant 12% reduction in the incidence of hip fractures. A sensitivity analysis of participants adherent to the treatment demonstrated a 29% decrease in the risk of hip fractures, as has been seen in other trials of Ca with vitamin D supplementation, illustrating another difficulty in interpreting study results.[170]

Many of the referenced studies included women in the early postmenopausal years in addition to elderly men and women, suggesting that Ca supplementation can prevent bone loss at the hip and spine in both young and older postmenopausal women and men.[83,171] In a 24-month RCT of 323 healthy men assigned to calcium supplementation (600 mg/d, 1200 mg/d, or placebo), BMD increased at all sites in the 1200 mg/d group, whereas the subjects taking 600 mg/d were no different from the placebo group at any BMD site.[172] A downward, nonsignificant trend in fractures was noted. A consistent finding in many studies is that the effect of Ca/vitamin D supplementation is greater in the elderly (>70 years), the institutionalized, and those with vitamin D and/or Ca insufficiency. Much of the available data from several meta-analyses suggest that Ca intake of approximately 1200 mg or more per day in conjunction with vitamin D (800 IU/d) reduces fractures, particularly of the hip, in this high-risk population.

The relationship of Ca, vitamin D, and PTH to cortical bone and the correlation of BMD with nonvertebral fracture risk lend support to these fracture data. In interpreting studies involving Ca treatment, one must consider that a reduction in PTH secretion can lead to fewer bone-remodeling loci and thus a suppression of bone resorption, while mineralization of previously activated sites continues, creating a temporary imbalance resulting in an increase in bone mass for a period of time. This phenomenon has been referred to as a remodeling transient, the effect of which can last from 3 to 6 months in children and as long as 12 to 18 months in mature adults and the elderly.[173] It is clear that long-term dose-ranging RCTs of Ca and vitamin D would be required to ultimately answer these concerns, a scenario which is unlikely to occur. High Ca intake has been demonstrated to enhance the effect of estrogen replacement therapy in postmenopausal women, and potentiated the effect of calcitonin on the lumbar spine BMD.[84] Bonnick and colleagues[174] demonstrated in 700 postmenopausal women with a mean intake of Ca 800 mg/d that alendronate plus 100 mg Ca reduced urinary N-terminal telopeptide significantly greater than alendronate alone, without significant changes in BMD over 2 years.

CALCIUM REQUIREMENTS

The basic requirement for daily Ca intake needs to, at the very least, satisfy calcium balance requirements and additionally consider available data referable to bone-health studies. The current recommended dietary allowances (RDAs) last reviewed by the Institute of Medicine (IOM) are noted in **Table 2**. Essentially these criteria are designed to be at approximately the 95th percentile of individual dietary calcium requirements. The assumption is that if everyone ingested the RDA, 95% of the population would be getting what they need. However, in an individual person, multiple comorbid conditions (see **Table 1**) that could interfere with Ca absorption and excretion, in addition to potential toxicities, need to be considered. Although various estimates exist, the average diet in the United States today contains between 600 and 700 mg Ca per day, thus falling far short of the recommended intake.

CALCIUM BALANCE

Obligatory loss of calcium includes insensible losses through the skin and its appendages (sweat, hair, nails, and shed skin), as well as urinary and endogenous fecal excretion. Cutaneous losses vary from an average of 16 mg/d in sedentary individuals to more than 250 mg/d with strenuous activity.[175,176] Endogenous fecal loss averages about 80 mg/d, which includes digestive secretions and calcium contained in mucosal shedding.[177] Urinary excretion in developed countries averages 160 to 200 mg per 24 hours, but is influenced by dietary factors including Ca, Na, and protein intake.[178] Sodium and calcium compete with the same mechanisms in the proximal convoluted

Table 2
Recommended dietary allowances for calcium

Age	Male (mg)	Female (mg)	Pregnant (mg)	Lactating (mg)
0–6 mo[a]	200	200		
7–12 mo[a]	260	260		
1–3 y	700	700		
4–8 y	1000	1000		
9–13 y	1300	1300		
14–18 y	1300	1300	1300	1300
19–50 y	1000	1000	1000	1000
51–70 y	1000	1200		
71+ y	1200	1200		

[a] Adequate intake.

Data from Committee to Review Dietary Reference Intakes for Vitamin D and Calcium, Food and Nutrition Board, Institute of Medicine. Dietary reference intakes for calcium and vitamin D. Washington, DC: National Academy Press; 2010. Reviewed August, 2011.

tubules and, as a result, modify the resorption of each other. This process was first demonstrated in dog experiments in 1961.[179] On average every 100 mmol of sodium excretion is accompanied by 1 mmol of urinary Ca excretion.[180] The significance of these findings is supported by studies in which rats fed high-sodium diets developed accelerated osteoporosis, and in which salt administration and restriction led to changes in markers of bone turnover in postmenopausal women.[181–183] Low sodium intakes were associated with lower levels of bone-turnover markers in these studies and thus, salt restriction may be a factor in reducing bone resorption in postmenopausal women; conversely, high salt intakes may enhance bone resorption.

Calcium-balance studies have revealed increased Ca excretion with high-protein diets, quantitating Ca losses of 0.25 mmol for every 10 g of protein ingested.[184] Commensurate with this observation, a few studies have reported an adverse association of high protein intakes with bone health, whereas others have found the opposite.[185–187] Hypothesis-generating observational studies suggest that an increased incidence of fractures in subjects with high protein intake occurred mostly among those consuming nondairy animal protein, possibly because of a metabolic acidosis leading to enhanced bone resorption.[188,189]

Despite many theoretical mechanisms to explain the hypercalciuria, the source of this increased Ca excretion seems to be multifactorial and is clearly influenced by protein ingestion.[190] Animal studies strongly suggest that increasing dietary protein increases intestinal calcium absorption, and tends to shift calcium excretion from the intestinal tract to the urine.[191] Balance studies in healthy women have more recently demonstrated that higher protein intakes are associated with increased Ca intestinal absorption, which may explain much of the increased calciuria, particularly because the high protein diet in this study was associated with a significant decrease in the fraction of urinary calcium of bone origin.[192] The dietary calcium in this study (20 mmol/d) was not adequate to maintain positive bone balance even when the intestinal Ca absorption was highest during the high protein diet. In addition, protein supplementation increased production of insulin-like growth factor 1 (IGF-1), particularly in elderly subjects who were deficient in IGF-1, which had a positive effect on bone.[193] IGF-1 regulates osteoblastic recruitment and differentiation, and has been demonstrated in elderly women to have an anabolic effect at a low dose, whereas it increased markers of both formation and resorption at a higher dose, providing another theoretical basis for Ca need.[194]

Heaney[195] suggested that "protein and calcium act synergistically on bone if both are present in adequate quantities in the diet, but that protein may seem effectively antagonistic toward bone (because of its calciuric effect) when calcium intake is low." This proposal is somewhat supported by a French study that found no association between total protein intake and fracture risk in postmenopausal women on a fairly high calcium intake, but evidence that a high protein–high acid ash diet was associated with an increased risk of fracture when calcium intake was low (<400 mg/1000 kcal).[196] The study by Meyer and colleagues[189] also found a higher incidence of hip fractures in the subjects with the highest nondairy protein intake in combination with the lowest calcium intake. A recent study examining an association between protein intake and hip-fracture risk in 946 men and women from the Framingham Osteoporosis Study, with a mean age of approximately 75 years and calcium intake of 800 mg/d, found a reduced risk for hip fracture with a higher protein intake.[197]

While magnesium plays a role in bone health, its presence in virtually all food groups, especially those of cellular origin, make a deficiency of it rare in the absence of a severe defect in intestinal or renal function. Phosphorus is a nutrient that complexes with calcium in the intestine, whose importance relies more on its ratio with calcium than in its absolute intake level. A high calcium intake without a correspondingly high phosphorus intake could result in a low enough phosphorus level to augment osteoclastic bone resorption and interfere with osteoblastic function.[198,199] In recent years most osteoporosis studies have required high-dose cotherapy with calcium, which is often in the form of carbonate or citrate rather than phosphate compounds. Coupled with the fact that a substantial percentage of the elderly population consumes less than the suggested amount of phosphorus, this can result in a level of absorbed phosphorus that is too low to support tissue-phosphorus needs as well as new bone mineralization (which consumes mineral at a Ca/phosphorus molar ratio of approximately 1.6:1).[200] Tricalcium phosphate was used in one of the most impressive calcium supplementation studies in the elderly.[201] The investigators suggested that the extra phosphorus may have been a factor in the magnitude of effect. It seems reasonable intuitively to include at least one of the calcium phosphate salts for a portion of a supplementation regimen.

CALCIUM DOSAGE

Considering the fact that calcium does not exist in a nutritional vacuum, the factors discussed up to this point need to be addressed when advising calcium intake for an individual patient. It seems prudent to consider low-fat dairy or other calcium-fortified foods for the primary maintenance of calcium balance because of the other nutrients present in food including, but not limited to, protein, magnesium, phosphorus, and potassium. Although a high-fat meal has been demonstrated to slow the progression of chyme through the intestine and thus prolong contact with the intestinal mucosa, resulting in augmented Ca absorption, the cost/benefit ratio may not support such a recommendation.[113] If adequate dietary Ca intake is not possible, supplementation will be necessary. It has been a long-held belief that Ca absorption requires the presence of gastric acid secretions or gastric acidity, particularly for food calcium or calcium carbonate. Bo-Linn and colleagues[202] demonstrated that dietary Ca or $CaCO_3$ is equally absorbed in the presence of achlorhydria when taken with a meal. This finding tends to circumvent the concern of diminished Ca absorption in the presence of achlorhydria/atrophic gastritis, whether due to protein-pump inhibitors, pernicious anemia, or idiopathic etiology in the elderly. If a person has achlorhydria and must rely on Ca supplements without concomitant food ingestion, calcium citrate would be the better choice. It is advisable to limit a single dose of Ca to 500 mg, which is the approximate dose-absorptive saturation point. A second dose, if necessary, should be separated by 6 to 8 hours ideally.

Based on the available data, including the suggestion of potential cardiovascular issues, in an otherwise healthy adult, there is unlikely to be any additional benefit in exceeding a 1200 mg/d Ca intake, particularly because it is a threshold nutrient (see **Table 2**). In addition, given the racial differences in efficiency of Ca absorption and excretion, it may be a reasonable assumption that blacks might require up to 300 mg/d less Ca intake than whites.[203] A significant proportion of patients hold the belief that while taking the current medications for osteoporosis (ie, bisphosphonates), Ca supplementation is unnecessary, and is discontinued; thus compliance and adherence are problematic, requiring frequent reinforcement by health professionals.

POTENTIAL COMPLICATIONS OF CALCIUM SUPPLEMENTATION

Whether through the diet or dedicated supplements, calcium therapy is generally very well tolerated. Like many things in life, however, excess amounts can lead to adverse events. According to the IOM report on dietary reference levels, conditions that have been associated with excessive calcium intake include hypercalcemia, hypercalciuria, nephrolithiasis, constipation, vascular and soft-tissue calcification, interactions with zinc and iron, and prostate cancer.[204] Most, if not all, of these conditions are potential complications of therapy with supplements, and are seldom attributed to excess calcium intake from the diet. Some of the more common concerns of Ca supplementation are discussed further here.

Hypercalcemia

Hypercalcemia attributable to calcium intake is generally associated with daily ingestion of at least 3000–4000 mg of calcium, often in the setting of some degree of renal impairment, although toxic levels have rarely been reported in patients taking as little as 1500 mg per day.[205] Although excess absorbed calcium can often be buffered through storage in a young skeleton, in the postmenopausal population there is a net efflux of calcium from the bones, preventing this buffer and predisposing patients to hypercalcemia. Care needs to be taken to avoid excessive calcium intake in certain populations at risk for hypercalcemia, such as pregnant women, those on thiazide diuretics, and patients with advanced kidney disease or sarcoidosis.[206–208]

Hypercalciuria and Nephrolithiasis

Another concern with calcium therapy is the development of calcium-containing kidney stones primarily caused by hypercalciuria. In addition to pain on stone passage, the morbidity of nephrolithiasis includes predisposition to infections of the urinary system, as well as risk of renal damage and ongoing insufficiency. Despite the fact that the vast majority of kidney stones contain calcium, factors well beyond the simple intake and absorption of calcium are involved in their pathogenesis, making the determination of the role of individual factors very nuanced.[209]

In an effort to further investigate the role of Ca intake on kidney stones, Jackson and colleagues[169] analyzed data from 36,000 postmenopausal women aged 50 to 79 years as part of the Women's Health Initiative trial. The women were randomized to either placebo or 1000 mg of supplemental calcium carbonate per day plus 400 units of vitamin D3. The mean baseline dietary intake of calcium for the subjects was

1100 mg per day, thereby making the total daily intake of calcium around 2100 mg in the experimental group. Kidney stones were reported by 449 women taking the supplemental calcium and vitamin D, and by 381 in the placebo group. This difference was significant, indicating possible increased risk of kidney stones in postmenopausal women when consuming at least 2100 mg of calcium per day.

A smaller study by Riggs and colleagues[210] followed 236 postmenopausal women for the development of hypercalciuria or nephrolithiasis during 1 year of supplementation with calcium or placebo. Baseline dietary Ca intake was 800 mg/d among the women, and the experimental group received 1600 mg/d of supplemental Ca for a total of nearly 2400 mg of Ca per day. Nearly 50% of the experimental group developed urinary Ca greater than 350 mg/d, compared with 8% of those in the control group; no patients in either group developed kidney stones during the study. Intake of Ca at high amounts, such as greater than 2000 mg/d, appears to be associated with hypercalciuria and, to some extent, nephrolithiasis.

Using data of women aged 34 to 59 years from the Nurses' Health Study, Curhan and colleagues[211] showed an inverse relationship between dietary Ca intake and kidney stone formation, with a positive association of stones with supplemental Ca use. Other studies involving younger women and men[212,213] have shown the same trend of decreased nephrolithiasis with increased dietary Ca intake, although they did not demonstrate any association with use of Ca supplement. Overall, it appears that calcium obtained in the diet is not associated with increased risk of kidney stones, and in many series has actually been protective.

Increased absorption of oxalate, and subsequent increased levels in the urine, are known risk factors for development of calcium-containing stones. In fact, Robertson and Peacock[214] provided evidence that even small rises in urinary oxalate concentrations are more important than large increases in calcium levels for crystallization of calcium oxalate in urine. The main proposed reason why Ca obtained in the diet may be associated with decreased stone formation is that Ca binds dietary oxalate in the gastrointestinal tract, thereby reducing the absorption of oxalate. Hess and colleagues[215] demonstrated that sufficient calcium intake along with even a 20-fold increased oxalate load can prevent the hyperoxaluria that occurs in healthy subjects. These data suggest that calcium supplements taken with food, rather than in between meals or at bedtime, may therefore have less risk of increasing nephrolithiasis rates, although this remains unproven, and underscore the importance of obtaining Ca from the diet when possible.

Cardiovascular Disease

The risk of atherosclerotic vascular disease with calcium supplementation has been the subject of numerous recent observational and epidemiologic studies. Calcium has many potential biological effects on risk factors for cardiovascular disease (CVD) that have been documented over the years. These effects include downregulation of the renin-angiotensin system and decreasing vascular smooth muscle tone, both of which could have potential beneficial effects on regulation of blood pressure.[216,217] Favorable changes in lipid profiles have been seen in older women with Ca supplementation, with animal and human studies showing the binding of Ca to fatty acids and bile acids in the gut, resulting in malabsorption of fat and decreased serum lipid levels.[218,219] In addition, changes in intracellular Ca levels can affect lipolysis in adipocytes, and insulin secretion by pancreatic β cells, modifying other CVD risk factors.[220] On the other hand, calcium supplementation has been shown to lead to transient elevations in serum Ca, potentially contributing to vascular calcification, a known marker of atherosclerotic vascular disease.[221]

Several studies have allowed the examination of dietary calcium intake and the risk of atherosclerotic vascular disease, such as the Iowa Women's Health Study of 34,486 postmenopausal women in the United States.[222] In this study, women in the highest versus lowest quartile of calcium intake had a lower relative risk of mortality from coronary artery disease (CAD). The Boston Nurses' Health Study showed a decreased risk of ischemic stroke in those with the highest quintile of Ca intake compared with the lowest quintile, and a 10-year population-based cohort of Swedish men showed a lower rate of CVD mortality in those with higher dietary Ca intake.[223,224] Other cohorts, however, have not shown an association between dietary Ca intake and CAD.[225]

Bolland and colleagues[226] conducted a randomized, placebo-controlled trial of calcium supplementation of 1471 postmenopausal women to primarily assess effects on BMD and fracture risk, with myocardial infarction (MI), stroke, and sudden death as prespecified secondary outcomes. Baseline dietary calcium use was more than 800 mg/d, and subjects were randomized to either a total of 1000 mg of calcium citrate per day or placebo, for a total of nearly 1900 mg/d of Ca in the calcium group. An MI was more commonly reported in the calcium group than in the placebo group, as was the composite end point of MI, stroke, or sudden death. This trial was among the first to demonstrate a possible increase in risk of MI or other CAD events among women taking calcium supplements for the purposes of bone health. Subsequently, in a pooled analysis of nearly 12,000 patients (including men and women) from 11 clinical trials of calcium supplementation, Bolland and colleagues[5] showed a 30% increased risk of an MI and smaller, statistically insignificant increases in the risks of stroke and death in those receiving calcium rather than placebo.

Lewis and colleagues,[227] using a database from a trial of 1460 women randomized to either 1200 mg of calcium carbonate per day or placebo, analyzed mortality or first-time hospital admission data for atherosclerotic vascular disease over a 5-year period. There was no significant increase in mortality or hospitalization rate for atherosclerotic disease in the calcium intervention group during the 5-year RCT or over 9.5 years of observational study, compared with those receiving placebo.

Of course, there are cohorts and observational studies yielding conflicting conclusions on the potential contribution of calcium supplementation to CAD risk. The bulk of the literature is derived from secondary analyses of existing trial data. There is tremendous heterogeneity of these studies in terms of forms and dosage of calcium supplementation, dietary amounts of vitamin D therapy, reporting and adjudication of CAD events, and controlling for other CAD risk factors and concomitant medications. In many of the trials the numbers of CAD-related events were very low, making it more difficult to draw definitive conclusions. Overall, there is a lack of RCTs specifically designed to address the effect of calcium use on incident atherosclerotic vascular disease, and until these are able to be accomplished, the available data remain hypothesis generating and in no way conclusive of the harm of calcium supplementation at currently recommended doses (see **Table 2**).

SUMMARY

Calcium is a very important element, involved in bone health as well as various cellular functions in humans. Despite these needs and enormous resources directed at increasing Ca intake in our population, the mean daily intake in the United States is significantly lower than the suggested RDA. As a result Ca insufficiency continues to be a problem, and can lead to bone loss via mechanisms discussed in this article. Great progress has been made in the understanding of both genomic and nongenomic mechanisms of absorption, as well as in understanding the effects of various factors and racial differences in absorption and excretion of Ca. These contributions have enabled physicians to individualize therapy appropriately and to better understand the pathophysiology of bone loss relative to entities altering Ca absorption, including poor nutrition. While Ca and vitamin D have been demonstrated to reduce fractures, the precise influence of each component is difficult to discern. The ability to perform large meta-analyses of osteoporosis RCTs and observational studies, in addition to many excellent and basic Ca-balance studies, have provided investigators and clinicians with the tools to make reasonable assumptions about the current therapeutic recommendations cited herein. Additional efforts to discriminate more specific levels of Ca intake and Ca/vitamin D intake ratios (levels), to determine more simple and precise methods of clinically assessing Ca absorption, and to understand pertinent vitamin D polymorphisms will be areas of important research in the future. Certainly randomized controlled studies would be helpful in elucidating the significance of the recent cardiovascular observations suggesting a possible relationship of cardiovascular events to levels of Ca intake. Based on these early observations, the data available are too insubstantial to recommend altering the current RDA for Ca at present.

REFERENCES

1. Eaton SB, Nelson DA. Calcium in evolutionary perspective. Am J Clin Nutr 1991; 54:S281–7.
2. Nelson DA. An anthropological perspective on optimizing calcium consumption for the prevention of osteoporosis. Osteoporos Int 1996;6:325–8.
3. Smith P, Bloom RA, Berkowitz J. Diachronic trends in humeral cortical thickness of Near Eastern populations. J Hum Evol 1984;13:603–11.
4. Heaney RP. Calcium. In: Bilezikian JP, Raisz LG, Rodan GA, editors. Principles of bone biology. 2nd edition. San Diego (CA): Academic Press; 2002. p. 1325–37.
5. Bolland MJ, Avenell A, Baron JA, et al. Effect of calcium supplements on risk of myocardial infarction and cardiovascular events: meta-analysis. BMJ 2010;341: c3691.
6. Mursu J, Robien K, Harnack LJ, et al. Dietary supplements and mortality rate in older women. Arch Intern Med 2011;171(18):1625–33.
7. Wang L, Manson JE, Song V, et al. Systematic review: vitamin D and calcium supplementation in prevention of cardiovascular event. Ann Intern Med 2010; 152:315–23.
8. Avioli LV, Birge SJ. Mechanisms of calcium absorption: a reappraisal. In: Andreoli TE, Hoffman JF, Fanestil DD, editors. Physiology of membrane disorders. New York: Plenum; 1978. p. 919–40.
9. Krall EA, Dawson-Hughes B. Relation of fractional ^{47}Ca retention to season and rates of bone loss in healthy postmenopausal women. J Bone Miner Res 1991;6: 1323–9.
10. Malm OJ. Calcium requirement and adaptation in adult men. Scand J Clin Lab Invest 1958;10(Suppl 36):1–280.
11. Bronner F, Pansu D. Nutritional aspects of calcium absorption. J Nutr 1999;129: 9–12.
12. Hoenderop JG, Nilius B, Bindels RJ. Calcium absorption across epithelia. Physiol Rev 2005;85:373–422.
13. Peng JB, Chen XZ, Vassilev PM, et al. Molecular cloning and characterization of a channel-like transporter mediating intestinal calcium absorption. J Biol Chem 1999;274(32):22739–46.

14. O'Doherty PJ. 1,25 Dihydroxyvitamin D increases the activity of the intestinal phosphatidylcholine deacylation-acylation cycle. Lipids 1979;14:75.

15. Brasitus TA, Dudeja PK, Eby B, et al. Correction by 1,25(OH)2D3 of the abnormal fluidity and lipid composition of enterocyte brush border membranes in vitamin D-deprived rats. J Biol Chem 1981;256:3354–60.

16. Max EE, Goodman DB, Rasmussen H. Purification and characterization of chick intestine brush border membrane. Effects of 1alpha(OH) vitamin D3 treatment. Biochim Biophys Acta 1978;511:224–39.

17. Matsumoto T, Fontaine O, Rasmussen H. Effect of 1,25-dihydroxyvitamin D3 on phospholipid metabolism in chick duodenal mucosal cell. Relationship to its mechanism of action. J Biol Chem 1981;256:3354–60.

18. Peng JB, Chen XZ, Berger UV, et al. Human calcium transport protein CaT1. Biochem Biophys Res Commun 2000;278(2):326–32.

19. Muller D, Hoenderop JG, Meij IC, et al. Molecular cloning, tissue distribution, and chromosomal mapping of the human epithelial Ca^{2+} channel(ECaC1). Genomics 2000;67(1):48–53.

20. Zhuang L, Peng JB, Tou L, et al. Calcium-selective ion channel, CaT1, is apically localized in gastrointestinal tract epithelia and is aberrantly expressed in human malignancies. Lab Invest 2002;82(12):1755–64.

21. Barley NF, Howard A, O'Callaghan D, et al. Epithelial calcium transporter expression in human duodenum. Am J Physiol 2001;280(2):G285–90.

22. Song Y, Peng X, Porta A, et al. Calcium transporter 1 and epithelial calcium channel messenger ribonucleic acid are differentially regulated by 1,25 dihydroxyvitamin D3 in the intestine and kidney of mice. Endocrinology 2003;144: 3885–94.

23. Peng JB, Brown EM, Hediger MA. Apical entry channels in calcium-transporting epithelia. News Physiol Sci 2003;18(4):158–63.

24. Wood RJ, Tchack L, Tapania S. 1,25-Dihydroxyvitamin D3 increases the expression of the CaT1 epithelial calcium channel in the Caco-2 human intestinal cell line. BMC Physiol 2001;1:11.

25. Walters JR, Barley NF, Khanju M, et al. Duodenal expression of the epithelial calcium transporter gene TRPV6: is there evidence for Vitamin D-dependence in humans? J Steroid Biochem Mol Biol 2004;89–90(1–5):317–9.

26. Walters JR, Balesaria S, Chavele KM, et al. Calcium channel TRPV6 expression in human duodenum: different relationships to the vitamin D system and aging in Men and women. J Bone Miner Res 2006;21(11):1770–7.

27. Bouillon R, Van Cromphout S, Carmeliet G. Intestinal calcium absorption: molecular vitamin D mediated mechanisms. J Cell Biochem 2003;88(2):332–9.

28. Glenney JR Jr, Glenney P. Comparison of Ca^{++}-regulated events in the intestinal brush border. J Cell Biol 1985;100(3):754–63.

29. Christakos S, Gabrielides C, Rhoten WB. Vitamin D-dependent calcium binding proteins: chemistry, distribution, functional considerations, and molecular biology. Endocr Rev 1989;10(1):3–26.

30. Wasserman RH, Taylor AN. Vitamin D-dependent calcium-binding protein. Response to some physiological and nutritional variables. J Biol Chem 1968; 243:3987–93.

31. Bikle DD, Munson S, Chafouleas J. Calmodulin may mediate 1,25-dihydroxyvitamin D-stimulated intestinal calcium transport. FEBS Lett 1984;174(1):30–3.

32. Bikle DD, Munson W, Christakos S, et al. Calmodulin binding to the intestinal brush-border membrane: comparison with other calcium-binding proteins. Biochim Biophys Acta 1989;1010(1):122–7.

33. Bikle DD, Munson S. The villus gradient of brush border membrane calmodulin and the calcium-independent calmodulin-binding protein parallels that of calcium-accumulating ability. Endocrinology 1986;118:727–32.

34. Yue L, Peng JB, Hediger MA, et al. CaT1 manifests the pore properties of the calcium-release-activated calcium channel. Nature 2001;410(6829):705–9.

35. Hoenderop JG, Nilius B, Bindels RJ. EcaC: the gatekeeper of transepithelial Ca^{2+} transport. Biochim Biophys Acta 2002;1600(1–2):6–11.

36. Bronner F, Pansu D, Stein WD. An analysis of intestinal calcium transport across the rat intestine. Am J Physiol 1986;250(1):G561–9.

37. Feher JJ, Fullmer CS, Wasserman RH. Role of facilitated diffusion of calcium by calbindin in intestinal calcium absorption. Am J Physiol 1992;262(6Pt.1): C517–26.

38. Wasserman RH, Chandler JS, Meyer SA, et al. Intestinal calcium transport and calcium extrusion processes at the basolateral membrane. J Nutr 1992;122: 662–71.

39. Ghijsen WE, De Jong MD, Van Os CH. ATP-dependent calcium transport and its correlation with Ca^{2+}-ATPase activity in basolateral plasma membranes of rat duodenum. Biochim Biophys Acta 1982;689:327–36.

40. Van Os CH. Transcellular calcium transport in intestinal and renal epithelial cells. Biochim Biophys Acta 1987;906:195–222.

41. Cai Q, Chandler JS, Wasserman RH, et al. Vitamin D and adaptation to dietary calcium and phosphate deficiencies increase intestinal plasma membrane calcium pump gene expression. Proc Natl Acad Sci U S A 1993;90:1345–9.

42. Ghijsen WE, De Jong MD, Van Os CH. Kinetic properties of Na^+/Ca^{2+} exchange in basolateral plasma membranes of rat small intestine. Biochim Biophys Acta 1983;730:85–94.

43. Nemere I, Norman AW. Transcaltachia, vesicular calcium transport, and microtubule-associated calbindin-D28K. Emerging views of 1,25-dihydroxyvitamin D3-mdiated intestinal calcium absorption. Miner Electrolyte Metab 1990;16: 109–14.

44. Goodenough DA. Plugging the leaks. Proc Natl Acad Sci U S A 1999;96:319–21.

45. Kutuzova GD, DeLuca JF. Gene expression profiles in rat intestine identify pathways for 1,25-dihydroxyvitamin D3 stimulated calcium absorption and clarify its immunomodulatory properties. Arch Biochem Biophys 2004;432: 152–66.

46. Fujita H, Sugimoto K, Inatomi S, et al. Tight junction proteins claudin-2 and -12 are critical for vitamin D-dependent Ca^{2+} absorption between enterocytes. Mol Biol Cell 2008;19:1912–21.

47. Stenson WF, Essom RA, Riehl TE, et al. Regulation of paracellular permeability in Caco-2 cell monolayers by protein kinase C. Am J Physiol 1993; 265:G955–62.

48. Morgan EL, Mace OJ, Helliwell PA, et al. A role for Cav1.3 in rat intestinal calcium absorption. Biochem Biophys Res Commun 2003;312:487–93.

49. Wood RJ, Tchack L, Angelo G, et al. DNA microarray analysis of vitamin D-induced gene expression in a human colon carcinoma cell line. Physiol Genomics 2004;17:122–9.

50. Meyers MB, Puri TS, Chien AJ, et al. Sorcin associates with pore-forming subunit of voltage-dependent L-type Ca^{2+} channels. J Biol Chem 1998;273:18930–5.

51. Christakos S, Dhawan P, Ajibade D, et al. Mechanisms involved in vitamin D mediated intestinal calcium absorption and in non-classical actions of vitamin D. J Steroid Biochem Mol Biol 2010;121(1–2):183–7.

52. Pansu D, Bellaton C, Bronner F. The effects of calcium intake on the saturable and non-saturable components of duodenal calcium transport. Am J Physiol 1981;240:G32–7.

53. Pansu D, Bellaton C, Bronner F. Effect of lactose on duodenal calcium-binding protein and calcium absorption. J Nutr 1979;109:509–12.

54. Cassidy MM, Tidball CS. Cellular mechanisms of intestinal permeability alterations produced by chelation depletion. J Cell Biol 1967;32:685–98.

55. Heaney RP, Recker RR, Stegman MR, et al. Calcium absorption in women: relationships to calcium intake, estrogen status, and age. J Bone Miner Res 1989; 4(4):469–75.

56. van Cromphaut SJ, Dewerchin M, Hoenderop JG, et al. Duodenal calcium absorption in vitamin D receptor-knockout mice: functional and molecular aspects. Proc Natl Acad Sci U S A 2001;98:13324–9.

57. Heaney RP, Saville PD, Recker RR. Calcium absorption as a function of calcium intake. J Lab Clin Med 1975;85:881–90.

58. Dawson-Hughes B, Harris S, Kramich C, et al. Calcium retention and hormone levels in black and white women on high- and low-calcium diets. J Bone Miner Res 1993;8(7):779–87.

59. Sernka TJ, Borle AB. Calcium in the intestinal contents of rats on different calcium diets. Proc Soc Exp Biol Med 1969;131:1420–3.

60. Barger-Lux MJ, Heaney RP, Lanspa SJ, et al. An investigation of sources of variation in calcium absorption efficiency. J Clin Endocrinol Metab 1995;80:406–11.

61. Favus MJ, Goltzman D. Regulation of calcium and magnesium. In: Rosen CJ, editor. Primer on the metabolic bone diseases and disorders of mineral metabolism. 7th edition. Washington, DC: ASBMR; 2008. p. 104–8.

62. Epstein S, Bryce G, Hinman JW. The influence of age on bone mineral regulating hormones. Bone 1986;7:421–5.

63. Sherman SS, Hollis BW, Tobin JD. Vitamin D status and related parameters in a healthy population: the effects of age, sex and season. J Clin Endocrinol Metab 1990;71:405–13.

64. Prince TL, Dick I, Garcia WP, et al. The effects of the menopause on calcitriol and PTH: responses to a low dietary calcium stress test. J Clin Endocrinol Metab 1990;70:1119–23.

65. Orwoll ES, Meier D. Alterations in calcium, vitamin D and PTH physiology in normal men with aging. J Clin Endocrinol Metab 1986;63:1262–9.

66. Lund B, Sornensen OH, Lund B, et al. Serum 1,25(OH)2D in normal subjects and inpatients with postmenopausal osteopenia. Horm Metab Res 1982;14:271–4.

67. Halloran BP, Portale AA, Lonergan ET, et al. Production and metabolic clearance of 1,25(OH)2D in men: effect of advancing age. J Clin Endocrinol Metab 1990; 70:318–23.

68. Rowe JW, Anders R, Tobin JR, et al. The effect of age on creatinine clearance in man: a cross-sectional and longitudinal study. J Gerontol 1976;31:155–63.

69. Lindeman RE, Tobin J, Schock NW. Longitudinal studies on the rate of decline in renal function with age. J Am Geriatr Soc 1985;33:278–85.

70. Pattanaungkul S, Riggs BL, Yergey AL, et al. Relationship of intestinal calcium absorption to 1,25-dihydroxyvitamin D levels in young versus elderly women: evidence for age-related intestinal resistance to 1,25(OH)2D action. J Clin Endocrinol Metab 2000;85:4023–7.

71. Wood RJ, Fleet JC, Cashman K, et al. Intestinal calcium absorption in the aged rat: evidence of intestinal resistance to 1,25(OH)2D. Endocrinology 1998;139: 3843–8.

72. Ebeling PR, Sandgren ME, DiMagno EP, et al. Evidence of an age-related decrease in intestinal responsiveness to vitamin D: relationship between serum 1,25-dihydroxyvitamin D and intestinal vitamin D receptor concentrations in normal women. J Clin Endocrinol Metab 1992;75:176–82.

73. Horst TL, Goff JP, Reinhardt TA. Advancing age results in reduction of intestinal bone 1,25-dihydroxyvitamin D receptor. Endocrinology 1990;126:1053–7.

74. van AM, Huybers S, Hoenderop JG, et al. Age-dependent alterations in Ca^{2+} homoeostasis: role of TRPV5 and TRPF6. Am J Physiol Renal Physiol 2006; 291(6):F1177–83.

75. Heaney RP, Recker RR, Saville PD. Menopausal changes in calcium balance performance. J Lab Clin Med 1978;92:953–63.

76. Arjandi BH, Salih MA, Herbert DC, et al. Evidence for estrogen receptor-linked calcium transport in the intestine. Bone Miner 1993;21:63–74.

77. Dick IM, Liu J, Glendenning P, et al. Estrogen and androgen regulation of plasma membrane calcium pump activity in immortalized distal tubule kidney cells. Mol Cell Endocrinol 2003;212:11–8.

78. Van Cromphaut SJ, Rummens K, Stockmans I, et al. Intestinal calcium transporter genes are upregulated by estrogens and the reproductive cycle through vitamin D receptor-independent mechanisms. J Bone Miner Res 2003;18: 1725–36.

79. Gallagher JC, Riggs L, DeLuca H. Effect of estrogen on calcium absorption and serum vitamin D metabolites in postmenopausal Osteoporosis. J Clin Endocrinol Metab 1980;51(6):1359–64.

80. Reid IR. Primer on the metabolic bone diseases and disorders of mineral metabolism. 7th edition. Washington, DC: Menopause; 2009. p. 95–7.

81. Cerda D, Peris P, Monegal A, et al. Increase of PTH in post-menopausal osteoporosis. Rev Clin Esp 2011;211(7):338–43.

82. Rejnmark L, Vestergaard P, Brot C, et al. Increased fracture risk in normocalcemic postmenopausal women with high parathyroid hormone levels: a 16-year follow-up study. Calcif Tissue Int 2011;88:238–45.

83. Shea B, Wells G, Cranney A, et al. VII. Meta-analysis of calcium supplementation for the prevention of postmenopausal osteoporosis. Endocr Rev 2002; 23(4):552–9.

84. Nieves JW, Komar L, Cosman F, et al. Calcium potentiates the effect of estrogen and calcitonin on bone mass: review and analysis. Am J Clin Nutr 1998;67:18–24.

85. Huybers S, Naber TH, Bindels RJ, et al. Prednisolone-induced Ca^{2+} malabsorption is caused by diminished expression of the epithelial Ca^{2+} channel TRPV6. Am J Physiol Gastrointest Liver Physiol 2006;292:G92–7.

86. Lee GS, Choi KC, Jeung EB. Glucocorticoids differentially regulate expression of duodenal and renal calbindin-D9k through glucocorticoid receptor-mediated pathway in mouse model. Am J Physiol Endocrinol Metab 2005;290:E299–307.

87. Kovacs CS, Kronenberg HM. Maternal-fetal calcium and bone metabolism during pregnancy, puerperium, and lactation. Endocr Rev 1997;18(6):832–72.

88. Quan-Sheng D, Miller SC. Calciotrophic hormone levels and calcium absorption during pregnancy in rats. Am J Physiol 1989;257:E118–23.

89. Halloran BP, DeLuca HF. Calcium transport in small intestine during pregnancy and lactation. Am J Physiol 1980;239:E64–8.

90. Ajibade DV, Dhaqan P, Fechner AJ, et al. Evidence for a role of prolactin in calcium homeostasis: regulation of intestinal transient receptor potential vanilloid type 6, intestinal calcium absorption, and the 25-hydroxyvitamin D3, 1 alpha hydroxylase gene by prolactin. Endocrinology 2010;151(7):2974–84.

91. Kalkwarf HJ, Specker BL, Heuby JE, et al. Intestinal calcium absorption of women during lactation and after weaning. Am J Clin Nutr 1996;63:526–31.
92. Sharma OP, Vucinic V. Sarcoidosis of the thyroid and kidneys and calcium metabolism. Semin Respir Crit Care Med 2002;23(6):579–88.
93. Sharma OP. Hypercalcemia in granulomatous disorders: a critical review. Curr Opin Pulm Med 2000;6:442–7.
94. Stoffels K, Overbergh L, Bouillon R, et al. Immune regulation of 1 alpha-hydroxylase in murine peritoneal macrophages: unravelling the IFNgamma pathway. J Steroid Biochem Mol Biol 2007;103:567–71.
95. Esteban L, Vidal M, Dusso A. 1 alpha-hydroxylase transactivation by gamma-interferon in murine macrophages requires enhanced C/EBPbeta expression and activation. J Steroid Biochem Mol Biol 2004;89–90:131–7.
96. Papapoulos S, Clemens T, Fraher L, et al. 1,25-Dihydroxycholecalciferol in the pathogenesis of the hypercalcemia of sarcoidosis. Lancet 1979;1:627–30.
97. Bryant RJ, Wastney ME, Martin BR, et al. Racial differences in bone turnover and calcium metabolism in adolescent females. J Clin Endocrinol Metab 2003;88: 1043–7.
98. Abrams SA, O'Brien KO, Liang LK, et al. Differences in calcium absorption and kinetics between black and white girls aged 5-16 years. J Bone Miner Res 1995; 10(5):829–33.
99. Braun M, Palacious C, Wigertz K, et al. Racial differences in skeletal calcium retention in adolescent girls with varied controlled calcium intakes. Am J Clin Nutr 2007;85:1657–63.
100. Shapses SA, Riedt CS. Bone, body weight, and weight reduction: what are the concerns? J Nutr 2006;136:1453–6.
101. Shapses SA, Sukumar D, Schneider SH. Hormonal and dietary influences on true fractional calcium absorption in women: role of obesity. Osteoporos Int 2012. [Epub ahead of print].
102. Bolland MJ, Grey AB, Ames RW, et al. Fat mass is an important predictor of parathyroid hormone levels in postmenopausal women. Bone 2006;38:317–21.
103. Pitroda AP, Harris SS, Dawson-Hughes B. The association of adiposity with parathyroid hormone in healthy older adults. Endocrine 2009;36:218–23.
104. Armstrong ME, Spencer EA, Cairns BJ, et al. Body mass index and physical activity in relation to the incidence of hip fracture in postmenopausal women. J Bone Miner Res 2011;26:1330–8.
105. Baker AR, McDonell DP, Hughes M, et al. Cloning and expression of full-length cDNA encoding human vitamin D receptor. Proc Natl Acad Sci U S A 1988;85: 3294–8.
106. Miyamoto KI, Kesterson RA, Yamamoto H, et al. Structural organization of the human vitamin D receptor chromosomal gene and its promoter. Mol Endocrinol 1997;11:1165–79.
107. Morrison NA, Qi JC, Tokita A, et al. Prediction of bone density from vitamin D receptor alleles. Nature 1994;367:284–7.
108. Dawson-Hughes B, Harris SS, Finneran S. Calcium absorption on high and low calcium intakes in relation to vitamin D receptor genotype. J Clin Endocrinol Metab 1995;80:3657–61.
109. Gennari L, Becherini L, Masi L, et al. Vitamin D receptor genotypes and intestinal calcium absorption in postmenopausal women. Calcif Tissue Int 1997;61:460–3.
110. Wishart JM, Horowitz M, Need AG, et al. Relations between calcium intake, calcitriol, polymorphisms of the vitamin D receptor gene, and calcium absorption in premenopausal women. Am J Clin Nutr 1997;65:798–802.

111. Ames SK, Ellis KJ, Gunn SK, et al. Vitamin D receptor gene Fok1 polymorphism predicts calcium absorption and bone mineral density in children. J Bone Miner Res 1999;14:740–6.

112. Francis RM, Harrington F, Turner E, et al. Vitamin D receptor gene polymorphism in men and its effect on bone density and calcium absorption. Clin Endocrinol 1997;46:83–6.

113. Wolf RL, Cauley JA, Baker CE, et al. Factors associated with calcium absorption efficiency in pre- and perimenopausal women. Am J Clin Nutr 2000;72:466–71.

114. Laaksonen M, Karkkainen M, Outila T, et al. Vitamin D receptor gene Bsml-polymorphism in Finnish premenopausal and postmenopausal women: its association with bone mineral density, markers of bone turnover, and intestinal calcium absorption with adjustment for lifestyle factors. J Bone Miner Metab 2002;20:383–90.

115. Hagenau T, Vest R, Gissel TN, et al. Global vitamin D levels in relation to age, gender, skin pigmentation and latitude: an ecologic meta-regression analysis. Osteoporos Int 2009;20:133–40.

116. Shafer RB, Gregory DH. Calcium malabsorption in hyperthyroidism. Gastroenterology 1972;63:235.

117. Singhelakis P, Alevizaki CC, Ikkos DG. Intestinal calcium absorption in hyperthyroidism. Metabolism 1974;23:311.

118. Friedland JA, Williams GA, Bowser EN, et al. Effect of hyperthyroidism on intestinal absorption of calcium in the rat. Exp Biol Med 1965;120(1):20–3.

119. Peerenboom H, Keck E, Kruskemper HL, et al. The defect of intestinal calcium transport in hyperthyroidism and its response to therapy. J Clin Endocrinol Metab 1984;59:936.

120. Pazianas M, Butcher GP, Subhani JM, et al. Calcium absorption and bone mineral density in celiacs after long term treatment with gluten-free diet and adequate calcium intake. Osteoporos Int 2005;16(1):56–63.

121. Molteni N, Bardella MT, Vezzoli G, et al. Intestinal calcium absorption as shown by stable strontium test in celiac disease before and after gluten-free diet. Am J Gastroenterol 1995;909(11):2025–8.

122. Strohmayer E, Via MA, Yanagisawa R. Metabolic management following bariatric surgery. Mt Sinai J Med 2010;77:431–45.

123. Heaney RP, Smith KP, Recker RR, et al. Meal effects on calcium absorption. Am J Clin Nutr 1989;49:372–6.

124. Recker RR. Calcium absorption and achlorhydria. N Engl J Med 1965;313:70–3.

125. Buzinaro ER, Almeida RN, Mazeto GM. Bioavailability of dietary calcium. Arq Bras Endocrinol Metabol 2006;50:852–61.

126. Jewel C, Cashman KD. The effect of conjugated linoleic acid and medium-chain fatty acids on transepithelial calcium transport in human intestinal-like Caco-2 cells. Br J Nutr 2003;89:639–47.

127. Jewell C, Cusack S, Cashman RD. The effect of conjugated linoleic acid on transepithelial calcium transport and mediators of paracellular permeability in human intestinal-like caco-2 cells. Prostaglandins Leukot Essent Fatty Acids 2005;72:29–39.

128. Vagata C, Bagao Y, Shibuya C, et al. Fat intake is associated with serum estrogen and androgen concentrations in postmenopausal Japanese women. J Nutr 2005;135:2862–5.

129. Wu AH, Pike MC, Stram DO. Meta-analysis: dietary fat intake, serum estrogen levels, and the risk of breast cancer. J Natl Cancer Inst 1999; 91:529–34.

130. Heaney RP, Weaver CM, Barger-Lux MJ. Food factors influencing calcium availability. Challenges Mod Med 1995;7:229–41.
131. Zitterman A, Bock P, Drummer C, et al. Lactose does not enhance calcium bioavailability in lactose-tolerant, healthy adults. Am J Clin Nutr 2000;71:931–6.
132. Teramoto F, Rokutan K, Sugano Y, et al. Long-term administration of 4G-beta-galactosylsucrose(lactosucrose) enhances intestinal calcium absorption in young women: a randomized, placebo-controlled 96-wk study. J Nutr Sci Vitaminol 2006;52:337–46.
133. Scholz-Ahrens KE, Ade P, Marten B, et al. Prebiotics, probiotics, and symbiotics affect mineral absorption, bone mineral content, and bone structure. J Nutr 2007;137:S838–46.
134. Abrams S, Griffin I, Hawthorne K, et al. A combination of prebiotic short- and long-chain inulin-type fructans enhances calcium absorption and bone mineralization in young adolescents. Am J Clin Nutr 2005;82(2):471–6.
135. Weaver CM, Heaney RP, Martin BR, et al. Human calcium absorption from whole wheat products. J Nutr 1991;121:1769–75.
136. Heaney RP. Nutritional factors in osteoporosis. Annu Rev Nutr 1993;73:287–316.
137. Heaney RP, Weaver CM. Oxalate in vegetables. Effect on calcium absorbability. J Bone Miner Res 1993;8:S333.
138. Heaney RP, Weaver CM, Hinders SM, et al. Absorbability of calcium from spinach. Am J Clin Nutr 1988;47:707–9.
139. Barger-Lux MJ, Heaney RP. Caffeine and the calcium economy revisited. Osteoporos Int 1995;5:97–102.
140. Barrett-Connor E, Chang JC, Edelstein SL. Coffee-associated osteoporosis offset by daily milk consumption. JAMA 1994;271:280–3.
141. Jung TT, Davie M, Hunter JO, et al. Abnormal vitamin D metabolism in cirrhosis. Gut 1978;19:290–3.
142. Need AG, Kemp A, Giles N, et al. Relationships between intestinal calcium absorption, serum vitamin D metabolites and smoking in postmenopausal women. Osteoporos Int 2002;1:83–8.
143. Jorde R, Saleh F, Figenschau Y, et al. Serum parathyroid Hormone(PTH) levels in smokers and non-smokers. The fifth Tromso study. Eur J Endocrinol 2005;152:39–45.
144. Barbieri J, Gochberg J, Ryan KJ. Nicotine, cotinine, and anabasine inhibit aromatase in human trophoblast in vitro. J Clin Invest 1986;77:1727–33.
145. Michnovicz J, Hershcopf FJ, Naganuma H, et al. Increased 2-hydroxylation of estradiol as a possible mechanism for the anti-estrogenic effect of cigarette smoking. N Engl J Med 1986;315:1305–9.
146. Christakos S, Dhawan P, Liu Y, et al. New insights into the mechanisms of vitamin D action. J Cell Biochem 2003;88(4):695–705.
147. Jowsey J, Gershon-Cohen J. Effect of dietary calcium levels on production and reversal of experimental osteoporosis in cats. Proc Soc Exp Biol Med 1964;116:437–41.
148. Jowsey J, Raisz LG. Experimental osteoporosis and parathyroid activity. Endocrinology 1968;82:384–96.
149. Matkovic V, Jelic T, Wardlaw GM, et al. Timing of peak bone mass in Caucasian females and its implication for the prevention of osteoporosis. J Clin Invest 1994;93:799–808.
150. Johnston CC Jr, Miller JZ, Slemenda CW, et al. Calcium supplementation and increases in bone mineral density in children. N Engl J Med 1992;327(2):82–7.

151. Nowson CA, Green RM, Hopper JL, et al. A co-twin study of the effect of calcium supplementation on bone density during adolescence. Osteoporos Int 1997; 7(3):219–25.
152. Lloyd T, Martel JK, Rollings N, et al. The effect of calcium supplementation and Tanner stage on bone density, content and area in teenage women. Osteoporos Int 1996;6:276–83.
153. Nieves JW, Golden AL, Sitis E, et al. Teenage and current calcium intake are related to bone mineral density of the hip and forearm in women aged 30-39 years. Am J Epidemiol 1995;141(4):342–51.
154. Murphy S, Khaw KT, May H, et al. Milk consumption and bone mineral density in middle aged and elderly women. BMJ 1994;308:939–41.
155. Sandler RB, Slemenda CW, La Porte RE, et al. Postmenopausal bone density and milk consumption in childhood and adolescence. Am J Clin Nutr 1985;42:270–4.
156. Soroko S, Hobrook TL, Edelstein S, et al. Lifetime milk consumption and bone mineral density in older women. Am J Public Health 1994;84:1319–22.
157. Kalkwarf HJ, Khoury JC, Lanphear BP. Milk intake during childhood and adolescence, adult bone density, and osteoporotic fractures in US women. Am J Clin Nutr 2003;77:257–65.
158. Barr SI, McKay HA. Nutrition, exercise and bone status in youth. Int J Sport Nutr 1998;8:124–42.
159. Matkovic V, Ilitch JZ. Calcium requirements for growth: are current recommendations adequate? Nutr Rev 1993;51:171–80.
160. Chevally T, Rizzoli R, Nydegger V, et al. Effects of calcium supplements on femoral bone mineral density and fracture rate in vitamin d replete elderly patients. Osteoporos Int 1994;4(5):245–52.
161. Recker RR, Hinders S, Davies KM, et al. Correcting calcium nutritional deficiency prevents spine fractures in elderly women. J Bone Miner Res 1996; 11(12):1961–6.
162. Peacock M, Liu G, Carey M, et al. Effect of calcium or 25(OH)vitamin D3 dietary supplementation on bone loss at the hip in men and women over the age of 60. J Clin Endocrinol Metab 2000;85(9):3011–9.
163. Bischoff-Ferrari HA, Willett WC, Wong JB, et al. Fracture prevention with vitamin D supplementation: meta-analysis of randomized controlled trials. JAMA 2005; 293(18):2257–64.
164. Boonen S, Lips P, Bouillon R, et al. Need for additional calcium to reduce the risk of hip fracture with vitamin D supplementation: evidence from a comparative metaanalysis of randomized controlled trials. J Clin Endocrinol Metab 2007; 92(4):1415–23.
165. Bischoff-Ferrari HA, Dawson-Hughes B, Baron JA, et al. Calcium intake and hip fracture risk in men and women: a meta-analysis of prospective cohort studies and randomized controlled trials. Am J Clin Nutr 2007;86(6):1780–90.
166. Heaney RP. Calcium, dairy products, and osteoporosis. J Am Coll Nutr 2000; 19(2):83s–99s.
167. Avenell A, Gillespie WJ, Gillespie LD, et al. Vitamin D and vitamin D analogues for preventing fractures associated with involutional postmenopausal osteoporosis. Cochrane Database Syst Rev 2005;(3):CD000227.
168. Tang BM, Eslick GD, Nowson C, et al. Use of calcium or calcium in combination with vitamin D supplementation to prevent fractures and bone loss in people aged 50 years and older: a meta-analysis. Lancet 2007;370(9588):657–66.
169. Jackson RD, LaCroix AZ, Gass M, et al. Calcium plus vitamin D supplementation and the risk of fractures. N Engl J Med 2006;354(7):669–83.

170. Chapuy MC, Arlot ME, Delmas PD, et al. Effect of calcium and cholecalciferol treatment for three years on hip fractures in elderly women. BMJ 1994; 308(6936):1081–2.
171. Aloia JF, Vaswani A, Yeth JK, et al. Calcium supplementation with and without hormone replacement therapy to prevent postmenopausal bone loss. Ann Intern Med 1994;120(2):97–103.
172. Reid IR, Ames R, Mason B, et al. Randomized controlled trial of calcium in healthy, non-osteoporotic men. Arch Intern Med 2008;168(20):2276–82.
173. Heaney RP. The bone remodeling transient: implications for the interpretation of clinical studies of bone mass change. J Bone Miner Res 1994;9:1515–23.
174. Bonnick S, Broy S, Kaiser F, et al. Treatment with alendronate plus calcium, alendronate alone, or calcium alone for postmenopausal low bone mineral density. Curr Med Res Opin 2007;23(6):1341–9.
175. Rianon N, Feeback D, Wood R, et al. Monitoring sweat calcium using skin patches. Calcif Tissue Int 2003;72:694–7.
176. Klesges RC, Ward KD, Shelton ML, et al. Changes in bone mineral content in male athletes. Mechanisms of action and intervention effects. JAMA 1996;276: 226–30.
177. Heaney RP, Recker RR. Determinant of endogenous fecal calcium in healthy women. J Bone Miner Res 1994;9:1621–7.
178. MacFadyen IJ, Nordin BE, Smith DA, et al. Effect of variation in dietary calcium on plasma concentration and urinary excretion of calcium. BMJ 1965;1:161–4.
179. Walser M. Calcium clearance as a function of sodium clearance in the dog. Am J Physiol 1961;200:769–73.
180. Nordin BE, Need AG, Morris HA, et al. The nature and significance of the relationship between urinary sodium and urinary calcium in women. J Nutr 1993; 123:1615–22.
181. Goulding A, Campbell D. Dietary NaCl loads promote calciuria and bone loss in adult oophorectomized rats consuming a low calcium diet. J Nutr 1983;113: 1409–14.
182. McParland BE, Goulding A, Campbell AJ. Dietary salt affects biochemical markers of resorption and formation of bone in elderly women. BMJ 1989;299:834–5.
183. Need AG, Morris HA, Cleghorn DB, et al. Effect of salt restriction on urine hydroxyproline excretion in postmenopausal women. Arch Intern Med 1991;151: 757–9.
184. Heaney RP, Recker RR. Effects of nitrogen, phosphorus, and caffeine on calcium balance in women. J Lab Clin Med 1982;99:46–55.
185. Sellmeyer DL, Stone KL, Sebastian A, et al. A high ratio of dietary animal to vegetable protein increases the rate of bone loss and the risk of fracture in postmenopausal women. Am J Clin Nutr 2001;73:118–22.
186. Munger RG, Cerhan JR, Chiu BC. Prospective study of dietary protein intake and risk of hip fracture in postmenopausal women. Am J Clin Nutr 1999;69:147–52.
187. Hannan MT, Tucher KL, Dawson-Hughes B, et al. Effect of dietary protein on bone loss in elderly men and women: the Framingham Osteoporosis Study. J Bone Miner Res 2000;15:2504–12.
188. Abelow BJ, Holford TR, Insogna KL. Cross-cultural association between dietary animal protein and hip fracture: a hypothesis. Calcif Tissue Int 1992;50:14–8.
189. Meyer HE, Pedersen JI, Loken EB, et al. Dietary factors and the incidence of hip fracture in middle-aged Norwegians. A prospective study. Am J Epidemiol 1997; 145:117–23.

190. Roughead ZK, Johnson LK, Lykken GI, et al. Controlled high meat diets do not affect calcium retention or indices of bone status in healthy postmenopausal women. J Nutr 2003;133:1020–6.
191. Calvo MS, Bell RR, Forges RM. Effect of protein-induced calciuria on calcium metabolism and bone status in adult rats. J Nutr 1982;112:1401–13.
192. Kerstetter JE, O'Brien KO, Caseria DM, et al. The impact of dietary protein on calcium absorption and kinetic measures of bone turnover in women. J Clin Endocrinol Metab 2005;90:26–31.
193. Schurch MA, Rizzoli R, Slosman D, et al. Protein supplements increase serum insulin-like growth factor-1 levels and attenuate proximal femur bone loss in patients with recent hip fracture: a randomized, double-blind, placebo-controlled trial. Ann Intern Med 1998;128(10):801–9.
194. Ghiron L, Thompson J, Halloway L. Effects of rhGH and IGF-1 on bone turnover in elderly women. J Bone Miner Res 1995;10:1844–52.
195. Heaney RP. Protein and calcium: antagonists or synergists? Am J Clin Nutr 2002;75:609–10.
196. Dargent-Molina P, Sabia S, Touvier M, et al. Proteins, dietary acid load, and calcium and risk of postmenopausal fractures in the E3N French women prospective study. J Bone Miner Res 2008;23(12):1915–22.
197. Misra D, Berry SD, Broe KE, et al. Does dietary protein reduce hip fracture risk in elders? The Framingham osteoporosis study. Osteoporos Int 2011;22:345–9.
198. Raisz LG, Niemann I. Effect of phosphate, calcium and magnesium on bone resorption and hormonal responses in tissue culture. Endocrinology 1969;85:446–52.
199. Lotz M, Zisman E, Bartter FC. Evidence for a phosphorus-depletion syndrome in man. N Engl J Med 1968;278:409–15.
200. Heaney RP, Nordin BE. Calcium effects on phosphorus absorption: implications for the prevention and co-therapy of osteoporosis. J Am Coll Nutr 2002;21(3):239–44.
201. Chapuy MC, Arlot ME, Duboeuf F, et al. Vitamin D3 and calcium to prevent hip fractures in the elderly women. N Engl J Med 1992;327:1637–42.
202. Bo-Linn GW, Davis GR, Buddnus DJ, et al. An evaluation of the importance of gastric acid secretion in the absorption of dietary calcium. J Clin Invest 1984;73:640–7.
203. Heaney RP. Ethnicity, bone status, and the Ca requirement. Nutr Res 2002;22:153–78.
204. IOM (Institute of Medicine). Dietary reference intakes for calcium and vitamin D. Washington, DC: The National Academies Press; 2011.
205. Nabhan FA, Sizemore GW, Camacho PM. Milk alkali syndrome from ingestion of calcium carbonate in a patient with hypoparathyroidism. Endocr Pract 2004;10(4):372–5.
206. Picolos MK, Sims CR, Mastrobattista JM, et al. Milk alkali syndrome in pregnancy. Obstet Gynecol 2004;104(5):1201–4.
207. Picolos MS, Lavis VR, Orlander PR. Milk alkali syndrome is a major cause of hypercalcemia among non-end-stage renal disease inpatients. Clin Endocrinol 2005;63(5):566–76.
208. Burke RR, Rybicki BA, Rao DS. Calcium and vitamin D in sarcoidosis: how to assess and manage. Semin Respir Crit Care Med 2010;31(4):474–84.
209. Coe FL, Parks JH, Asplin JR. The pathogenesis and treatment of kidney stones. N Engl J Med 1992;327:1141–52.
210. Riggs BL, O'Fallon WM, Muhs J, et al. Long term effects of calcium supplementation on serum parathyroid hormone level, bone turnover, and bone loss in elderly women. J Bone Miner Res 1998;13(2):168–74.

211. Curhan GC, Willett WC, Speizer FE, et al. Comparison of dietary calcium with supplemental calcium and other nutrients as factors affecting risk for kidney stones in women. Ann Intern Med 1997;126(7):497–504.

212. Curhan GC, Willett WC, Knight EL, et al. Dietary factors and the risk of incident kidney stones in younger women: Nurses Health Study II. Arch Intern Med 2004; 164(8):885–91.

213. Curhan GC, Willett WC, Rimm EB, et al. A prospective study of dietary calcium and other nutrients and the risk of symptomatic kidney stones. N Engl J Med 1993;328(12):833–8.

214. Robertson WG, Peacock M. Stone disease of the urinary tract. Practitioner 1981; 225(1357):961–9.

215. Hess B, Jost C, Zipperle L, et al. High calcium intake abolishes hyperoxaluria and reduces urinary crystallization during a 20-fold normal oxalate load in humans. Nephrol Dial Transplant 1998;13(9):2241–7.

216. Resnick LM, Laragh JH, Sealey JE, et al. Divalent cations in essential hypertension. Relations between serum ionized calcium, magnesium, and plasma renin activity. N Engl J Med 1983;309(15):888–91.

217. Bohr DF. Vascular smooth muscle: dual effect of calcium. Science 1963; 139(3555):197–9.

218. Reid IR, Mason B, Horne A, et al. Effects of calcium supplementation on serum lipid concentrations in normal older women: a randomized controlled trial. Am J Med 2002;112(5):343–7.

219. Denke MA, Fox MM, Schulte MC. Short-term dietary calcium fortification increases fecal saturated fat content and reduces serum lipids in men. J Nutr 1993;123(6):1047–53.

220. Draznin B, Sussman KE, Eckel RH, et al. Possible role of cytosolic free calcium concentrations in mediating insulin resistance of obesity and hyperinsulinemia. J Clin Invest 1988;82(6):1848–52.

221. Reid IR, Schooler BA, Hannan SF, et al. The acute biochemical effects of four proprietary calcium preparations. Aust N Z J Med 1986;16(2):193–7.

222. Bostick RM, Kushi LH, Wu Y, et al. Relation of calcium, vitamin D, and dairy food intake to ischemic heart disease mortality among postmenopausal women. Am J Epidemiol 1999;149(2):151–61.

223. Iso H, Stampfer MJ, Manson JE, et al. Prospective study of calcium, potassium, and magnesium intake and risk of stroke in women. Stroke 1999;30(9):1772–9.

224. Kaluza J, Orsini N, Levitan EB, et al. Dietary calcium and magnesium intake and mortality: a prospective study of men. Am J Epidemiol 2010;171(7):801–7.

225. Al-Delaimy WK, Rimm E, Willett WC, et al. A prospective study of calcium intake from diet and supplements and risk of ischemic heart disease among men. Am J Clin Nutr 2003;77(4):814–8.

226. Bolland MJ, Barber PA, Doughty RN, et al. Vascular events in healthy older women receiving calcium supplementation: randomised controlled trial. BMJ 2008;336(7638):262–6.

227. Lewis JR, Calver J, Zhu K, et al. Calcium supplementation and the risks of atherosclerotic vascular disease in older women: results of a 5-year RCT and a 4.5-year follow-up. J Bone Miner Res 2011;26(1):35–41.

How Vitamin D Works on Bone

Tomohiko Yoshida, MD, PhD[a], Paula H. Stern, PhD[b],*

KEYWORDS

- Vitamin D • Mineralization • Bone resorption • Rickets • Osteomalacia • Fracture
- Analogues

KEY POINTS

- Vitamin D is important for the normal development and maintenance of bone.
- Our understanding of the actions of vitamin D on bone has been advanced by the elucidation of its activation pathway and the cloning of the vitamin D receptor.
- The preponderance of evidence indicates that $1,25(OH)_2D_3$ enhances bone mineralization through its effects to promote calcium and phosphate absorption.
- Although $1,25(OH)_2D_3$ stimulates bone resorption in vitro, treatment in vivo can prevent bone loss and fracture, through several potential mechanisms.
- The development of vitamin D analogues has provided new therapeutic options.

INTRODUCTION

Vitamin D is involved in calcium and phosphate metabolism in bone, intestine, and kidney. Several clinical and animal studies indicate that the physiologic effects of vitamin D extend beyond these tissue sites. Adequate vitamin D levels have a role in muscle integrity,[1–4] cancer prevention,[5–8] innate and acquired immune responses,[9,10] and cardiovascular morbidity and mortality.[11–14] Although these extraskeletal effects of vitamin D have recently attracted attention, the actions on bone, which have been recognized for many years, are still not fully understood. This article summarizes the effects of vitamin D on bone and highlights issues that are not yet resolved.

VITAMIN D METABOLISM AND ACTIONS

Vitamin D is produced from previtamin D_3, and is in part provided by dietary sources. Previtamin D_3 is generated from the vitamin D_3 precursor, 7-dehydrocholesterol, in the skin after sunlight exposure (ultraviolet B light),[15–17] and is then readily converted

[a] Division of Endocrinology, Diabetes and Metabolism, Chiba University Hospital, 1-8-1 Inohana, Chuo-ku, Chiba-shi, Chiba 260-8670, Japan; [b] Department of Molecular Pharmacology and Biological Chemistry, Northwestern University Feinberg School of Medicine, 303 East Chicago Avenue, Chicago, IL 60611, USA
* Corresponding author.
E-mail address: p-stern@northwestern.edu

Endocrinol Metab Clin N Am 41 (2012) 557–569
doi:10.1016/j.ecl.2012.04.003
0889-8529/12/$ – see front matter © 2012 Elsevier Inc. All rights reserved.

endo.theclinics.com

to vitamin D_3. Vitamin D_3 is hydroxylated in the liver to make 25-hydroxyvitamin D_3 (25(OH)D_3), and further hydroxylated in the kidney to 1,25-dihydroxyvitamin D_3 (1,25(OH)$_2D_3$, calcitriol), the active form.[18]

In book III of *The Persian Wars* (500–600 BC), the beneficial effect of physiologically produced vitamin D on bone was indirectly implicated by the description of the difference in skulls between the Egyptians and the Persians.[19] The skulls of the Persians were weaker than those of the Egyptians, and the explanation for this was that the Persians had their heads covered by turbans, whereas the heads of the Egyptians were more exposed to sunlight because they had their heads shaved. Later, in the early twentieth century, ultraviolet light came into use as a treatment of rickets.[20] Around the same time, specific dietary deficiencies in phosphorous and photosynthesized fat-soluble vitamins were found to have a causal role in the development of rickets.[21–25] After the discovery that irradiation of some dietary components conferred antirachitic properties,[26,27] the metabolism of vitamin D was investigated,[28,29] providing a basis of our current understanding of the dietary and metabolic mechanisms of osteomalacia.

VITAMIN D RECEPTOR AND ITS EFFECTS ON BONE MINERALIZATION

Before the cloning of vitamin D receptor (VDR), the action was predicted by the observation of hereditary vitamin-D–resistant rickets, or vitamin-D–dependent rickets type II (VDDRII) (OMIM 277440).[30,31] A brother and sister presented with hypocalcemia caused by calcium malabsorption, and manifested secondary hyperparathyroidism with hypophosphatemia and high serum concentrations of 1,25(OH)$_2D_3$. The male proband failed to walk unsupported by age 20 months, possibly because of muscular weakness. High doses of ergocalciferol or 1,25-dihydroxycholecalciferol were required to obtain radiographic healing, but the bowing deformities of the tibias and femurs were remarkable (genu varum) and required corrective surgery. Radiologic pictures of the patient showed diffusely decreased bone mineral density (BMD), subperiosteal resorption, and a pseudofracture of the left ischiopubic ramus.

The skeletal action of vitamin D became more evident after the discovery, cloning, and expression of VDR.[32–35] Through the screening of human intestine (jejunum) and T47D (human ductal breast epithelial tumor cell line) cell cDNA libraries, complementary DNA clones encoding the human VDR were isolated. The cloned sequences were transfected into COS-1 cells, and the protein encoded by the cDNA was comparable with the native receptor in terms of the binding affinity to 1,25(OH)$_2D_3$, binding preferences for other vitamin D metabolites, and sedimentation characteristics with VDR antibody.[35] Vitamin D and its metabolites have a unique characteristic as to flexibility in structure, and the VDR have had to adapt to the conformational mobility of its ligand. Five carbon-carbon single bonds in the intact 8-carbon side chain,[36] the chair-chair inversion of the cyclohexanelike A-ring,[37] and the rotation around B-ring[38] allow 1,25(OH)$_2D_3$ to be highly conformationally mobile.

VDR belongs to the steroid hormone nuclear receptor superfamily, and has been shown to regulate both gene transcription as well as rapid responses such as the opening of voltage-gated Ca^{2+} channels,[39] and stimulation of intestinal Ca^{2+} absorption.[40] These rapid responses of VDR seem to be mediated through the membrane-bound VDR in caveolae[41,42] or through a variety of receptor types located within or near the plasma membrane or caveolae.[43] Protein-disulfide isomerase-associated 3 is hypothesized to be one of these receptors, and was shown to directly inhibit mineralization in osteoblastlike MC3T3-E1 cells through phospholipase A_2-dependent rapid release of prostaglandin E_2 (PGE$_2$), activation of protein kinase C, and regulation of bone-related gene transcription.[44]

A mouse model of VDDRII, in which the second zinc finger of the VDR DNA-binding domain was ablated, showed hypocalcemia, hyperparathyroidism, rickets, and osteomalacia. Alopecia was seen in some kindreds, although it is not a common feature of vitamin D deficiency.[45] VDR null mutant mice showed no defects in development and growth before weaning, irrespective of reduced expression of vitamin D target genes.[46] However, after weaning, mutants failed to thrive, and presented with alopecia, hypocalcemia, infertility, and severely reduced bone formation. It was previously shown that parenteral calcium infusions could cure the osteomalacic lesions in children or rodent with mutant VDRs,[47,48] but a proper ratio of dietary phosphorous (0.25%) to calcium (0.5%) was shown to be critical for mineralization,[49] suggesting that VDR-mediated effect on bone is achieved mainly through the intestinal calcium and phosphorous absorption. Experimental studies supporting this theory include the observation that infusion of calcium and phosphate to vitamin-D–deficient rats induced growth and mineralization as effectively as vitamin D replacement.[50] Also, VDR−/− mouse bone transplanted into WT mice showed even greater density and mineralization after 4 weeks than transplanted WT bone.[51] On the other hand, recent findings have suggested that $1,25(OH)_2D_3$ can directly accelerate osteoblast-mediated mineralization by stimulating the production of ALP-positive mature matrix vesicles in the period before mineralization in the human preosteoblastic cell line SV-HFO,[52] although it is still unclear how VDR is involved in the direct acceleration of mineralization.

VITAMIN D ACTIONS ON BONE RESORPTION

Contrary to the effect on mineralization, $1,25(OH)_2D_3$ has clear direct effects on bone resorption. Addition of $1,25(OH)_2D_3$ to cocultures of mouse osteoblasts and bone marrow cells induces osteoclast differentiation in vitro.[53] $1,25(OH)_2D_3$ acts as a calcium-regulating hormone and induces receptor activator of nuclear factor κB ligand (RANKL) expression in osteoblasts, which results in an increase in serum calcium levels by stimulating osteoclastogenesis and bone resorption.[54] RANKL is a member of the tumor necrosis α family, and its interaction with the receptor RANK on osteoclast precursor cells leads to their differentiation into multinucleated cells capable of resorbing bone.[55] Vitamin-D–induced osteoclastogenesis seems to be effected through a VDR-mediated increase in RANKL expression in osteoblasts, because VDR-deficient osteoblasts were not able to induce osteoclastogenesis in response to $1,25(OH)_2D_3$.[56] $1,25(OH)_2D_3$-stimulated osteoclast formation in spleen-osteoblast cocultures was suggested to be mediated in part by enhanced interleukin 1α-stimulated RANKL production in osteoblasts.[57,58] PGE_2 production from hematopoietic cells was suggested to be involved in $1,25(OH)_2D_3$-dependent calcitonin-receptor positive cell formation and bone resorption.[59] SC-19220, a PGE_2 antagonist, inhibits $1,25(OH)_2D_3$-stimulated osteoclastogenesis in bone marrow cultures.[60]

VDR can bind to DNA response elements as homodimers and as heterodimers with RAR, RXR, and T3R,[61,62] and the ability to form heterodimers with other receptors allows a diverse range of physiologic effects.[63] It is therefore likely that vitamin D actions on bone could be affected by other ligands for nuclear receptors. In 21-day cultures of peripheral blood mononuclear cells, the number of tartrate-resistant acid phosphatase-positive and vitronectin-positive multinucleated cells and the area of lacunar resorption were shown to be decreased when $1,25(OH)_2D_3$ alone was added at concentrations of 10^{-9} M and higher. A marked increase in resorption pit formation was noted when the combination of $1,25(OH)_2D_3$ and dexamethasone was added to peripheral blood mononuclear cell cultures.[64] 3,5,3'-Triiodo-L-thyronine (T3) weakly induced mRNA expression of RANKL in primary osteoblasts. This effect was amplified in the copresence of $1,25(OH)_2D_3$.[65]

Osteoprotegerin (OPG), a soluble member of the tumor necrosis factor receptor family and the decoy receptor for RANKL, prevents $1,25(OH)_2D_3$-stimulated bone resorption as shown by its antagonism of the $1,25(OH)_2D_3$-mediated increase of calcium concentration,[66,67] osteoclast number,[67] and serum cross-linked N-telopeptides.[68] OPG expression is also regulated by vitamin D analogues; however, there are differences in the effects observed. $1,25(OH)_2D_3$ at a concentration of 10^{-7} M increased OPG mRNA levels by 50% in normal trabecular osteoblast cells and increased OPG mRNA 90% and OPG protein 60% in a fetal osteoblast cell line.[69] In another study, the highly potent $1,25(OH)_2D_3$ analogue 2-methylene-19-nor-(20S)-1,25-dihydroxyvitamin D_3 and $1,25(OH)_2D_3$ at concentrations of approximately 10^{-8} M inhibited OPG production by osteoblastic cells.[70]

Although earlier studies using tracer kinetics revealed that physiologic replacement doses of vitamin D caused mobilization of calcium from bone,[71] it has been unclear whether vitamin-D–stimulated calcium release from bone is a physiologic event. Coculture systems are widely used in osteoclastogenesis studies, but higher concentration (10^{-8}–10^{-9} M) of $1,25(OH)_2D_3$ compared with that normally seen in serum (10^{-10} M) are required for the induction of osteoclast formation in these models.[46,53] However, in organ cultures we could clearly show that $1,25(OH)_2D_3$ effectively stimulates ^{45}Ca release from fetal rat radii and ulnae at a concentration as low as 10^{-11} M,[18,72] which is at the low end of the physiologic range. We also found that $1,25(OH)_2D_3$-stimulated ^{45}Ca release from bone was significantly inhibited by partially purified serum extract, whereas further purified serum extract using high-pressure liquid chromatography did not significantly affect the responses of the bones to $1,25(OH)_2D_3$.[72] This finding suggests that other serum factors, possibly OPG, could modulate the effects on osteoclastogenesis in vivo. In an in vivo rat model, supraphysiologic doses of $1,25(OH)_2D_3$ increased serum Ca and expression of RANKL, but parathyroid hormone (PTH)-induced expression of RANKL mRNA was inhibited by physiologic doses of $1,25(OH)_2D_3$.[73] The proven effect of 1α-OH-D to decrease serum PTH and PTH effects on bone turnover[74] suggests this as a mechanism of decreased bone turnover in response to vitamin D treatment. The osteolytic response and hypercalcemic effects of vitamin D become increasingly apparent at higher concentrations or when metabolites and analogues that bypass critical regulatory steps are used therapeutically. The dietary vitamin D levels that cause vitamin D intoxication were estimated at 50,000 units or more in a person with normal parathyroid function and sensitivity to vitamin D.[75]

VITAMIN D SIGNALING IN BONE AND ITS MODULATION

In short-term cultures of human bone-derived cells obtained from surgical bone biopsies, $1,25(OH)_2D_3$ increased insulin-like growth factor 1 levels time-dependently and dose-dependently, and also dose-dependently stimulated osteocalcin secretion and alkaline phosphate activity in bone cell supernatants.[76] $1,25(OH)_2D_3$ promotes osteoblast differentiation by regulating the transcription of several genes associated with the osteoblast phenotype.[77,78] Inducible nitric oxide synthase (iNOS) was shown to be stimulated by $1,25(OH)_2D_3$ in osteoblasts.[79] Nitric oxide (NO) affects bone mass during mechanical loading,[80,81] and $1,25(OH)_2D_3$ stimulates iNOS expression and NO production by osteoblasts in the absence of mechanical stimulation, likely via genomic VDR action.[79] $1,25(OH)_2D_3$ may also affect mechanical loading-induced NO production independent of genomic VDR action, because $1,25(OH)_2D_3$ diminished pulsating fluid flow-induced NO production in VDR-knockout bone cells. In osteo-blastic cells, VDR shows a nuclear punctate signal distribution that is significantly enhanced on ligand stimulation.[82,83] This interaction of VDR with the nuclear matrix occurs rapidly after the treatment of $1,25(OH)_2D_3$ and does not require a functional VDR DNA-binding domain.[84] VDR transcriptional coactivators of DRIP205[84] as well as NcoA62/Ski[85] are bound to the nuclear matrix of osteoblastic cells in the absence of $1,25(OH)_2D_3$, indicating that after ligand stimulation, the VDR rapidly enters the nucleus and associates with the nuclear matrix preceding VDR-dependent transcriptional activation. It has recently been proposed that the tumor suppressor BRCA1 is involved in the VDR accumulation in the nucleus.[86] In osteoblastic cells in which BRCA1 expression is depleted, $1,25(OH)_2D_3$-dependent accumulation of VDR in the nucleus is significantly reduced. Moreover, physiologic concentrations of prolactin block increased osteocalcin and VDR expression in response to $1,25(OH)_2D_3$.

THE ROLE OF OSTEOCYTES IN VITAMIN D ACTIONS IN BONE

Actions of vitamin D have been believed to be mediated mainly through osteoblasts, but osteocytes may also be involved. Ultrastructural immunocytochemical localization of endogenous $1,25(OH)_2D_3$ and its receptors in osteocytes from neonatal mouse and rat calvaria was shown.[87] Nongenomic antiapoptotic effects of $1,25(OH)_2D_3$ were observed in murine osteocytic cells.[88] The antiapoptotic effects of $1,25(OH)_2D_3$ were blocked by cytoplasmic kinase inhibitors of Src, phosphatidylinositol 3 kinase, or JNK. Further, actinomycin D or cycloheximide prevented the antiapoptotic effect of $1,25(OH)_2D_3$, indicating that transcriptional events are also required.

INVOLVEMENT OF VITAMIN D IN COLLAGEN CROSS-LINKING

Collagen cross-linking is considered as one of the determinants of bone quality. Alfa-calcidol, or 1α-hydroxyvitamin D_3, at doses of 0.1 or 0.2 µg/kg increased bone mass and mechanical strength of the lumbar spine as well as the femur in a 3-month treatment period in ovariectomized female Wistar rats. Alfacalcidol treatment increased interconnections and platelike structures, and caused a significant suppression of bone resorption, whereas it maintained formation in the endocortical perimeter, and also stimulated bone formation in the periosteal perimeter.[89] Lysyl hydroxylases (LH1-3) and lysyl oxidases (LOX, LOXL1-4) are collagen cross-linking and related enzymes. Gene expressions of LH1, LH2b, and LOXL2 were significantly increased by $1,25(OH)_2D_3$ up to 72 hours of culture. In addition, hydroxylysine (Hyl), Hyl aldehyde (Hyl^{ald}), Hyl^{ald}-derived cross-links, and a total number of cross-links of collagen were significantly higher and the cross-link maturation was accelerated in the $1,25(OH)_2D_3$-treated group.[90]

RICKETS AND OSTEOMALACIA

Osteomalacia is characterized by decreased longitudinal growth, widening of the epiphyseal zones, and painful swelling in the region caused by defective bone mineralization of the growing skeleton.[91] Rickets differs from osteomalacia in that it occurs before fusion of growth plate, and it often presents with a more severe skeletal phenotype, muscular weakness, and symptoms of low serum calcium levels, such as tetany and convulsions. These features are mainly caused by inadequate amounts of available calcium and phosphorus.

Fibroblast growth factor-23 (FGF-23) reduces the serum concentration of phosphorus and inhibits the activation of vitamin D.[92] Excess FGF-23 is being recognized as having a role in some forms of rickets and osteomalacias.[93] In patients with osteomalacia caused by vitamin D deficiency or by resistance to the action of vitamin D, serum FGF-23 levels are low.

VITAMIN D ANALOGUES

Many vitamin D analogues are available. Several analogues with differential activities have been approved for clinical use, although this varies in different countries. A potent analogue of $1,25(OH)_2D_3$, 2-methylene-19-nor-(20S)-$1,25(OH)_2D_3$ (2MD), selectively induces bone formation. Selectivity for bone was first shown through the observation that 2MD is at least 30-fold more effective than $1,25(OH)_2D_3$ in stimulating osteoblast-mediated bone calcium mobilization and is only slightly more potent in supporting intestinal calcium transport. 2MD is also highly potent in promoting osteoblast-mediated osteoclast formation in vitro. 2MD (7 pmol/d) causes a substantial increase (9%) in total body bone mass in ovariectomized rats over a 23-week period.[94] Eldecalcitol (ED-71), a novel analogue of $1,25(OH)_2D_3$, increases bone mass to a greater extent than alfacalcidol in a murine bone marrow ablation model,[95] and also increases BMD by suppressing RANKL expression in mouse trabecular bone.[96] Eldecalcitol is an orally administered analogue of $1,25(OH)_2D_3$, and is now available in Japan for the treatment of osteoporosis. In a randomized, double-blind, placebo-controlled, dose-ranging trial, eldecalcitol reduced markers of bone turnover more than placebo. Similarly, in a randomized, double-blind comparison with 1.0 μg/d of alfacalcidol, eldecalcitol 0.75 μg/d produced significantly greater reductions in markers of bone turnover. In both trials, eldecalcitol treatment was associated with an increase in BMD, whereas patients who received the comparators generally had a reduction in BMD. Eldecalcitol significantly reduced the 3-year incidence of vertebral fractures, with a relative risk reduction of 26%.[97]

DIFFERENCES IN BIOLOGIC ACTIVITY BETWEEN VITAMIN D_2 AND D_3

Vitamin D_2, or ergocalciferol, is derived from fungus or yeast, and there has been debate as to whether it is equipotent with vitamin D_3 (cholecalciferol). It is well known that serum 25(OH)D levels correlate better with calcium absorption than $1,25(OH)_2D$[98,99] and that 25(OH)D affects calcium metabolism without changes in circulating total $1,25(OH)_2D$.[100] Although a few reports have indicated that ergocalciferol is as effective as cholecalciferol,[101] several reports found that ergocalciferol is less potent in increasing or sustaining serum 25(OH)D than cholecalciferol.[102–106]

EPIDEMIOLOGY

Although it has a smaller effect on the increase in BMD than nitrogen-containing bisphosphonates, vitamin D has been shown to reduce the incidence of vertebral fracture more than would be predicted from the effect on BMD.[107] This beneficial effect of vitamin D might be achieved through the effects on muscle or bone quality. Patients with a mean 25(OH)D 33 ng/mL or greater had a ~4.5-fold greater odds of a favorable bisphosphonate response. The 25(OH)D level was significantly associated with response; a 1 ng/mL decrease in 25(OH)D was associated with a ~5% decrease in odds of responding.[108] Vitamin D deficiency is prevalent in individuals who have increased skin pigmentation or always wear sun protection or spend little time outdoors. Vitamin D deficiency is often treated or prevented by high intermittent doses of vitamin D, but treatment outcomes have been inconsistent, and even a transient increase in fracture and fall risk was reported. Rossini and colleagues[109] have investigated the short-term effects on bone turnover markers of a single bolus vitamin D.

Twelve elderly people were given a single oral bolus of 600,000 IU vitamin D. Serum osteo-calcin, a bone formation marker, increased slightly within the first 3 days and then declined by day 60, possibly explaining the negative clinical results obtained by using intermittent high doses of vitamin D to treat or prevent vitamin D deficiency. The Institute of Medicine published in 2011 new dietary requirements for vitamin D. Based on bone health, recommended dietary allowances (RDAs; covering requirements of $\geq$97.5% of the population) for vitamin D were 600 IU/d for ages 1 to 70 years and 800 IU/d for ages 71 years and older, corresponding to a serum 25-hydroxyvitamin D level of at least 20 ng/mL. RDAs for vitamin D were based on conditions of minimal sun exposure caused by wide variability in vitamin D synthesis from ultraviolet light and the risks of skin cancer. Higher values were not consistently associated with greater benefit, and for some outcomes, U-shaped associations were observed, with risks at both low and high levels.[110]

SUMMARY

Adequate vitamin D levels clearly contribute to maintaining skeletal integrity, as shown by epidemiologic studies. The mechanisms of this process are still unclear, with some inconsistencies between in vitro findings and in vivo results. Although most evidence indicates that the stimulation of intestinal calcium and phosphate absorption is the mechanism by which vitamin D increases bone mineralization, effects on matrix vesicles and other mechanisms could conceivably contribute to the response. Vitamin D metabolites and analogues can stimulate bone resorption in vitro, but decrease bone loss in vivo. The roles of dose, of effects on the parathyroid glands, of other ligands that interact with receptors that heterodimerize or otherwise affect the VDR, and the contribution of effects on inhibitors including OPG still need to be defined. Also, anti-apoptotic effects on osteocytes and stimulatory actions on collagen cross-linking could contribute to the beneficial effects of vitamin D on bone. Although there is much new knowledge, a full understanding of how vitamin D achieves its beneficial effects on bone is still elusive.

REFERENCES

1. Prineas JW, Mason AS, Henson RA. Myopathy in metabolic bone disease. BMJ 1965;1(5441):1034–6.
2. Schott GD, Wills MR. Muscle weakness in osteomalacia. Lancet 1976;1(7960): 626–9.
3. Sorensen OH, Lund B, Saltin B, et al. Myopathy in bone loss of ageing: improvement by treatment with 1 alpha-hydroxycholecalciferol and calcium. Clin Sci (Lond) 1979;56(2):157–61.
4. Visser M, Deeg DJ, Lips P. Low vitamin D and high parathyroid hormone levels as determinants of loss of muscle strength and muscle mass (sarcopenia): the Longitudinal Aging Study Amsterdam. J Clin Endocrinol Metab 2003;88(12): 5766–72.
5. Garland CF, Garland FC. Do sunlight and vitamin D reduce the likelihood of colon cancer? Int J Epidemiol 1980;9(3):227–31.
6. Krishnan AV, Peehl DM, Feldman D. Inhibition of prostate cancer growth by vitamin D: regulation of target gene expression. J Cell Biochem 2003;88(2): 363–71.
7. Welsh J. Vitamin D and breast cancer: insights from animal models. Am J Clin Nutr 2004;80(Suppl 6):1721S–4S.
8. Harris DM, Go VL. Vitamin D and colon carcinogenesis. J Nutr 2004;134(Suppl 12):3463S–71S.

9. Liu PT, Stenger S, Li H, et al. Toll-like receptor triggering of a vitamin D-mediated human antimicrobial response. Science 2006;311(5768):1770–3.

10. Lalor MK, Floyd S, Gorak-Stolinska P, et al. BCG vaccination: a role for vitamin D? PLoS One 2011;6(1):e16709.

11. Dobnig H, Pilz S, Scharnagl H, et al. Independent association of low serum 25-hydroxyvitamin d and 1,25-dihydroxyvitamin d levels with all-cause and cardiovascular mortality. Arch Intern Med 2008;168(12):1340–9.

12. Giovannucci E, Liu Y, Hollis BW, et al. 25-hydroxyvitamin D and risk of myocardial infarction in men: a prospective study. Arch Intern Med 2008;168(11):1174–80.

13. Wang TJ, Pencina MJ, Booth SL, et al. Vitamin D deficiency and risk of cardiovascular disease. Circulation 2008;117(4):503–11.

14. Ginde AA, Scragg R, Schwartz RS, et al. Prospective study of serum 25-hydroxyvitamin D level, cardiovascular disease mortality, and all-cause mortality in older U.S. adults. J Am Geriatr Soc 2009;57(9):1595–603.

15. Rajakumar K, Greenspan SL, Thomas SB, et al. SOLAR ultraviolet radiation and vitamin D: a historical perspective. Am J Public Health 2007;97(10):1746–54.

16. Holick MF. Resurrection of vitamin D deficiency and rickets. J Clin Invest 2006; 116(8):2062–72.

17. Holick MF. McCollum Award Lecture, 1994: vitamin D–new horizons for the 21st century. Am J Clin Nutr 1994;60(4):619–30.

18. Stern PH, Phillips TE, Mavreas T. Bioassay of 1,25-dihydroxyvitamin D in human plasma purified by partition, alkaline extraction, and high-pressure chromatography. Anal Biochem 1980;102(1):22–30.

19. Herodotus. The Persian Wars, Book III. New York: Random House; 1942.

20. Huldschinsky K. Heilung von Rachitis durch kunstliche Hohensonne. Deutsche Med Wochenschr 1919;45:712–3.

21. Mellanby E. The part played by an "accessory factor" in the production of experimental rickets. J Physiol 1918;52:liii–lvi.

22. McCollum EV, Simmonds N, Shipley PG, et al. The production of rachitis and similar diseases in the rat by deficient diets. J Biol Chem 1921;45:333–41.

23. Sherman HC, Pappenheimer AM. A dietetic production of rickets in rats and its prevention by an inorganic salt. Proc Soc Exp Biol Med 1921;18:193–7.

24. Shipley PG, Park EA, McCollum EV, et al. Studies on experimental rickets III. A pathological condition bearing fundamental resemblances to rickets of the human being resulting from diets low in phosphorus and fat soluble A: the phosphate ion in its prevention. Bull Johns Hopkins Hosp 1921;32:160–6.

25. Shipley PG, Park EA, McCollum EV, et al. Studies on experimental rickets II. The effect of cod liver oil administered to rats with experimental rickets. J Biol Chem 1921;45:343–8.

26. Steenbock H, Black A. Fat-soluble vitamins. XVII. The induction of growth-promoting and calcifying properties in a ration by exposure to ultra-violet light. J Biol Chem 1924;61:405–22.

27. Hess AF, Weinstock M. Antirachitic properties imparted to inert fluids and to green vegetables by ultraviolet irradiation. J Biol Chem 1924;62:301–13.

28. Holick MF, DeLuca HF. Vitamin D metabolism. Annu Rev Med 1974;25:349–67.

29. DeLuca HF, Zierold C. Mechanisms and functions of vitamin D. Nutr Rev 1998; 56(2 Pt 2):S4–10 [discussion: S 54–75].

30. Marx SJ, Spiegel AM, Brown EM, et al. A familial syndrome of decrease in sensitivity to 1,25-dihydroxyvitamin D. J Clin Endocrinol Metab 1978;47(6):1303–10.

31. Marx SJ, Liberman UA, Eil C, et al. Hereditary resistance to 1,25-dihydroxyvitamin D. Recent Prog Horm Res 1984;40:589–620.

32. Haussler MR, Norman AW. Chromosomal receptor for a vitamin D metabolite. Proc Natl Acad Sci U S A 1969;62(1):155–62.

33. Tsai HC, Wong RG, Norman AW. Studies on calciferol metabolism. IV. Subcellular localization of 1,25-dihydroxy-vitamin D 3 in intestinal mucosa and correlation with increased calcium transport. J Biol Chem 1972;247(17):5511–9.

34. McDonnell DP, Mangelsdorf DJ, Pike JW, et al. Molecular cloning of complementary DNA encoding the avian receptor for vitamin D. Science 1987;235(4793): 1214–7.

35. Baker AR, McDonnell DP, Hughes M, et al. Cloning and expression of full-length cDNA encoding human vitamin D receptor. Proc Natl Acad Sci U S A 1988; 85(10):3294–8.

36. Okamura WH, Palenzuela JA, Plumet J, et al. Vitamin D: structure-function analyses and the design of analogs. J Cell Biochem 1992;49(1):10–8.

37. Wing RM, Okamura WH, Pirio MR, et al. Vitamin D in solution: conformations of vitamin D3, 1alpha,25-dihydroxyvitamin D3, and dihydrotachysterol3. Science 1974;186(4167):939–41.

38. Norman AW, Okamura WH, Farach-Carson MC, et al. Structure-function studies of 1,25-dihydroxyvitamin D3 and the vitamin D endocrine system. 1,25-dihydroxy-pentadeuterio-previtamin D3 (as a 6-s-cis analog) stimulates nongenomic but not genomic biological responses. J Biol Chem 1993;268(19):13811–9.

39. Caffrey JM, Farach-Carson MC. Vitamin D3 metabolites modulate dihydropyridine-sensitive calcium currents in clonal rat osteosarcoma cells. J Biol Chem 1989;264(34):20265–74.

40. Nemere I, Yoshimoto Y, Norman AW. Calcium transport in perfused duodena from normal chicks: enhancement within fourteen minutes of exposure to 1,25-dihydroxyvitamin D3. Endocrinology 1984;115(4):1476–83.

41. Norman AW, Olivera CJ, Barreto Silva FR, et al. A specific binding protein/receptor for 1alpha,25-dihydroxyvitamin D(3) is present in an intestinal caveolae membrane fraction. Biochem Biophys Res Commun 2002;298(3):414–9.

42. Huhtakangas JA, Olivera CJ, Bishop JE, et al. The vitamin D receptor is present in caveolae-enriched plasma membranes and binds 1 alpha,25(OH)2-vitamin D3 in vivo and in vitro. Mol Endocrinol 2004;18(11):2660–71.

43. Norman AW, Mizwicki MT, Norman DP. Steroid-hormone rapid actions, membrane receptors and a conformational ensemble model. Nat Rev Drug Discov 2004;3(1):27–41.

44. Chen J, Olivares-Navarrete R, Wang Y, et al. Protein-disulfide isomerase-associated 3 (Pdia3) mediates the membrane response to 1,25-dihydroxyvitamin D3 in osteoblasts. J Biol Chem 2010;285(47):37041–50.

45. Li YC, Pirro AE, Amling M, et al. Targeted ablation of the vitamin D receptor: an animal model of vitamin D-dependent rickets type II with alopecia. Proc Natl Acad Sci U S A 1997;94(18):9831–5.

46. Yoshizawa T, Handa Y, Uematsu Y, et al. Mice lacking the vitamin D receptor exhibit impaired bone formation, uterine hypoplasia and growth retardation after weaning. Nat Genet 1997;16(4):391–6.

47. Balsan S, Garabedian M, Larchet M, et al. Long-term nocturnal calcium infusions can cure rickets and promote normal mineralization in hereditary resistance to 1,25-dihydroxyvitamin D. J Clin Invest 1986;77(5):1661–7.

48. Amling M, Priemel M, Holzmann T, et al. Rescue of the skeletal phenotype of vitamin D receptor-ablated mice in the setting of normal mineral ion homeostasis: formal histomorphometric and biomechanical analyses. Endocrinology 1999;140(11):4982–7.

49. Masuyama R, Nakaya Y, Tanaka S, et al. Dietary phosphorus restriction reverses the impaired bone mineralization in vitamin D receptor knockout mice. Endocrinology 2001;142(1):494–7.

50. Underwood JL, DeLuca HF. Vitamin D is not directly necessary for bone growth and mineralization. Am J Physiol 1984;246(6 Pt 1):E493–8.

51. Tanaka H, Seino Y. Direct action of 1,25-dihydroxyvitamin D on bone: VDRKO bone shows excessive bone formation in normal mineral condition. J Steroid Biochem Mol Biol 2004;89–90(1–5):343–5.

52. Woeckel VJ, Alves RD, Swagemakers SM, et al. 1Alpha,25-(OH)2D3 acts in the early phase of osteoblast differentiation to enhance mineralization via accelerated production of mature matrix vesicles. J Cell Physiol 2010;225(2):593–600.

53. Takahashi N, Akatsu T, Sasaki T, et al. Induction of calcitonin receptors by 1 alpha, 25-dihydroxyvitamin D3 in osteoclast-like multinucleated cells formed from mouse bone marrow cells. Endocrinology 1988;123(3):1504–10.

54. Suda T, Takahashi N, Udagawa N, et al. Modulation of osteoclast differentiation and function by the new members of the tumor necrosis factor receptor and ligand families. Endocr Rev 1999;20(3):345–57.

55. Takahashi N, Udagawa N, Takami M, et al. Cells of bone: osteoclast generation. In: Bilezikian JP, Raisz LG, Rodan GA, editors. Principles of bone biology. San Diego (CA): Academic Press; 2002. p. 109–26, 1.

56. Takeda S, Yoshizawa T, Nagai Y, et al. Stimulation of osteoclast formation by 1,25-dihydroxyvitamin D requires its binding to vitamin D receptor (VDR) in osteoblastic cells: studies using VDR knockout mice. Endocrinology 1999;140(2):1005–8.

57. Tsukii K, Shima N, Mochizuki S, et al. Osteoclast differentiation factor mediates an essential signal for bone resorption induced by 1 alpha,25-dihydroxyvitamin D3, prostaglandin E2, or parathyroid hormone in the microenvironment of bone. Biochem Biophys Res Commun 1998;246(2):337–41.

58. Lee SK, Kalinowski J, Jastrzebski S, et al. 1,25(OH)2 vitamin D3-stimulated osteoclast formation in spleen-osteoblast cocultures is mediated in part by enhanced IL-1 alpha and receptor activator of NF-kappa B ligand production in osteoblasts. J Immunol 2002;169(5):2374–80.

59. Collins DA, Chambers TJ. Prostaglandin E2 promotes osteoclast formation in murine hematopoietic cultures through an action on hematopoietic cells. J Bone Miner Res 1992;7(5):555–61.

60. Inoue H, Tsujisawa T, Fukuizumi T, et al. SC-19220, a prostaglandin E2 antagonist, inhibits osteoclast formation by 1,25-dihydroxyvitamin D3 in cell cultures. J Endocrinol 1999;161(2):231–6.

61. Schrader M, Bendik I, Becker-Andre M, et al. Interaction between retinoic acid and vitamin D signaling pathways. J Biol Chem 1993;268(24):17830–6.

62. Carlberg C. RXR-independent action of the receptors for thyroid hormone, retinoid acid and vitamin D on inverted palindromes. Biochem Biophys Res Commun 1993;195(3):1345–53.

63. Norman AW. 1α,25(OH)2 vitamin D3: vitamin D nuclear receptor (VDR) and plasma vitamin D-binding protein (DBP) structures and ligand shape preferences for genomic and rapid biological responses. In: Bilezikian JP, Raisz LG, Martin TJ, editors. Principles of bone biology. 3rd edition. San Diego: Academic Press; 2008. p. 749–78.

64. Itonaga I, Sabokbar A, Neale SD, et al. 1,25-Dihydroxyvitamin D(3) and prostaglandin E(2) act directly on circulating human osteoclast precursors. Biochem Biophys Res Commun 1999;264(2):590–5.

65. Miura M, Tanaka K, Komatsu Y, et al. A novel interaction between thyroid hormones and 1,25(OH)(2)D(3) in osteoclast formation. Biochem Biophys Res Commun 2002;291(4):987–94.
66. Yamamoto M, Murakami T, Nishikawa M, et al. Hypocalcemic effect of osteoclastogenesis inhibitory factor/osteoprotegerin in the thyroparathyroidectomized rat. Endocrinology 1998;139(9):4012–5.
67. Morony S, Capparelli C, Lee R, et al. A chimeric form of osteoprotegerin inhibits hypercalcemia and bone resorption induced by IL-1beta, TNF-alpha, PTH, PTHrP, and 1, 25(OH)2D3. J Bone Miner Res 1999;14(9):1478–85.
68. Price PA, June HH, Buckley JR, et al. Osteoprotegerin inhibits artery calcification induced by warfarin and by vitamin D. Arterioscler Thromb Vasc Biol 2001;21(10):1610–6.
69. Hofbauer LC, Dunstan CR, Spelsberg TC, et al. Osteoprotegerin production by human osteoblast lineage cells is stimulated by vitamin D, bone morphogenetic protein-2, and cytokines. Biochem Biophys Res Commun 1998;250(3):776–81.
70. Yamamoto H, Shevde NK, Warrier A, et al. 2-Methylene-19-nor-(20S)-1,25-dihydroxyvitamin D3 potently stimulates gene-specific DNA binding of the vitamin D receptor in osteoblasts. J Biol Chem 2003;278(34):31756–65.
71. Carlsson A. Tracer experiments on the effect of vitamin D on the skeletal metabolism of calcium and phosphorus. Acta Physiol Scand 1952;26(2–3):212–20.
72. Stern PH, Hamstra AJ, DeLuca HF, et al. A bioassay capable of measuring 1 picogram of 1,25-dihydroxyvitamin D3. J Clin Endocrinol Metab 1978;46(6):891–6.
73. Suda T, Ueno Y, Fujii K, et al. Vitamin D and bone. J Cell Biochem 2003;88(2): 259–66.
74. Shiraki M, Fukuchi M, Kiriyama T, et al. Alfacalcidol reduces accelerated bone turnover in elderly women with osteoporosis. J Bone Miner Metab 2004;22(4): 352–9.
75. Marcus R. Agents affecting calcification and bone turnover. In: Hardman JG, Limbird LE, editors. Goodman & Gilman's the pharmacological basis of therapeutics. 10th edition. New York: McGraw-Hill; 2001. p. 1715–43.
76. Chenu C, Valentin-Opran A, Chavassieux P, et al. Insulin like growth factor I hormonal regulation by growth hormone and by 1,25(OH)2D3 and activity on human osteoblast-like cells in short-term cultures. Bone 1990;11(2):81–6.
77. van Driel M, Pols HA, van Leeuwen JP. Osteoblast differentiation and control by vitamin D and vitamin D metabolites. Curr Pharm Des 2004;10(21):2535–55.
78. Montecino M, Stein GS, Cruzat F, et al. An architectural perspective of vitamin D responsiveness. Arch Biochem Biophys 2007;460(2):293–9.
79. Willems HM, van den Heuvel EG, Carmeliet G, et al. VDR dependent and independent effects of 1,25-dihydroxyvitamin D3 on nitric oxide production by osteoblasts. Steroids 2012;77(1–2):126–31.
80. Vatsa A, Mizuno D, Smit TH, et al. Bio imaging of intracellular NO production in single bone cells after mechanical stimulation. J Bone Miner Res 2006;21(11): 1722–8.
81. Kunnel JG, Igarashi K, Gilbert JL, et al. Bone anabolic responses to mechanical load in vitro involve COX-2 and constitutive NOS. Connect Tissue Res 2004; 45(1):40–9.
82. Barsony J, Renyi I, McKoy W. Subcellular distribution of normal and mutant vitamin D receptors in living cells. Studies with a novel fluorescent ligand. J Biol Chem 1997;272(9):5774–82.
83. Paredes R, Arriagada G, Cruzat F, et al. Bone-specific transcription factor Runx2 interacts with the 1alpha,25-dihydroxyvitamin D3 receptor to up-regulate rat

osteocalcin gene expression in osteoblastic cells. Mol Cell Biol 2004;24(20): 8847–61.

84. Arriagada G, Paredes R, van Wijnen AJ, et al. 1alpha,25-dihydroxy vitamin D(3) induces nuclear matrix association of the 1alpha,25-dihydroxy vitamin D(3) receptor in osteoblasts independently of its ability to bind DNA. J Cell Physiol 2010;222(2):336–46.

85. Zhang C, Dowd DR, Staal A, et al. Nuclear coactivator-62 kDa/Ski-interacting protein is a nuclear matrix-associated coactivator that may couple vitamin D receptor-mediated transcription and RNA splicing. J Biol Chem 2003;278(37):35325–36.

86. Deng C, Ueda E, Chen KE, et al. Prolactin blocks nuclear translocation of VDR by regulating its interaction with BRCA1 in osteosarcoma cells. Mol Endocrinol 2009;23(2):226–36.

87. Boivin G, Mesguich P, Pike JW, et al. Ultrastructural immunocytochemical localization of endogenous 1,25-dihydroxyvitamin D3 and its receptors in osteoblasts and osteocytes from neonatal mouse and rat calvaria. Bone Miner 1987;3(2):125–36.

88. Vertino AM, Bula CM, Chen JR, et al. Nongenotropic, anti-apoptotic signaling of 1alpha,25(OH)2-vitamin D3 and analogs through the ligand binding domain of the vitamin D receptor in osteoblasts and osteocytes. Mediation by Src, phosphatidylinositol 3-, and JNK kinases. J Biol Chem 2005;280(14):14130–7.

89. Shiraishi A, Higashi S, Masaki T, et al. A comparison of alfacalcidol and menatetrenone for the treatment of bone loss in an ovariectomized rat model of osteoporosis. Calcif Tissue Int 2002;71(1):69–79.

90. Nagaoka H, Mochida Y, Atsawasuwan P, et al. 1,25(OH)2D3 regulates collagen quality in an osteoblastic cell culture system. Biochem Biophys Res Commun 2008;377(2):674–8.

91. Lips P, VanSchoor NM, Bravenboer N. Vitamin D-related disorders. In: Rosen CJ, editor. Primer on the metabolic bone diseases and disorders of mineral metabolism. 7th edition. Washington DC: American Society for Bone and Mineral Research; 2008. p. 329–35.

92. Hasegawa H, Nagano N, Urakawa I, et al. Direct evidence for a causative role of FGF23 in the abnormal renal phosphate handling and vitamin D metabolism in rats with early-stage chronic kidney disease. Kidney Int 2010;78(10):975–80.

93. Fukumoto S. Actions and mode of actions of FGF19 subfamily members. Endocr J 2008;55(1):23–31.

94. Shevde NK, Plum LA, Clagett-Dame M, et al. A potent analog of 1alpha,25-dihydroxyvitamin D3 selectively induces bone formation. Proc Natl Acad Sci U S A 2002;99(21):13487–91.

95. Okuda N, Takeda S, Shinomiya K, et al. ED-71, a novel vitamin D analog, promotes bone formation and angiogenesis and inhibits bone resorption after bone marrow ablation. Bone 2007;40(2):281–92.

96. Harada S, Mizoguchi T, Kobayashi Y, et al. Daily administration of eldecalcitol (ED-71), an active vitamin D analog, increases bone mineral density by suppressing RANKL expression in mouse trabecular bone. J Bone Miner Res 2012;27(2):461–73.

97. Sanford M, McCormack PL. Spotlight on eldecalcitol in osteoporosis. Drugs Aging 2012;29(1):69–71.

98. Bell NH, Epstein S, Shary J, et al. Evidence of a probable role for 25-hydroxyvitamin D in the regulation of human calcium metabolism. J Bone Miner Res 1988; 3(5):489–95.

99. Barger-Lux MJ, Heaney RP, Lanspa SJ, et al. An investigation of sources of variation in calcium absorption efficiency. J Clin Endocrinol Metab 1995;80(2):406–11.

100. Heaney RP, Barger-Lux MJ, Dowell MS, et al. Calcium absorptive effects of vitamin D and its major metabolites. J Clin Endocrinol Metab 1997;82(12):4111–6.
101. Holick MF, Biancuzzo RM, Chen TC, et al. Vitamin D2 is as effective as vitamin D3 in maintaining circulating concentrations of 25-hydroxyvitamin D. J Clin Endocrinol Metab 2008;93(3):677–81.
102. Trang HM, Cole DE, Rubin LA, et al. Evidence that vitamin D3 increases serum 25-hydroxyvitamin D more efficiently than does vitamin D2. Am J Clin Nutr 1998; 68(4):854–8.
103. Armas LA, Hollis BW, Heaney RP. Vitamin D2 is much less effective than vitamin D3 in humans. J Clin Endocrinol Metab 2004;89(11):5387–91.
104. Romagnoli E, Mascia ML, Cipriani C, et al. Short and long-term variations in serum calciotropic hormones after a single very large dose of ergocalciferol (vitamin D2) or cholecalciferol (vitamin D3) in the elderly. J Clin Endocrinol Metab 2008;93(8):3015–20.
105. Glendenning P, Chew GT, Seymour HM, et al. Serum 25-hydroxyvitamin D levels in vitamin D-insufficient hip fracture patients after supplementation with ergocalciferol and cholecalciferol. Bone 2009;45(5):870–5.
106. Heaney RP, Recker RR, Grote J, et al. Vitamin D(3) is more potent than vitamin D(2) in humans. J Clin Endocrinol Metab 2011;96(3):E447–52.
107. Papadimitropoulos E, Wells G, Shea B, et al. Meta-analyses of therapies for postmenopausal osteoporosis. VIII: Meta-analysis of the efficacy of vitamin D treatment in preventing osteoporosis in postmenopausal women. Endocr Rev 2002;23(4):560–9.
108. Carmel AS, Shieh A, Bang H, et al. The 25(OH)D level needed to maintain a favorable bisphosphonate response is >/=33 ng/ml. Osteoporos Int 2012. [Epub ahead of print].
109. Rossini M, Gatti D, Viapiana O, et al. Short-term effects on bone turnover markers of a single high dose of oral vitamin D3. J Clin Endocrinol Metab 2012;97(4):E622–6.
110. Ross AC, Manson JE, Abrams SA, et al. The 2011 report on dietary reference intakes for calcium and vitamin D from the Institute of Medicine: what clinicians need to know. J Clin Endocrinol Metab 2011;96(1):53–8.

Extraskeletal Effects of Vitamin D

Heidi Wolden-Kirk, MSc, Conny Gysemans, PhD,
Annemieke Verstuyf, PhD, Chantal Mathieu, MD, PhD*

KEYWORDS

- Vitamin D • Diabetes • Immune system • Cancer • Cardiovascular disease

KEY POINTS

- The active metabolite of vitamin D, 1,25-dihydroxyvitamin D_3, exerts its biological actions by binding to a nuclear receptor, the vitamin D receptor.
- A possible role for vitamin D in immune or infectious diseases was known for many years, in fact dating from the nineteenth century.
- In recent years, the study of vitamin D has extended beyond the possible beneficial effects in infectious defenses and has moved toward a possible role of vitamin D in protecting against noncommunicable diseases.

INTRODUCTION

The active metabolite of vitamin D, 1,25-dihydroxyvitamin D_3 ($1,25(OH)_2D_3$), exerts its biological actions by binding to a nuclear receptor, the vitamin D receptor (VDR). Since the discovery of VDRs in organs outside the calcium and bone system, including immune system, muscle, and myocardium, extraskeletal effects of $1,25(OH)_2D_3$ have been suggested (**Fig. 1**). The discovery of the machinery for local production and inactivation of $1,25(OH)_2D_3$ in many tissues, including hair follicles, lymph nodes, tonsils, colon, adrenal gland, insulin-secreting pancreatic β cells, the brain, and the vasculature, have even generated the hypothesis of a physiologic role for vitamin D and its metabolites in general health.[1]

A possible role for vitamin D in immune or infectious diseases was known for many years. As early as the nineteenth century, the detrimental effects of vitamin D deficiency (or lack of sunlight exposure) on the clearing of infectious agents was well recognized, culminating in the construction of sanatoria in sun-rich areas or the administration of cod-liver oil to children not only to avoid the skeletal consequences of rickets but also to enhance resistance against infections such as tuberculosis.

In recent years, the study of vitamin D has extended beyond the possible beneficial effects in infectious defenses and has moved toward a possible role for vitamin D in protecting against noncommunicable diseases. This article focuses on the possible

Laboratory for Clinical and Experimental Endocrinology, Catholic University Leuven (KUL), O&N I Herestraat 49 - bus 902, Leuven 3000, Belgium
* Corresponding author.
E-mail address: chantal.mathieu@med.kuleuven.be

Endocrinol Metab Clin N Am 41 (2012) 571–594
http://dx.doi.org/10.1016/j.ecl.2012.05.004
0889-8529/12/$ – see front matter © 2012 Elsevier Inc. All rights reserved.

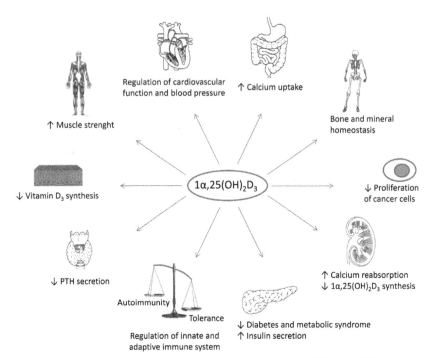

Fig. 1. Major targets and actions of active vitamin D₃ on peripheral tissues. PTH, parathyroid hormone.

role of vitamin D in the immune system, focusing on infectious defenses and autoimmune diseases, diabetes, cardiovascular disease (CVD), and cancer.

VITAMIN D AND THE IMMUNE SYSTEM: INFECTIONS AND AUTOIMMUNE DISEASES

The awareness of a role for vitamin D in the regulation of immune responses was triggered by the discovery of VDRs in almost all immune cells of the innate and adaptive immune compartment, including activated CD4⁺ and CD8⁺ T cells, B cells, neutrophils, and antigen-presenting cells, such as macrophages and dendritic cells (DCs).[2] Moreover, immune signals can regulate expression levels of the VDR and the enzymes involved in vitamin D metabolism.[3] In vitro, 1,25(OH)₂D₃ influences innate immune responses by enhancing chemotaxis and phagocytosis by macrophages isolated from vitamin D–deficient mice. An important observation is the induction of secretion of antimicrobial proteins such as cathelicidin LL-37[4] or β-defensin by 1,25(OH)₂D₃.

In the adaptive immune system, the DC is the most important target of 1,25(OH)₂D₃, with the induction of tolerogenic DCs, as 1,25(OH)₂D₃ inhibits the surface expression of major histocompatibility complex (MHC)-II–complexed antigen, costimulatory molecules, and the production of the cytokines interleukin (IL)-12 and IL-23.[5,6] Thus, DCs are created with less antigen-presenting capacity but, more importantly, this gives rise to a DC that induces a shift in T-cell polarization from a T-helper (Th)1 and Th17 phenotype toward a Th2 and a T-regulatory (Treg) phenotype.[6,7] These dramatic effects in DCs are observed in human as well as murine DCs and are accompanied by important alterations in the proteomic and metabolic profile of these cells.[8,9]

T lymphocytes are also direct target cells for 1,25(OH)₂D₃, but start to express VDR only after immune activation, in contrast to DCs or macrophages, which have measurable VDR expression also in resting conditions.[10] Direct effects of $1,25(OH)_2D_3$ on T lymphocytes include a modest inhibition in T-cell proliferation, but more importantly an alteration in the expression of chemokine receptors, thus determining the direction in which these cells will move in the body. The chemokine receptor profile induced by $1,25(OH)_2D_3$ or some of its structural analogues promotes the migration of T cells to sites of inflammation.[11] In addition, $1,25(OH)_2D_3$ directly affects T-cell responses, by inhibiting the production of Th1 cytokines (IL-2 and interferon [IFN]-γ), Th9 cytokines (IL-9), and Th17 cytokines (IL-17 and IL-21),[12] and by stimulating Th2 cytokine production (IL-4).[13] Finally, $1,25(OH)_2D_3$ favors Treg cell development via modulation of DCs but also by directly targeting T cells.[11,14] The effect of $1,25(OH)_2D_3$ on B lymphocytes is less clear cut, but inhibition of plasma-cell differentiation, immunoglobulin (Ig)G and IgM production, and B-cell proliferation have been described.[15]

In vivo, 3 levels of evidence exist in the relationship between vitamin D and the immune system: animal models of infectious diseases and autoimmunity, association studies and, most importantly, intervention studies in humans.

Defenses Against Infections

Data correlating vitamin D deficiency and susceptibility to respiratory infections are most solid in the context of tuberculosis (TB). Data on known VDR gene polymorphisms as a host genetic susceptibility factor for TB are conflicting.[16] A recent study showed complex associations of methylation status with *Taq I* genotype, highlighting the need to consider both genetic and epigenetic variants in genetic studies.[17] In addition, analysis of a large cohort of white individuals identified an association between single-nucleotide polymorphisms (SNPs) in the vitamin D–binding protein gene and the risk of serum vitamin D insufficiency.[18,19] In the context of TB, therefore, genetic variations in the vitamin D–binding protein gene and epigenetic rather than genetic variations in the VDR gene seem to associate with disease susceptibility.

In vitamin D–deficient mice, disease progression following infection with *Mycobacterium tuberculosis* was severely aggravated,[20] and in humans a higher susceptibility to TB was seen in subjects with vitamin D deficiency or lower vitamin D levels, including the elderly, uremic patients, and dark-skinned persons.[21] Although TB has become the most studied aspect of vitamin D and antibacterial activity, only a limited number of clinical trials of vitamin D supplementation have been reported in patients with this disease. Promising is the increased frequency sputum conversion and radiologic improvements in patients with moderate TB treated with a combination of vitamin D supplementation and conventional antituberculosis drugs.[22] However, robust intervention trials to date have failed to demonstrate any beneficial effect on intervention with large doses of vitamin D in TB-infected patients on top of standard TB therapy. Of particular interest was the trial in which 3 high doses of vitamin D_3 (100,000 IU at inclusion, months 5 and 8) could not alter the clinical outcome in TB patients treated with regular standard of care in anti-TB medications.[23] These findings were confirmed in a randomized, placebo-controlled study in which 4 high doses of vitamin D_3 (100,000 IU at 0, 14, 28, and 42 days) were administered in a severely vitamin D–deficient TB-infected population, and again, no difference in sputum culture conversion or clinical outcome was observed. Of note, in participants with the tt genotype of the *Taq I* VDR polymorphism, a positive effect of the vitamin D supplements was observed.[24]

Data on viral or fungal infections are scarce. Seasonal changes in serum $25(OH)D_3$ levels have been associated with seasonal variations in the incidence of influenza, suggesting a potential role for vitamin D. However, there was no benefit of vitamin D_3 supplementation (2000 IU daily for 12 weeks) in decreasing the incidence or severity of symptomatic upper respiratory tract infection (URI) during winter.[25] Low vitamin D levels have also been reported in patients infected with human immunodeficiency virus (HIV)-1,[26] and vitamin D levels are positively associated with CD4$^+$ T-cell numbers.[26] In vitro, the antimicrobial peptide LL-37 inhibits HIV-1 replication.[27] Nevertheless, because antiviral treatment itself can affect vitamin D metabolism, the clinical implication of low vitamin D levels in HIV patients is not clear. Data on fungal infections are even less clear, with some reports suggesting a link between hypocalcaemia and fungal infections, but only a fraction of these patients show elevated levels of vitamin D$_3$ metabolites,[28,29] so the relation between vitamin D levels and fungal infections remains unclear.

Genetic Variants in Vitamin D Pathway Genes, Vitamin D Deficiency, and Autoimmune Diseases

In many studies, correlations between polymorphisms in genes involved in vitamin D signaling or metabolism and autoimmune disease prevalence have been looked for. In type 1 diabetes (T1D) the search for genetic polymorphisms in the VDR has yielded conflicting results, with positive correlations in most published studies,[30] with a recent meta-analysis concluding there was no such evidence.[31] Recent studies have confirmed the absence of a relationship between VDR polymorphisms and β-cell autoimmunity, but did identify T1D-associated polymorphisms in 3 key enzymes involved in vitamin D metabolism, namely CYP27B1, 7-dehydrocholesterol reductase (DHCR7), and CYP2R1.[32,33] In multiple sclerosis (MS), a study in Swedish patients confirmed the association that was previously identified in an Australian and New Zealand population[34] for SNPs on chromosomes 12q13-14, the region containing the CYP27B1 (1α-hydroxylase). Moreover, the strongest known MS susceptibility gene, HLA-DRB1*15, includes a putative VDR responsive element in its promoter.[35] Associations of polymorphisms in the VDR gene with inflammatory bowel disease (IBD) susceptibility have been found, but show ethnic differences. The VDR gene polymorphisms *Taq I* and *Fok I* are associated with Crohn disease susceptibility in European Caucasian[36] and in Iranian patients, respectively. In Han Chinese, the *Bsm I* polymorphism of the VDR gene is associated with ulcerative colitis susceptibility.

Epidemiology and association studies are very suggestive for a promoting role of vitamin D deficiency in autoimmune diseases.[37] In particular, T1D, MS, and IBD have been studied extensively. Most autoimmune diseases have a striking geographic variance in prevalence, with prevalences rising with increasing latitude in both hemispheres. For MS, for instance, this changes from a low of 1 to 2 cases per 10^5 people near the equator to a high of more than 200 cases per 10^5 people at latitudes higher than 50°.[38] However, a recent study suggested that ultraviolet (UV) light may have an ameliorating effect on this disorder, independent of vitamin D levels. Nevertheless, in white American adolescents, a low 25(OH)D$_3$ level has been found to be associated with a higher MS incidence in comparison with high 25(OH)D$_3$ levels.[39] A correlation between increased outdoor activities in childhood and adolescence, which might also increase 25(OH)D$_3$ levels, and a decreased risk of developing MS has been found in Norwegian, Tasmanian, and North American populations.[40–42] Indeed, many MS patients also have low serum levels of 25(OH)D$_3$ (<50 nmol/L in 77% of patients),[43] and some correlations between 25(OH)D$_3$ serum levels and disease activity parameters have been found.[44]

In T1D, the incidence follows a seasonal pattern[45,46] and a clear North-South gradient exists in the northern hemisphere (and vice versa in the Southern hemisphere), suggesting an influence of the amount of UV exposure (and thus vitamin D production) on T1D presentation.[47] Furthermore, several observational studies have revealed a worldwide association between vitamin D deficiency and the prevalence of T1D. In 4 studies North Indian,[48] Italian,[49] Swedish,[50] and British[33] children or young adults with newly diagnosed T1D, in comparison with healthy controls, displayed lower levels of serum 25(OH)D$_3$. Of interest are the studies whereby correlations between vitamin D deficiency or supplements in early life and later T1D were described, with rickets in the first year of life leading to a 3-fold increase in the risk for later T1D.[51,52]

A higher prevalence of IBD is found in areas with decreased sunlight exposure, such as North America and northern Europe,[53,54] whereas patients with IBD have low serum levels of 25(OH)D$_3$.[55] Vitamin D deficiency might occur more frequently in IBD because of the combined effects of, for example, low vitamin D intake, malabsorption of many nutrients including vitamin D, and decreased outdoor activities with decreased exposure to sunlight. Nevertheless, newly diagnosed patients already have lower 25(OH)D$_3$ levels than controls.

Animal models of autoimmune diseases confirm the negative relationship between vitamin D and autoimmunity, with vitamin D–deficient genetically at-risk mice having a higher risk of T1D (NOD mice) and a greater susceptibility to induction of experimental autoimmune encephalomyelitis (EAE; the model for MS) or IBD.[56]

The greatest disappointment of the potential of vitamin D as an immune modulator lies in the absence of positive intervention trials that are large, blinded, placebo-controlled, and randomized, in which the beneficial effect of avoiding vitamin D deficiency on the occurrence of autoimmune diseases has been evaluated.

Vitamin D Metabolites as Immune Modulators in Autoimmune Diseases

Considering the presence of VDR in all cells of the immune system, the possibility of applying vitamin D or, even better, its active form 1,25(OH)$_2$D$_3$, as a pharmacologic immune modulator has been tested and confirmed in animal models of autoimmune disease over many years.[2] As such, administering 1,25(OH)$_2$D$_3$ as high doses (5 μg/kg/2 d intraperitoneally) was able to prevent both EAE[57] and T1D in mouse models of the disease.[58] The price to pay, however, was hypercalcemia and hypercalciuria. These predictable side effects could be avoided by applying a diet low in calcium that, however, in turn induced severe bone decalcification. A suggested solution was the synthesis of analogues of 1,25(OH)$_2$D$_3$ that share (or exceed) the immunomodulatory properties of 1,25(OH)$_2$D$_3$, but have a dissociation in their calcemic and osseous effects, allowing administration in mice in doses that are immunomodulatory but do not affect calcium levels or bone calcification.[59] The effects of several of these analogues have been studied in mouse models of MS, rheumatoid arthritis, T1D, IBD, and asthma.[60] Several of these analogues can prevent the autoimmune disease studied, but to achieve a cure in already diseased mice, combination with other immune modulators is often necessary.[61] Despite the great promise of these products, to date none has been marketed for application in patients with autoimmune diseases.

VITAMIN D AND DIABETES
Type 1 Diabetes and the Influence of Vitamin D Deficiency and Supplementation

As previously mentioned, observational studies suggest a worldwide association between vitamin D deficiency and the prevalence of T1D.[48,50] Moreover, polymorphisms in key vitamin D–related genes may be linked to T1D, including CYP27B1,[32] DHCR7, CYP2R1,[33] and VDR.[30,31] In vivo studies examining the influence of early-onset, long-term vitamin D deficiency in a mouse model of T1D (NOD) support the existence of an inverse relationship between vitamin D levels and the incidence of T1D.[62,63] However, in contrast to animal studies of vitamin D deficiency, no compelling evidence has been provided that the lack of the VDR in mice is associated with impaired glucose tolerance or the development of diabetes.

In two large-scale trials, vitamin D supplementation from early in life was capable of reducing the incidence of T1D.[51,64] The conclusions of these studies were supported by a meta-analysis of 4 case-control studies and 1 cohort study.[65] On the other hand, a few studies were not able to confirm this effect.[66,67] However, the conclusions drawn from these studies were compromised by long recall periods for the involved mothers and low doses of vitamin D. By contrast, an effect of maternal vitamin D intake on T1D risk in the offspring is still to be proved.[52,68] However, some of these latter studies may suffer from limitations such as low doses and the use of questionnaires that overestimate the intake of vitamin D. Studies of animal models of T1D appear to confirm the conclusion drawn from prevention and intervention studies in human T1D. For instance, $1,25(OH)_2D_3$ or nonhypercalcemic analogues were able to inhibit the development of insulitis and prevent the onset of diabetes in NOD and NOD-SCID mice[58,63,69] as well as in streptozotocin-induced diabetic mice.[70]

Type 2 Diabetes and the Influence of Vitamin D Deficiency and Supplementation

Variations in UV exposure and seasonal timing may correlate with the incidence and prevalence of impaired glucose tolerance and type 2 diabetes (T2D), suggesting a role for vitamin D. Furthermore, a correlation between vitamin D deficiency and decreased β-cell function, impaired glucose tolerance, T2D, or mortality from T2D has been observed across age and ethnic groups.[71–73] However, contrasting results have been published on the importance of allelic variations of vitamin D–related genes on glucose tolerance and T2D; these include the vitamin D–binding protein gene[74,75] and VDR[76,77] Moreover, clear evidence for a negative correlation of serum $25(OH)D_3$ levels with insulin resistance is still warranted.[71,78,79] Nevertheless, there is evidence to suggest that VDR polymorphisms are linked to the occurrence of insulin resistance.[76,80] Likewise, studies in animal models have contributed to the current knowledge on a role for vitamin D deficiency in T2D. Vitamin D deficiency has been linked to impaired glucose clearance and insulin secretion in rats and rabbits, with amelioration after vitamin D repletion independently of dietary intake and calcium homeostasis.[81–83] However, convincing evidence for an association between the absence of VDR and impaired glucose tolerance or T2D is lacking.

A large prospective study from 2006, and other trials using relatively high doses of vitamin D, suggests preventive actions of vitamin D against T2D.[84,85] Another large-scale trial could not confirm these findings; however, significantly lower doses were applied in this study.[86] By contrast, evidence for a beneficial effect of vitamin D against established T2D is scarce and contrasting. Most of these intervention trials have involved a very limited number of participants with a short duration of treatment.[87] Finally, a few intervention studies in rodent experimental models of T2D support the hypothesis that vitamin D treatment could contribute to improved glucose homeostasis and T2D.[88,89]

Effects of Vitamin D on the β-Cell and Insulin Target Tissues

The nearly ubiquitous expression pattern of VDR includes cell types of special importance to diabetes, including insulin-producing β cells of the pancreas[90] and insulin target cells, as described in a later section.

Effect of Vitamin D Deficiency and Treatment on Insulin Secretion

In several studies, islets from vitamin D–deficient mice displayed impaired in vitro insulin secretion in response to glucose, whereas in vivo and in vitro vitamin D supplementation ameliorated this condition.[91–93] However, such results should be interpreted with caution because hypocalcaemia is an important feature of vitamin D deficiency in vivo, which can impair β-cell function substantially unless normocalcemia is maintained by dietary measures. A few studies offer contrasting results; however, these were performed with $1,25(OH)_2D_3$-treated insulinoma-cell lines and vitamin D–replete islets.[94]

Protection of the β-Cell Against Immune and Metabolic Stress by Vitamin D

T1D and T2D islets are exposed to various kinds of stress compromising insulin release and β-cell survival. For instance, in T2D islets can be exposed to high levels of glucose and fatty acids over extended periods of time. Indeed, a decline in insulin secretion in response to a short glucose stimulus was observed in C57BL/6J mouse islets cultured in vitro for 7 days in 28 mM glucose. This effect, however, was significantly ameliorated on cotreatment with $1,25(OH)_2D_3$.[95]

Whereas T1D is well known to be an autoimmune disease with local inflammation of islets, systemic inflammation is likely to contribute to the compromised β-cell function and survival occurring in T2D. Thus, in both diseases proinflammatory cytokines such as IL-1β, IFN-γ, and tumor necrosis factor (TNF)-α are expected to play important roles. Combinations of these cytokines have been shown to impair β cells functionally and to increase apoptosis of primary islets and β-cell lines in vitro.[96] Although the actions of $1,25(OH)_2D_3$ on cells of the immune system most likely constitute a crucial part of its protective actions toward immune-mediated damage during T1D (see section on immune effects), a direct protection of β cells against immune mediators may contribute as well. So far, studies on the ability of $1,25(OH)_2D_3$ or analogues to ameliorate the damaging effects of cytokines on in vitro insulin secretion are rather conflicting.[97–100] Similarly, it remains controversial whether $1,25(OH)_2D_3$ can exert a beneficial effect against cytokine-induced β-cell death as well as NO production.[101,102] The lack of compelling evidence for a direct protective effect of $1,25(OH)_2D_3$ in terms of β-cell insulin secretion and cell death is likely due to the use of different experimental conditions and animal models.

Moreover, some investigators have reported an antagonizing effect of $1,25(OH)_2D_3$ and analogues on cytokine-triggered expression of nuclear factor (NF)-κB family members and regulatory kinases, as well as nuclear translocation of NF-κB complexes in primary islets and β-cell lines.[69,102] A few studies have reported that the mRNA expression and secretion of a selection of chemokines and cytokines by β cells themselves in response to in vitro cytokine exposure, or in vivo in NOD and NOD-SCID mice, can be prevented to some degree by $1,25(OH)_2D_3$.[69,98,101] Similarly, a few reports on a partial inhibition of cytokine-induced MHC-I expression on primary rat β cells and human islets have been published.[98,103] Such actions of $1,25(OH)_2D_3$ might suppress the recruitment and activation of immune cells in islets, limiting insulitis in early diabetes.

Effects on the Liver, Muscle, and Adipose Tissue

In addition to β cells, $1,25(OH)_2D_3$ may affect other cell types of interest in a T2D perspective. For instance, VDR mRNA and protein expression has been reported in rat and human liver. In streptozotocin-induced diabetic rats, insulin receptors were upregulated in liver and adipose tissue. However, this effect was antagonized by $1,25(OH)_2D_3$ without alterations in receptor affinity.[104] By contrast, other investigators later demonstrated a decline in insulin receptor gene expression in the liver of streptozotocin-induced diabetic rats, which were almost fully normalized by vitamin D_3 treatment.[105] These investigators further reported that vitamin D_3 treatment improved the impairments observed in hepatic glucose uptake, malate dehydrogenase activity, glycogen content, and expression levels of the antioxidant enzymes superoxide dismutase and glutathione peroxidase. The finding of Vitamin D response element (VDRE) in the human insulin receptor gene further supports the theory that $1,25(OH)_2D_3$ can modulate insulin sensitivity.[106]

Another insulin target tissue, skeletal muscle, also seems to be a target of vitamin D actions. In vitro culture of myotubes with free fatty acids (FFA) was demonstrated to induce insulin resistance and atrophy. However, $1,25(OH)_2D_3$ protected against the FFA actions, causing an improvement in insulin-stimulated glucose uptake in a dose-dependent and time-dependent manner, and completely prevented atrophy.[107] Another important issue may be the modulation of calcium levels by vitamin D. Apart from playing a pivotal role in insulin release in β cells, appropriate cytosolic calcium concentrations are crucial for the transport of glucose in muscle cells.[108,109] Moreover, the peroxisome proliferator-activated receptor δ (PPARδ) may be a target of vitamin D_3 in humans[110]; indeed, PPARδ activation was shown to improve insulin secretion in INS-1e cells[111] as well as FFA-induced insulin resistance in skeletal muscle.[112] Furthermore, systemic inflammation is believed to play a role in the compromised insulin sensitivity in T2D.[113–115] Of note, inflammation of adipose tissue predisposes to insulin resistance. However, $1,25(OH)_2D_3$ seems to protect against inflammation in this tissue by reducing cytokine-induced secretion of monocyte chemotactic protein 1 and recruitment of monocytes.[116]

In conclusion, interpretation of data on glucose intolerance and diabetes in animal models and humans with vitamin D deficiency requires caution, because this condition is characterized not only by low vitamin D levels but also by altered caloric intake, modified parathyroid hormone (PTH) levels and, very importantly, hypocalcemia, which by itself causes a dramatic alteration in β-cell function. However, evidence points to vitamin D deficiency as a probable risk factor in the development of both T1D and T2D. Polymorphisms in vitamin D–related genes are likely candidates as well, although results differ significantly between studies. By contrast, no compelling evidence exists that absence of the VDR increases the susceptibility to either of these diseases.

VITAMIN D AND CARDIOVASCULAR DISEASE

CVD, including heart failure and coronary artery disease, is a major cause of morbidity and mortality worldwide. The occurrence of VDRs and vitamin D–metabolizing enzymes in both the vasculature and the heart including cardiac myocytes, vascular smooth muscle cells, and endothelial cells has definitely fueled the awareness of the direct cardiovascular effects of vitamin D (reviewed in Ref.[117]). On the other hand, the model of direct VDR activation in the arterial wall was recently disputed, as VDRs could not be detected in all nucleated cells and was found to be absent from vascular smooth muscle and endothelial cells.[118] Nevertheless, vitamin D might still regulate the vascular system indirectly. VDR-deficient mice clearly suffer from hypertension, myocardial hypertrophy, and increased thrombogenicity, and even selective VDR deletion in cardiomyocytes leads to cardiac hypertrophy, which is related to an increase in renin.[119] Moreover, epidemiologic and clinical evidence supports a role for vitamin D in cardiovascular health, as hypovitaminosis D is associated with increased risk of CVD and increased mortality.[117,120]

Vitamin D Deficiency and the Cardiovascular System

Ecological studies have reported a higher incidence of coronary heart disease and hypertension during the winter months in both the northern and southern hemispheres. Moreover, based on several epidemiologic and clinical trial data, (mild) vitamin D deficiency is associated with increased cardiovascular risk (factors) such as hypertension,[121] insulin resistance,[78] metabolic syndrome, and diabetes, with markers of subclinical atherosclerosis such as extensive coronary calcium phosphate deposits[122] and with cardiovascular events such as stroke and sudden cardiac deaths.[123] It is striking that vitamin D deficiency was reported to be present in more than 90% of patients with acute myocardial infarction.[124] Just recently the Ludwigshafen Risk and Cardiovascular Health (LURIC) study reported a 75% and 69% decline in all-cause and CVD mortality, respectively, in those with optimal vitamin D levels compared with those with severe vitamin D deficiency. These associations were not driven by diabetes, a factor known to be related with reduced vitamin D levels.[125] To date, the number of cross-sectional and prospective cohort studies examining $25(OH)D_3$ levels and the incidence of cardiovascular events are limited and the results remain inconclusive.

Whether all these associations are causal definitely needs further study, but it is often demonstrated that vitamin D (metabolites) influences a variety of genes with great importance for overall and cardiovascular health, making causality a reasonable theory. Active vitamin D indeed plays a major role in the regulation of the renin-angiotensin-aldosterone system by directly suppressing renin biosynthesis. Moreover, vitamin D interacts with the more recently identified proteins, such as fibroblast growth factor 23 (FGF23) and Klotho. Disturbance of the vitamin D–FGF23–Klotho axis is associated with cardiovascular risk in several studies. Therefore, the interactions of this axis with the renin-angiotensin-aldosterone system may have therapeutic implications in both renal and cardiovascular outcomes (see also next section). Moreover, vitamin D deficiency has been shown to trigger secondary hyperparathyroidism, stimulates inflammatory cytokines, and promotes cardiac myocyte growth.[37] Elevated levels of PTH reflect, in part, inadequate biological vitamin D activity, increases intracellular calcium in target tissues, and is associated with hyperlipidemia and an increased risk of hypertension, cardiac valve calcification, and vascular disease. Based on these findings, it is therefore not surprising that administration of activated forms of vitamin D has the ability to reverse cardiac hypertrophy and decrease cardiovascular mortality in rats and in patients with end-stage renal disease and secondary hyperparathyroidism.[126–128] Several of the biological pathways through which the effects of $1,25(OH)_2D_3$ are regulated remain poorly understood, but may account for its role in cardiovascular health.

Only a limited number of interventional trials have linked (pure) vitamin D replenishment to beneficial effects on cardiovascular risk factors such as arterial hypertension. Indeed, vitamin D supplementation has been reported to reduce systolic blood pressure but not diastolic blood pressure. Subgroup analysis suggested that the change of blood pressure did not vary markedly across the dose of vitamin D supplementation, study length, or intervention.[129] On the other hand, vitamin D intake (>500 IU/d) in the Nurses' Health Study (NHS) I and II and the Health Professionals Follow-up Study (HPFS) in more than 200,000 men and women without hypertension at trial entrance had no effect on risk of hypertension during 8 years of follow-up.[130] In reality, the effect of vitamin D on blood pressure was often only present in patients in whom blood pressure was already elevated at baseline[131] and in patients with T2D. Moreover, a recent meta-analysis of 18 independent randomized controlled trials for vitamin D, including 57,311 participants, described that intake of regular vitamin D supplements (from 300 IU to 2000 IU) was associated with reduced mortality risk.[132] By contrast, data from the Randomized Evaluation of Calcium or Vitamin D (RECORD) trial failed to find any benefit or harm from daily vitamin D and/or calcium supplements (800 IU vitamin

D_3 and/or 1 g calcium per day) on overall mortality, vascular disease mortality, cancer mortality, or incidence after a 3-year follow-up.[133]

Unfortunately, several of these interventional studies are often limited by the extra calcium supplements, which may increase the risk of cardiovascular events. A recently reported meta-analysis of 15 randomized, placebo-controlled trials of calcium supplementation ($\geq$500 mg calcium per day) showed no significant increase in total CVD or stroke but a significant 27% increase in myocardial infarction.[134] Doses of more than 1.5 g of calcium per day from diet or supplements are not beneficial for reduction of fracture risk, and might certainly be unsafe in terms of increasing overall and cardiovascular mortality.[135] Moreover, one of the largest intervention trials with calcium and vitamin D (1 g calcium and 400 IU vitamin D per day, respectively) on cardiovascular risk in the Women's Health Initiative (WHI) revealed no change in coronary or cerebrovascular risk,[135,136] although he study design was heavily criticized because the dosage of the vitamin D supplements was low, adherence was problematic, and vitamin D supplementation was allowed in the control group.

At present, there is insufficient evidence to support vitamin D supplementation as a way of improving cardiovascular outcomes,[137] but larger studies are being initiated to answer the question as to whether vitamin D supplementation reduces CVD outcome (eg, http://www.vitalstudy.org). Nevertheless, many cardiovascular patients are in poor health, clearly vitamin D deficient, and at risk of developing osteoporosis and bone fractures. In such patients vitamin D replenishment can be justified to avoid vitamin D deficiency with its effect on musculoskeletal pain, myopathy, and accelerated bone loss.

Thus far, the results of the few randomized control trials with (pure) vitamin D supplementation on cardiovascular outcomes have been indecisive or contradictory. Carefully designed randomized controlled trials are critical for the evaluation of the role of vitamin D replenishment in reducing CVD.

VDR Deficiency and the Cardiovascular System

As already mentioned, $1,25(OH)_2D_3$ and other vitamin D analogues function as endocrine suppressors of renin gene expression via a VDRE that is present in the renin gene. VDR knockout mice, representing a mouse model of vitamin D–dependent rickets type II have, besides classic symptoms such as rickets, osteomalacia, and secondary hyperparathyroidism, also an overstimulation of the renin-angiotensin-aldosterone system, leading to high blood pressure and cardiac hypertrophy.[138] On the other hand, in wild-type mice, $1,25(OH)_2D_3$ reduces renal renin production. The negative regulation of renin by active vitamin D seems independent of calcium and PTH.[139] A study on the cardiac myocyte-specific deletion of the VDR extended these data and acknowledged that vitamin D and the VDR signaling system possessed antihypertrophic activity in the heart. Similar data were found in 1α-hydroxylase–deficient mice that developed hypertension, cardiac hypertrophy, and impaired cardiac function, along with an upregulation of the renin-angiotensin-aldosterone system in both renal and cardiac tissues.[140]

Not all previous findings from the VDR-deficient mice were completely reproduced by others,[141,142] but most groups confirmed the cardiac hypertrophic phenotype. In the latter study, VDR-deficient mice revealed a low expression of tissue inhibitors of metalloproteinases (TIMP) such as TIMP-1 and TIMP-3 in left ventricular tissue, whereas metalloproteinases such as matrix metalloproteinase (MMP)-2 and MMP-9 were high, suggesting the pivotal role of VDR in regulating gelatinase activities in cardiac hypertrophy. MMPs are important in extracellular matrix (ECM) remodeling, are major effector molecules of inflammatory immune cells, and contribute to progressive left ventricular remodeling, dilation, and heart failure. Recent in vitro studies indicate that vitamin D downregulates MMP-9 production by TNF-α. Moreover, MMP-2 and MMP-9 activation are associated with collagen deposition and cardiac fibrosis.

Vitamin D Metabolites as Immune Modulators in Cardiovascular Disease

The beneficial effects of active vitamin D on cardiovascular function have been shown to be initiated by its direct actions on cardiac myocytes and the renin-angiotensin system, but are also believed to stem in part from its immunomodulatory effects. Because inflammation is crucially involved in the processes leading to macrophage cholesterol uptake, plaque production, and atherosclerosis, the inhibitory effects of $1,25(OH)_2D_3$ on the production of several proinflammatory Th1 cytokines, such as IFN-γ, IL-6, and TNF-α, while stimulating the effects of Th2 lymphocytes and leading to a reduction in matrix metalloproteinase, are all factors proposed as mechanisms contributing to protective effects of vitamin D on the cardiovascular system. Active vitamin D also favors the induction of Tregs, partly through the induction of tolerance-inducing DCs. Furthermore, it has been shown to have immunosuppressive effects whereby it reduces the proliferation of lymphocytes and the production of cytokines, which have been identified as having an important role in atherogenesis.[143]

In summary, strong clinical trial data are lacking to lend support to raising intake requirements for vitamin D and target 25(OH)D levels based on a role for vitamin D in preventing cardiovascular and metabolic diseases. Nonetheless, the high prevalence of vitamin D deficiency in the general population remains alarming, and requires implementation of clear supplementation guidelines.

VITAMIN D AND CANCER
Mechanisms Involved in the Antineoplastic Activity of 1,25(OH)$_2$D$_3$

The growth-inhibitory effect of $1,25(OH)_2D_3$ was first shown in melanoma cells, of which the doubling time increased after incubation with $1,25(OH)_2D_3$.[144] Shortly thereafter, its differentiation-inducing capacity was demonstrated in human HL60 leukemia cells, which differentiate toward the macrophage lineage when treated with $1,25(OH)_2D_3$.[145] Since then, the antineoplastic activity of $1,25(OH)_2D_3$ has been shown in vitro as well as in vivo in a wide variety of cancer types, including leukemia and colon, breast, and prostate cancer.[146–149] Besides hampering cell proliferation and promoting cell differentiation, $1,25(OH)_2D_3$ exerts its antineoplastic effects by inducing programmed cell death and by inhibiting cellular migration and invasion.

Cell proliferation

The molecular mechanisms by which $1,25(OH)_2D_3$ mediates these anticancer effects involve multiple pathways and are in some cases cell type–specific. Nevertheless, in most cell types that express a functional VDR, exposure to $1,25(OH)_2D_3$ results in the accumulation of cells in the G_0/G_1 phase of the cell cycle and a concomitant decrease of cells in the S phase.[150] The transition from G_0/G_1 is controlled by the activity of retinoblastoma pocket proteins (pRb and p107/p130). Phosphorylation of pRb is inhibited in cells treated with $1,25(OH)_2D_3$ and, as a consequence, hypophosphorylated pRb will sequester the transcription factors E2F1, E2F2, and E2F3 and refrain them from activating genes that drive cell cycle progression. Cyclins and cyclin-dependent kinase (CDK) complexes phosphorylate pRb, and a loss of their kinase activity generates hypophosphorylated Rb. Both the expression of cyclins (D1, E, A) and CDKs^{2,4,6} can be decreased by $1,25(OH)_2D_3$, albeit in a cell-type–specific way. Moreover, $1,25(OH)_2D_3$ induces the expression of several cyclin-dependent kinase inhibitors, either at the transcriptional or translational level, which will further decrease the cyclin-CDK kinase activity.[151,152] Furthermore, $1,25(OH)_2D_3$

also interferes with other signaling cascades and, as such, slows down the cell-cycle progression. Indeed, $1,25(OH)_2D_3$ inhibits the epidermal growth factor–induced signaling cascade and downregulates the mitogenic insulin-like growth factors.[153–155]

Apoptosis

The ability of $1,25(OH)_2D_3$ to induce apoptosis has been demonstrated in breast, colon, and prostate cancer cells. Although the mechanisms of the apoptotic effect are not fully unraveled, $1,25(OH)_2D_3$ can trigger the intrinsic, mitochondria-dependent pathway that induces cell death. Depending on the cell type, $1,25(OH)_2D_3$ decreases the expression of the antiapoptotic factors (B-cell lymphoma 2 [Bcl-2], Bcl-X$_L$) and/or increases the proapoptotic equivalents (Bcl-2 Associated X protein [Bax], Bcl-2 Antagonist Killer [Bak]), thus directing the cells more toward apoptosis than to survival.[156] In addition, pretreatment with $1,25(OH)_2D_3$ sensitizes cancer cells to different cytotoxic substances, irradiation, and cryoablation, and results in increased cell death.[157–159]

Angiogenesis and metastasis

$1,25(OH)_2D_3$ also inhibits angiogenesis, a key process in malignant tumor growth, by inhibiting the proliferation of endothelial cells and/or by repressing the release of angiogenic factors such as TGF-α, epidermal growth factor, and vascular endothelial growth factor (VEGF). Downregulation of VEGF is mediated by repression of hypoxia-inducible factor 1–dependent transactivation.[160] Elimination of blood vessels is also important in reducing the possibility of cancer cells invading the circulatory system and metastasizing to secondary sites. In addition, $1,25(OH)_2D_3$ also directly reduces the migration and invasion capacity of cancer cells. These anti-invasive effects are accompanied by a decreased adhesion to the ECM, through reduced expression of laminin and the receptors integrins $\alpha6$ and $\beta4$, as well as by a diminished ECM breakdown, accomplished by decreased metalloproteinase and cathepsin activities.[161] An increased expression of E-cadherin after treatment with $1,25(OH)_2D_3$ reduces the adhesion of cancer cells to the endothelium and inhibits the invasiveness of cancer cells.[162]

Vitamin D Deficiency and VDR Ablation in Rodent Models

Vitamin D deficiency

A large number of epidemiologic reports suggest that an increased cancer risk is associated with vitamin D deficiency. Several recent in vitro studies have addressed this hypothesis directly by the use of a vitamin D_3–deficient diet. In prostate cancer, more proliferation and less programmed cell death is observed in mice that are kept on a vitamin D_3–deficient diet, whereas in breast-cancer models, a vitamin D_3–deficient diet enhances metastasis by promoting the growth of the cancer cells in the bones.[163,164] To mimic human Western dietary habits, which are believed to play a role in the development of colorectal cancer, a rodent diet high in fat and low in calcium and vitamin D was created. Feeding rodents this Western diet promotes formation of colonic tumor, a process that is reversed on supplementation of the Western diet with calcium and vitamin D.[165,166]

VDR knockout mice

Complete loss of $1,25(OH)_2D_3$-mediated growth control, attained by a knockout of the VDR, is accompanied by an increase in cell proliferation and oxidative stress. Sporadic tumor formation is not present in VDR knockout mice, but the susceptibility to chemical carcinogens is increased in a tissue-specific manner. Epidermal and lymphoid tissues of VDR-null mice are more sensitive to dimethylbenzanthracene (DMBA) treatment, while spontaneous cutaneous tumors are rarely detected in these mice.[167] In the absence of VDR expression, DMBA also promotes hyperplasia of mammary glands and induces a higher percentage of hormone-independent breast tumors with squamous differentiation.[168] The enhanced susceptibility for breast cancer in VDR-null mice is also proven in another model system whereby VDR knockout mice were crossed with mouse mammary tumor virus-*neu* mice that specifically overexpress the *c-neu* proto-oncogene in the mammary gland. Ablation of the VDR is accompanied by pathologic changes such as dysplasia of the mammary ductal epithelia, atrophy of the associated fat pad, and reduced survival. In an LPB-Tag model for prostate cancer, lack of VDR signaling leads to an enhanced cellular proliferation in prostate tumors.[169] The role of the VDR in colon cancer is also demonstrated in a mouse model expressing a mutated adenomatous polyposis coli (APC) allele in combination with loss of both VDR alleles. Lack of the VDR in these mice increases the number of aberrant crypt foci (ACF), but not of adenomas or carcinomas, in either small intestine or colon. However, the existing tumors are larger than tumors of mice in which VDR signaling was present.[170,171]

Epidemiologic and Interventional Studies in Humans

Epidemiologic studies

The findings that $1,25(OH)_2D_3$ is able to inhibit the proliferation of a wide variety of cancer cells and that some cell types in the VDR knockout mice are characterized by dysregulated cell proliferation support the hypothesis that vitamin D levels can be associated with cancer risk in humans. Garland and Garland[172] reported in 1980 that colorectal cancer mortality rates were higher in regions with less UV irradiation. Subsequently, a large number of studies confirmed a decreased cancer risk in regions with high UV irradiation. However, the measurement of serum $25(OH)D_3$ levels is a much better indicator of an individual's vitamin D status, as it combines vitamin D levels obtained by exposure to sunlight and through dietary/supplemental intake of vitamin D.[173] Numerous studies addressed the relationship between circulating $25(OH)D_3$ levels and cancer incidence. For colorectal cancer, many epidemiologic studies and meta-analysis of different large cohorts agree with the hypothesis that low serum $25(OH)D_3$ is associated with an increased risk of cancer.[174–176] However, for most other cancer types the results are more conflicting. As it is suggested that the inverse correlation between serum $25(OH)D_3$ is more pronounced in the deficiency region, it is possible that in populations with elevated circulating vitamin D levels, no beneficial effects on cancer incidence are observed. Moreover, these association studies are not able to decipher whether low $25(OH)D_3$ levels are a predictor or rather have a causal relationship with cancer risk.

Intervention studies

The WHI designed a randomized placebo-controlled clinical trial in which postmenopausal women received calcium (1 g) plus vitamin D (400 IU) or a matching placebo on a daily basis.[177] The number of skeletal fractures was evaluated as the primary end point while cancer incidence in general, and breast and colon cancer in particular, served as secondary end points. After a mean follow-up of 7 years, calcium and vitamin D supplementation did not significantly alter cancer incidence or overall mortality. However, some participants were already taking calcium (1 g) and vitamin D (600 IU) on their own initiative at the time of trial randomization. When these individuals were excluded from analysis, a decreased incidence of cancer in general, and more specifically of breast and colon cancer, was observed in the supplementation group.[136] In a smaller 4-year, population-based, double-blind, randomized placebo-controlled trial, calcium (1.4–1.5 g) and vitamin D supplementation (1100 IU) resulted in a decreased risk of breast cancer.[178] In a randomized placebo-controlled clinical trial in patients with colorectal adenoma, patients were supplemented during 6 months with calcium (2 g) and/or vitamin D (800 IU), and changes in the normal colorectal mucosa were monitored. Daily supplementation with vitamin D induced beneficial changes in the normal rectal tissue, which suggests that vitamin D can promote antineoplastic pathways such as enhanced activity of DNA mismatch repair mechanisms, decreased oxidative stress damage, and increased colorectal epithelial cell differentiation and apoptosis.[179]

In summary, these data demonstrate potent antineoplastic activity in a variety of cell and animal models. The advantages seen in these preclinical studies suggest that clinical trials in patients with cancer are warranted. Supplementation to optimum levels in vitamin D_3–deficient patients can lead to a chemopreventive effect and to decreased risk of cancer. Treatment with $1,25(OH)_2D_3$ or its analogues, either alone or in combination with other anticancer drugs, may be effective in preventing cancer initiation or might delay cancer progression.

SUMMARY

- In addition to its classic role in calcium and bone homeostasis, vitamin D has been identified as a central regulator of other cellular functions (eg, the immune system, pancreas, heart, and in cancer cells).
- Extraskeletal health effects of vitamin D are plausible, but a true causal link between poor vitamin D status and nearly all major diseases (autoimmune diseases, infections, cardiovascular and metabolic diseases, and cancer) has not been proved, so no guidelines can be defined for such effects.
- Larger clinical trials are needed to assess whether vitamin D replenishment holds promise for long-term prevention of chronic noncommunicable diseases such as infectious diseases, diabetes, CVD, and cancer, possibly as part of a combination therapy rather than a short-term preventive therapy or treatment of established disease.
- In the meantime, both vitamin D deficiency and vitamin D excess need to be circumvented, and a daily supplement of 400 to 800 IU of vitamin D_3 would bring serum 25(OH)D levels to within the normal range in most otherwise healthy adults.

REFERENCES

1. Verstuyf A, Carmeliet G, Bouillon R, et al. Vitamin D: a pleiotropic hormone. Kidney Int 2010;78:140–5.
2. Baeke F, Takiishi T, Korf H, et al. Vitamin D: modulator of the immune system. Curr Opin Pharmacol 2010;10:482–96.
3. Overbergh L, Stoffels K, Valckx D, et al. Regulation of 25-hydroxyvitamin d-1alpha-hydroxylase by IFNgamma in human monocytic THP1 cells. J Steroid Biochem Mol Biol 2004;89–90:453–5.
4. Martineau AR, Wilkinson KA, Newton SM, et al. IFN-gamma- and TNF-independent vitamin D-inducible human suppression of mycobacteria: the role of cathelicidin LL-37. J Immunol 2007;178:7190–8.
5. Pedersen AW, Holmstrom K, Jensen SS, et al. Phenotypic and functional markers for 1alpha,25-dihydroxyvitamin D(3)-modified regulatory dendritic cells. Clin Exp Immunol 2009;157:48–59.
6. van Halteren AG, Van EE, de Jong EC, et al. Redirection of human autoreactive T-cells upon interaction with dendritic cells modulated by TX527, an analog of 1,25 dihydroxyvitamin D(3). Diabetes 2002;51:2119–25.

7. Penna G, Roncari A, Amuchastegui S, et al. Expression of the inhibitory receptor ILT3 on dendritic cells is dispensable for induction of CD4+Foxp3+ regulatory T cells by 1,25-dihydroxyvitamin D3. Blood 2005;106:3490–7.
8. Ferreira GB, Kleijwegt FS, Waelkens E, et al. Differential protein pathways in 1,25-dihydroxyvitamin d(3) and dexamethasone modulated tolerogenic human dendritic cells. J Proteome Res 2012;11:941–71.
9. Ferreira GB, Van EE, Lage K, et al. Proteome analysis demonstrates profound alterations in human dendritic cell nature by TX527, an analogue of vitamin D. Proteomics 2009;9:3752–64.
10. Baeke F, Korf H, Overbergh L, et al. Human T lymphocytes are direct targets of 1,25-dihydroxyvitamin D3 in the immune system. J Steroid Biochem Mol Biol 2010;121:221–7.
11. Baeke F, Korf H, Overbergh L, et al. The vitamin D analog, TX527, promotes a human CD4+CD25highCD127low regulatory T cell profile and induces a migratory signature specific for homing to sites of inflammation. J Immunol 2011;186:132–42.
12. Tang J, Zhou R, Luger D, et al. Calcitriol suppresses antiretinal autoimmunity through inhibitory effects on the Th17 effector response. J Immunol 2009;182:4624–32.
13. Mahon BD, Wittke A, Weaver V, et al. The targets of vitamin D depend on the differentiation and activation status of CD4 positive T cells. J Cell Biochem 2003;89:922–32.
14. Jeffery LE, Burke F, Mura M, et al. 1,25-Dihydroxyvitamin D3 and IL-2 combine to inhibit T cell production of inflammatory cytokines and promote development of regulatory T cells expressing CTLA-4 and FoxP3. J Immunol 2009;183:5458–67.
15. Chen S, Sims GP, Chen XX, et al. Modulatory effects of 1,25-dihydroxyvitamin D3 on human B cell differentiation. J Immunol 2007;179:1634–47.
16. Chocano-Bedoya P, Ronnenberg AG. Vitamin D and tuberculosis. Nutr Rev 2009;67:289–93.
17. Andraos C, Koorsen G, Knight JC, et al. Vitamin D receptor gene methylation is associated with ethnicity, tuberculosis, and TaqI polymorphism. Hum Immunol 2011;72:262–8.
18. Hewison M, Freeman L, Hughes SV, et al. Differential regulation of vitamin D receptor and its ligand in human monocyte-derived dendritic cells. J Immunol 2003;170:5382–90.
19. Wang TJ, Zhang F, Richards JB, et al. Common genetic determinants of vitamin D insufficiency: a genome-wide association study. Lancet 2010;376:180–8.
20. Waters WR, Palmer MV, Nonnecke BJ, et al. Mycobacterium bovis infection of vitamin D-deficient NOS2-/- mice. Microb Pathog 2004;36:11–7.
21. Chan TY. Vitamin D deficiency and susceptibility to tuberculosis. Calcif Tissue Int 2000;66:476–8.
22. Nursyam EW, Amin Z, Rumende CM. The effect of vitamin D as supplementary treatment in patients with moderately advanced pulmonary tuberculous lesion. Acta Med Indones 2006;38:3–5.
23. Wejse C, Gomes VF, Rabna P, et al. Vitamin D as supplementary treatment for tuberculosis: a double-blind, randomized, placebo-controlled trial. Am J Respir Crit Care Med 2009;179:843–50.
24. Martineau AR, Timms PM, Bothamley GH, et al. High-dose vitamin D(3) during intensive-phase antimicrobial treatment of pulmonary tuberculosis: a double-blind randomised controlled trial. Lancet 2011;377:242–50.

25. Li-Ng M, Aloia JF, Pollack S, et al. A randomized controlled trial of vitamin D3 supplementation for the prevention of symptomatic upper respiratory tract infections. Epidemiol Infect 2009;137:1396–404.
26. Beard JA, Bearden A, Striker R. Vitamin D and the antiviral state. J Clin Virol 2011;50:194–200.
27. Bergman P, Walter-Jallow L, Broliden K, et al. The antimicrobial peptide LL-37 inhibits HIV-1 replication. Curr HIV Res 2007;5:410–5.
28. Ali MY, Gopal KV, Llerena LA, et al. Hypercalcemia associated with infection by *Cryptococcus neoformans* and *Coccidioides immitis*. Am J Med Sci 1999;318: 419–23.
29. Spindel SJ, Hamill RJ, Georghiou PR, et al. Case report: vitamin D-mediated hypercalcemia in fungal infections. Am J Med Sci 1995;310:71–6.
30. Mathieu C, Gysemans C, Giulietti A, et al. Vitamin D and diabetes. Diabetologia 2005;48:1247–57.
31. Guo SW, Magnuson VL, Schiller JJ, et al. Meta-analysis of vitamin D receptor polymorphisms and type 1 diabetes: a HuGE review of genetic association studies. Am J Epidemiol 2006;164:711–24.
32. Bailey R, Cooper JD, Zeitels L, et al. Association of the vitamin D metabolism gene CYP27B1 with type 1 diabetes. Diabetes 2007;56:2616–21.
33. Cooper JD, Smyth DJ, Walker NM, et al. Inherited variation in vitamin D genes is associated with predisposition to autoimmune disease type 1 diabetes. Diabetes 2011;60:1624–31.
34. Australia and New Zealand Multiple Sclerosis Genetics Consortium (ANZgene). Genome-wide association study identifies new multiple sclerosis susceptibility loci on chromosomes 12 and 20. Nat Genet 2009;41:824–8.
35. Ramagopalan SV, Maugeri NJ, Handunnetthi L, et al. Expression of the multiple sclerosis-associated MHC class II Allele HLA-DRB1*1501 is regulated by vitamin D. PLoS Genet 2009;5:e1000369.
36. Simmons JD, Mullighan C, Welsh KI, et al. Vitamin D receptor gene polymorphism: association with Crohn's disease susceptibility. Gut 2000;47:211–4.
37. Mathieu C, Van der Schueren BJ. Vitamin D deficiency is not good for you. Diabetes Care 2011;34:1245–6.
38. Hayes CE, Cantorna MT, DeLuca HF. Vitamin D and multiple sclerosis. Proc Soc Exp Biol Med 1997;216:21–7.
39. Munger KL, Levin LI, Hollis BW, et al. Serum 25-hydroxyvitamin D levels and risk of multiple sclerosis. JAMA 2006;296:2832–8.
40. Islam T, Gauderman WJ, Cozen W, et al. Childhood sun exposure influences risk of multiple sclerosis in monozygotic twins. Neurology 2007;69:381–8.
41. Kampman MT, Wilsgaard T, Mellgren SI. Outdoor activities and diet in childhood and adolescence relate to MS risk above the Arctic Circle. J Neurol 2007;254: 471–7.
42. van der Mei IA, Ponsonby AL, Dwyer T, et al. Vitamin D levels in people with multiple sclerosis and community controls in Tasmania, Australia. J Neurol 2007;254:581–90.
43. Nieves J, Cosman F, Herbert J, et al. High prevalence of vitamin D deficiency and reduced bone mass in multiple sclerosis. Neurology 1994;44:1687–92.
44. Smolders J, Menheere P, Kessels A, et al. Association of vitamin D metabolite levels with relapse rate and disability in multiple sclerosis. Mult Scler 2008;14: 1220–4.
45. Kalliora MI, Vazeou A, Delis D, et al. Seasonal variation of type 1 diabetes mellitus diagnosis in Greek children. Hormones (Athens) 2011;10:67–71.

46. Moltchanova EV, Schreier N, Lammi N, et al. Seasonal variation of diagnosis of Type 1 diabetes mellitus in children worldwide. Diabet Med 2009;26: 673–8.
47. Mohr SB, Garland CF, Gorham ED, et al. The association between ultraviolet B irradiance, vitamin D status and incidence rates of type 1 diabetes in 51 regions worldwide. Diabetologia 2008;51:1391–8.
48. Borkar VV, Devidayal, Verma S, et al. Low levels of vitamin D in North Indian children with newly diagnosed type 1 diabetes. Pediatr Diabetes 2010;11: 345–50.
49. Pozzilli P, Manfrini S, Crino A, et al. Low levels of 25-hydroxyvitamin D3 and 1,25-dihydroxyvitamin D3 in patients with newly diagnosed type 1 diabetes. Horm Metab Res 2005;37:680–3.
50. Littorin B, Blom P, Scholin A, et al. Lower levels of plasma 25-hydroxyvitamin D among young adults at diagnosis of autoimmune type 1 diabetes compared with control subjects: results from the nationwide Diabetes Incidence Study in Sweden (DISS). Diabetologia 2006;49:2847–52.
51. Hypponen E, Laara E, Reunanen A, et al. Intake of vitamin D and risk of type 1 diabetes: a birth-cohort study. Lancet 2001;358:1500–3.
52. Stene LC, Ulriksen J, Magnus P, et al. Use of cod liver oil during pregnancy associated with lower risk of Type I diabetes in the offspring. Diabetologia 2000;43:1093–8.
53. Cantorna MT. Vitamin D and its role in immunology: multiple sclerosis, and inflammatory bowel disease. Prog Biophys Mol Biol 2006;92:60–4.
54. Carrillo-Vico A, Guerrero JM, Lardone PJ, et al. A review of the multiple actions of melatonin on the immune system. Endocrine 2005;27:189–200.
55. Jahnsen J, Falch JA, Mowinckel P, et al. Vitamin D status, parathyroid hormone and bone mineral density in patients with inflammatory bowel disease. Scand J Gastroenterol 2002;37:192–9.
56. Van Belle TL, Gysemans C, Mathieu C. Vitamin D in autoimmune, infectious and allergic diseases: a vital player? Best Pract Res Clin Endocrinol Metab 2011;25: 617–32.
57. Lemire JM, Archer DC. 1,25-dihydroxyvitamin D3 prevents the in vivo induction of murine experimental autoimmune encephalomyelitis. J Clin Invest 1991;87: 1103–7.
58. Mathieu C, Waer M, Casteels K, et al. Prevention of type I diabetes in NOD mice by nonhypercalcemic doses of a new structural analog of 1,25-dihydroxyvitamin D3, KH1060. Endocrinology 1995;136:866–72.
59. Verstuyf A, Segaert S, Verlinden L, et al. Recent developments in the use of vitamin D analogues. Expert Opin Investig Drugs 2000;9:443–55.
60. Branisteanu DD, Waer M, Sobis H, et al. Prevention of murine experimental allergic encephalomyelitis: cooperative effects of cyclosporine and 1 alpha, 25-(OH)2D3. J Neuroimmunol 1995;61:151–60.
61. Van Etten E, Branisteanu DD, Verstuyf A, et al. Analogs of 1,25-dihydroxyvitamin D3 as dose-reducing agents for classical immunosuppressants. Transplantation 2000;69:1932–42.
62. Giulietti A, Gysemans C, Stoffels K, et al. Vitamin D deficiency in early life accelerates Type 1 diabetes in non-obese diabetic mice. Diabetologia 2004;47: 451–62.
63. Zella JB, McCary LC, DeLuca HF. Oral administration of 1,25-dihydroxyvitamin D3 completely protects NOD mice from insulin-dependent diabetes mellitus. Arch Biochem Biophys 2003;417:77–80.

64. EURODIAB Substudy 2 Study Group. Vitamin D supplement in early childhood and risk for Type I (insulin-dependent) diabetes mellitus. Diabetologia 1999;42: 51–4.

65. Zipitis CS, Akobeng AK. Vitamin D supplementation in early childhood and risk of type 1 diabetes: a systematic review and meta-analysis. Arch Dis Child 2008; 93:512–7.

66. Brekke HK, Ludvigsson J. Vitamin D supplementation and diabetes-related autoimmunity in the ABIS study. Pediatr Diabetes 2007;8:11–4.

67. Stene LC, Joner G. Use of cod liver oil during the first year of life is associated with lower risk of childhood-onset type 1 diabetes: a large, population-based, case-control study. Am J Clin Nutr 2003;78:1128–34.

68. Marjamaki L, Niinisto S, Kenward MG, et al. Maternal intake of vitamin D during pregnancy and risk of advanced beta cell autoimmunity and type 1 diabetes in offspring. Diabetologia 2010;53:1599–607.

69. Giarratana N, Penna G, Amuchastegui S, et al. A vitamin D analog down-regulates proinflammatory chemokine production by pancreatic islets inhibiting T cell recruitment and type 1 diabetes development. J Immunol 2004;173: 2280–7.

70. Inaba M, Nishizawa Y, Song K, et al. Partial protection of 1 alpha-hydroxyvitamin D3 against the development of diabetes induced by multiple low-dose strepto-zotocin injection in CD-1 mice. Metabolism 1992;41:631–5.

71. Gagnon C, Lu ZX, Magliano DJ, et al. Serum 25-hydroxyvitamin D, calcium intake, and risk of type 2 diabetes after 5 years: results from a national, population-based prospective study (the Australian Diabetes, Obesity and Life-style study). Diabetes Care 2011;34:1133–8.

72. Pittas AG, Lau J, Hu FB, et al. The role of vitamin D and calcium in type 2 diabetes. A systematic review and meta-analysis. J Clin Endocrinol Metab 2007;92: 2017–29.

73. Scragg R, Sowers M, Bell C. Serum 25-hydroxyvitamin D, diabetes, and ethnicity in the Third National Health and Nutrition Examination Survey. Diabetes Care 2004;27:2813–8.

74. Baier LJ, Dobberfuhl AM, Pratley RE, et al. Variations in the vitamin D-binding protein (Gc locus) are associated with oral glucose tolerance in nondiabetic Pima Indians. J Clin Endocrinol Metab 1998;83:2993–6.

75. Ye WZ, Dubois-Laforgue D, Bellanne-Chantelot C, et al. Variations in the vitamin D-binding protein (Gc locus) and risk of type 2 diabetes mellitus in French Caucasians. Metabolism 2001;50:366–9.

76. Oh JY, Barrett-Connor E. Association between vitamin D receptor polymorphism and type 2 diabetes or metabolic syndrome in community-dwelling older adults: the Rancho Bernardo Study. Metabolism 2002;51:356–9.

77. Ortlepp JR, Metrikat J, Albrecht M, et al. The vitamin D receptor gene variant and physical activity predicts fasting glucose levels in healthy young men. Diabet Med 2003;20:451–4.

78. Chiu KC, Chu A, Go VL, et al. Hypovitaminosis D is associated with insulin resistance and beta cell dysfunction. Am J Clin Nutr 2004;79:820–5.

79. Erdonmez D, Hatun S, Cizmecioglu FM, et al. No relationship between vitamin D status and insulin resistance in a group of high school students. J Clin Res Pediatr Endocrinol 2011;3:198–201.

80. Jain R, von Hurst PR, Stonehouse W, et al. Association of vitamin D receptor gene polymorphisms with insulin resistance and response to vitamin D. Metab-olism 2012;61:293–301.

81. Cade C, Norman AW. Vitamin D3 improves impaired glucose tolerance and insulin secretion in the vitamin D-deficient rat in vivo. Endocrinology 1986;119: 84–90.

82. Nyomba BL, Bouillon R, De MP. Influence of vitamin D status on insulin secretion and glucose tolerance in the rabbit. Endocrinology 1984;115:191–7.

83. Cade C, Norman AW. Rapid normalization/stimulation by 1,25-dihydroxyvitamin D3 of insulin secretion and glucose tolerance in the vitamin D-deficient rat. Endocrinology 1987;120:1490–7.

84. Nagpal J, Pande JN, Bhartia A. A double-blind, randomized, placebo-controlled trial of the short-term effect of vitamin D3 supplementation on insulin sensitivity in apparently healthy, middle-aged, centrally obese men. Diabet Med 2009;26: 19–27.

85. Pittas AG, Dawson-Hughes B, Li T, et al. Vitamin D and calcium intake in relation to type 2 diabetes in women. Diabetes Care 2006;29:650–6.

86. de Boer I, Tinker LF, Connelly S, et al. Calcium plus vitamin D supplementation and the risk of incident diabetes in the Women's Health Initiative. Diabetes Care 2008;31:701–7.

87. Orwoll E, Riddle M, Prince M. Effects of vitamin D on insulin and glucagon secretion in non-insulin-dependent diabetes mellitus. Am J Clin Nutr 1994;59:1083–7.

88. de Souza SR, Vianna LM. Effect of cholecalciferol supplementation on blood glucose in an experimental model of type 2 diabetes mellitus in spontaneously hypertensive rats and Wistar rats. Clin Chim Acta 2005;358:146–50.

89. Kawashima H, Castro A. Effect of 1 alpha-hydroxyvitamin D3 on the glucose and calcium metabolism in genetic obese mice. Res Commun Chem Pathol Pharmacol 1981;33:155–61.

90. Johnson JA, Grande JP, Roche PC, et al. Immunohistochemical localization of the 1,25(OH)2D3 receptor and calbindin D28k in human and rat pancreas. Am J Physiol 1994;267:E356–60.

91. Billaudel BJ, Faure AG, Sutter BC. Effect of 1,25 dihydroxyvitamin D3 on isolated islets from vitamin D3-deprived rats. Am J Physiol 1990;258:E643–8.

92. Kadowaki S, Norman AW. Dietary vitamin D is essential for normal insulin secretion from the perfused rat pancreas. J Clin Invest 1984;73:759–66.

93. Norman AW, Frankel JB, Heldt AM, et al. Vitamin D deficiency inhibits pancreatic secretion of insulin. Science 1980;209:823–5.

94. Lee S, Clark SA, Gill RK, et al. 1,25-Dihydroxyvitamin D3 and pancreatic beta-cell function: vitamin D receptors, gene expression, and insulin secretion. Endocrinology 1994;134:1602–10.

95. Cheng Q, Li YC, Boucher BJ, et al. A novel role for vitamin D: modulation of expression and function of the local renin-angiotensin system in mouse pancreatic islets. Diabetologia 2011;54:2077–81.

96. Eizirik DL, Mandrup-Poulsen T. A choice of death–the signal-transduction of immune-mediated beta-cell apoptosis. Diabetologia 2001;44:2115–33.

97. Mauricio D, Andersen HU, Larsen CM, et al. Dexamethasone prevents interleukin-1beta-mediated inhibition of rat islet insulin secretion without decreasing nitric oxide production. Cytokine 1997;9:563–9.

98. Riachy R, Vandewalle B, Belaich S, et al. Beneficial effect of 1,25 dihydroxyvitamin D3 on cytokine-treated human pancreatic islets. J Endocrinol 2001;169: 161–8.

99. Riachy R, Vandewalle B, Kerr CJ, et al. 1,25-dihydroxyvitamin D3 protects RINm5F and human islet cells against cytokine-induced apoptosis: implication of the antiapoptotic protein A20. Endocrinology 2002;143:4809–19.

100. Sandler S, Buschard K, Bendtzen K. Effects of 1,25-dihydroxyvitamin D3 and the analogues MC903 and KH1060 on interleukin-1 beta-induced inhibition of rat pancreatic islet beta-cell function in vitro. Immunol Lett 1994;41:73–7.
101. Gysemans CA, Cardozo AK, Callewaert H, et al. 1,25-Dihydroxyvitamin D3 modulates expression of chemokines and cytokines in pancreatic islets: implications for prevention of diabetes in nonobese diabetic mice. Endocrinology 2005;146:1956–64.
102. Riachy R, Vandewalle B, Moerman E, et al. 1,25-Dihydroxyvitamin D3 protects human pancreatic islets against cytokine-induced apoptosis via downregulation of the Fas receptor. Apoptosis 2006;11:151–9.
103. Hahn HJ, Kuttler B, Mathieu C, et al. 1,25-Dihydroxyvitamin D3 reduces MHC antigen expression on pancreatic beta-cells in vitro. Transplant Proc 1997;29: 2156–7.
104. Calle C, Maestro B, Garcia-Arencibia M. Genomic actions of 1,25-dihydroxyvitamin D3 on insulin receptor gene expression, insulin receptor number and insulin activity in the kidney, liver and adipose tissue of streptozotocin-induced diabetic rats. BMC Mol Biol 2008;9:65.
105. George N, Peeyush KT, Antony S, et al. Effect of vitamin D3 in reducing metabolic and oxidative stress in the liver of streptozotocin-induced diabetic rats. Br J Nutr 2012;1–9.
106. Maestro B, Davila N, Carranza MC, et al. Identification of a vitamin D response element in the human insulin receptor gene promoter. J Steroid Biochem Mol Biol 2003;84:223–30.
107. Zhou QG, Hou FF, Guo ZJ, et al. 1,25-Dihydroxyvitamin D improved the free fatty-acid-induced insulin resistance in cultured C2C12 cells. Diabetes Metab Res Rev 2008;24:459–64.
108. Ojuka EO. Role of calcium and AMP kinase in the regulation of mitochondrial biogenesis and GLUT4 levels in muscle. Proc Nutr Soc 2004;63:275–8.
109. Wright DC, Hucker KA, Holloszy JO, et al. Ca^{2+} and AMPK both mediate stimulation of glucose transport by muscle contractions. Diabetes 2004;53: 330–5.
110. Dunlop TW, Vaisanen S, Frank C, et al. The human peroxisome proliferator-activated receptor delta gene is a primary target of 1alpha,25-dihydroxyvitamin D3 and its nuclear receptor. J Mol Biol 2005;349:248–60.
111. Cohen G, Riahi Y, Shamni O, et al. Role of lipid peroxidation and PPAR-delta in amplifying glucose-stimulated insulin secretion. Diabetes 2011;60:2830–42.
112. Coll T, varez-Guardia D, Barroso E, et al. Activation of peroxisome proliferator-activated receptor-{delta} by GW501516 prevents fatty acid-induced nuclear factor-{kappa}B activation and insulin resistance in skeletal muscle cells. Endocrinology 2010;151:1560–9.
113. Duncan BB, Schmidt MI, Pankow JS, et al. Low-grade systemic inflammation and the development of type 2 diabetes: the atherosclerosis risk in communities study. Diabetes 2003;52:1799–805.
114. Hu FB, Meigs JB, Li TY, et al. Inflammatory markers and risk of developing type 2 diabetes in women. Diabetes 2004;53:693–700.
115. Pradhan AD, Manson JE, Rifai N, et al. C-reactive protein, interleukin 6, and risk of developing type 2 diabetes mellitus. JAMA 2001;286:327–34.
116. Gao D, Trayhurn P, Bing C. 1,25-Dihydroxyvitamin D(3) inhibits the cytokine-induced secretion of MCP-1 and reduces monocyte recruitment by human pre-adipocytes. Int J Obes 2012. [Epub ahead of print].

117. Judd SE, Tangpricha V. Vitamin D deficiency and risk for cardiovascular disease. Am J Med Sci 2009;338:40–4.
118. Wang Y, DeLuca HF. Is the vitamin d receptor found in muscle? Endocrinology 2011;152:354–63.
119. Bouillon R, Carmeliet G, Verlinden L, et al. Vitamin D and human health: lessons from vitamin D receptor null mice. Endocr Rev 2008;29:726–76.
120. Gouni-Berthold I, Krone W, Berthold HK. Vitamin D and cardiovascular disease. Curr Vasc Pharmacol 2009;7:414–22.
121. Bouillon R. Vitamin D as potential baseline therapy for blood pressure control. Am J Hypertens 2009;22:816.
122. de Boer I, Kestenbaum B, Shoben AB, et al. 25-hydroxyvitamin D levels inversely associate with risk for developing coronary artery calcification. J Am Soc Nephrol 2009;20:1805–12.
123. Pilz S, Marz W, Wellnitz B, et al. Association of vitamin D deficiency with heart failure and sudden cardiac death in a large cross-sectional study of patients referred for coronary angiography. J Clin Endocrinol Metab 2008;93:3927–35.
124. Lee JH, Gadi R, Spertus JA, et al. Prevalence of vitamin D deficiency in patients with acute myocardial infarction. Am J Cardiol 2011;107:1636–8.
125. Thomas GN, Hartaigh O, Bosch JA, et al. Vitamin D levels predict all-cause and cardiovascular disease mortality in subjects with the metabolic syndrome: the Ludwigshafen Risk and Cardiovascular Health (LURIC) study. Diabetes Care 2012;35:1158–64.
126. Gafter U, Battler A, Eldar M, et al. Effect of hyperparathyroidism on cardiac function in patients with end-stage renal disease. Nephron 1985;41:30–3.
127. Rostand SG, Drueke TB. Parathyroid hormone, vitamin D, and cardiovascular disease in chronic renal failure. Kidney Int 1999;56:383–92.
128. Shoji T, Shinohara K, Kimoto E, et al. Lower risk for cardiovascular mortality in oral 1alpha-hydroxy vitamin D3 users in a haemodialysis population. Nephrol Dial Transplant 2004;19:179–84.
129. Wu SH, Ho SC, Zhong L. Effects of vitamin D supplementation on blood pressure. South Med J 2010;103:729–37.
130. Forman JP, Bischoff-Ferrari HA, Willett WC, et al. Vitamin D intake and risk of incident hypertension: results from three large prospective cohort studies. Hypertension 2005;46:676–82.
131. Witham MD, Nadir MA, Struthers AD. Effect of vitamin D on blood pressure: a systematic review and meta-analysis. J Hypertens 2009;27:1948–54.
132. Autier P, Gandini S. Vitamin D supplementation and total mortality: a meta-analysis of randomized controlled trials. Arch Intern Med 2007;167:1730–7.
133. Avenell A, MacLennan GS, Jenkinson DJ, et al. Long-term follow-up for mortality and cancer in a randomized placebo-controlled trial of vitamin D(3) and/or calcium (RECORD trial). J Clin Endocrinol Metab 2012;97:614–22.
134. Hennekens CH, Barice EJ. Calcium supplements and risk of myocardial infarction: a hypothesis formulated but not yet adequately tested. Am J Med 2011;124:1097–8.
135. Bolland MJ, Avenell A, Baron JA, et al. Effect of calcium supplements on risk of myocardial infarction and cardiovascular events: meta-analysis. BMJ 2010;341:c3691.
136. Bolland MJ, Grey A, Gamble GD, et al. Calcium and vitamin D supplements and health outcomes: a reanalysis of the Women's Health Initiative (WHI) limited-access data set. Am J Clin Nutr 2011;94:1144–9.

137. Elamin MB, bu Elnour NO, Elamin KB, et al. Vitamin D and cardiovascular outcomes: a systematic review and meta-analysis. J Clin Endocrinol Metab 2011;96:1931–42.
138. Xiang W, Kong J, Chen S, et al. Cardiac hypertrophy in vitamin D receptor knockout mice: role of the systemic and cardiac renin-angiotensin systems. Am J Physiol Endocrinol Metab 2005;288:E125–32.
139. Kong J, Qiao G, Zhang Z, et al. Targeted vitamin D receptor expression in juxtaglomerular cells suppresses renin expression independent of parathyroid hormone and calcium. Kidney Int 2008;74:1577–81.
140. Zhou C, Lu F, Cao K, et al. Calcium-independent and 1,25(OH)2D3-dependent regulation of the renin-angiotensin system in 1alpha-hydroxylase knockout mice. Kidney Int 2008;74:170–9.
141. Rahman A, Hershey S, Ahmed S, et al. Heart extracellular matrix gene expression profile in the vitamin D receptor knockout mice. J Steroid Biochem Mol Biol 2007;103:416–9.
142. Simpson RU, Hershey SH, Nibbelink KA. Characterization of heart size and blood pressure in the vitamin D receptor knockout mouse. J Steroid Biochem Mol Biol 2007;103:521–4.
143. Baeke F, Gysemans C, Korf H, et al. Vitamin D insufficiency: implications for the immune system. Pediatr Nephrol 2010;25:1597–606.
144. Colston K, Colston MJ, Feldman D. 1,25-Dihydroxyvitamin D3 and malignant melanoma: the presence of receptors and inhibition of cell growth in culture. Endocrinology 1981;108:1083–6.
145. Abe E, Miyaura C, Sakagami H, et al. Differentiation of mouse myeloid leukemia cells induced by 1 alpha,25-dihydroxyvitamin D3. Proc Natl Acad Sci U S A 1981;78:4990–4.
146. Palmer HG, Gonzalez-Sancho JM, Espada J, et al. Vitamin D(3) promotes the differentiation of colon carcinoma cells by the induction of E-cadherin and the inhibition of beta-catenin signaling. J Cell Biol 2001;154:369–87.
147. Skowronski RJ, Peehl DM, Feldman D. Vitamin D and prostate cancer: 1,25 dihydroxyvitamin D3 receptors and actions in human prostate cancer cell lines. Endocrinology 1993;132:1952–60.
148. Studzinski GP, Rathod B, Wang QM, et al. Uncoupling of cell cycle arrest from the expression of monocytic differentiation markers in HL60 cell variants. Exp Cell Res 1997;232:376–87.
149. Vink-van WT, Pols HA, Buurman CJ, et al. Inhibition of insulin- and insulin-like growth factor-I-stimulated growth of human breast cancer cells by 1,25-dihydroxyvitamin D3 and the vitamin D3 analogue EB1089. Eur J Cancer 1996;32A:842–8.
150. Jensen SS, Madsen MW, Lukas J, et al. Inhibitory effects of 1alpha,25-dihydroxyvitamin D(3) on the G(1)-S phase-controlling machinery. Mol Endocrinol 2001;15:1370–80.
151. Liu M, Lee MH, Cohen M, et al. Transcriptional activation of the Cdk inhibitor p21 by vitamin D3 leads to the induced differentiation of the myelomonocytic cell line U937. Genes Dev 1996;10:142–53.
152. Wang QM, Jones JB, Studzinski GP. Cyclin-dependent kinase inhibitor p27 as a mediator of the G1-S phase block induced by 1,25-dihydroxyvitamin D3 in HL60 cells. Cancer Res 1996;56:264–7.
153. Belochitski O, Ariad S, Shany S, et al. Efficient dual treatment of the hormone-refractory prostate cancer cell line DU145 with cetuximab and 1,25-dihydroxyvitamin D3. In Vivo 2007;21:371–6.

154. Matilainen M, Malinen M, Saavalainen K, et al. Regulation of multiple insulin-like growth factor binding protein genes by 1alpha,25-dihydroxyvitamin D3. Nucleic Acids Res 2005;33:5521–32.

155. Peehl DM, Krishnan AV, Feldman D. Pathways mediating the growth-inhibitory actions of vitamin D in prostate cancer. J Nutr 2003;133:2461S–9S.

156. Kizildag S, Ates H, Kizildag S. Treatment of K562 cells with 1,25-dihydroxyvitamin D(3) induces distinct alterations in the expression of apoptosis-related genes BCL2, BAX, BCL(XL), and p21. Ann Hematol 2009;89:1–7.

157. Baust JM, Klossner DP, Robilotto A, et al. Vitamin D(3) cryosensitization increases prostate cancer susceptibility to cryoablation via mitochondrial-mediated apoptosis and necrosis. BJU Int 2012;109:949–58.

158. Santucci KL, Snyder KK, Baust JM, et al. Use of 1,25alpha dihydroxyvitamin D3 as a cryosensitizing agent in a murine prostate cancer model. Prostate Cancer Prostatic Dis 2011;14:97–104.

159. Wilson EN, Bristol ML, Di X, et al. A switch between cytoprotective and cytotoxic autophagy in the radiosensitization of breast tumor cells by chloroquine and vitamin D. Horm Cancer 2011;2:272–85.

160. Ben-Shoshan M, Amir S, Dang DT, et al. 1alpha,25-dihydroxyvitamin D3 (Calcitriol) inhibits hypoxia-inducible factor-1/vascular endothelial growth factor pathway in human cancer cells. Mol Cancer Ther 2007;6:1433–9.

161. Iglesias-Gato D, Zheng S, Flanagan JN, et al. Substitution at carbon 2 of 19-nor-1alpha,25-dihydroxyvitamin D3 with 3-hydroxypropyl group generates an analogue with enhanced chemotherapeutic potency in PC-3 prostate cancer cells. J Steroid Biochem Mol Biol 2011;127:269–75.

162. Kouchi Z, Fujiwara Y, Yamaguchi H, et al. Phosphatidylinositol 5-phosphate 4-kinase type II beta is required for vitamin D receptor-dependent E-cadherin expression in SW480 cells. Biochem Biophys Res Commun 2011;408:523–9.

163. Ooi LL, Zheng Y, Zhou H, et al. Vitamin D deficiency promotes growth of MCF-7 human breast cancer in a rodent model of osteosclerotic bone metastasis. Bone 2010;47:795–803.

164. Tangpricha V, Spina C, Yao M, et al. Vitamin D deficiency enhances the growth of MC-26 colon cancer xenografts in Balb/c mice. J Nutr 2005;135:2350–4.

165. Newmark HL, Yang K, Kurihara N, et al. Western-style diet-induced colonic tumors and their modulation by calcium and vitamin D in C57Bl/6 mice: a preclinical model for human sporadic colon cancer. Carcinogenesis 2009;30: 88–92.

166. Yang K, Kurihara N, Fan K, et al. Dietary induction of colonic tumors in a mouse model of sporadic colon cancer. Cancer Res 2008;68:7803–10.

167. Zinser GM, Sundberg JP, Welsh J. Vitamin D(3) receptor ablation sensitizes skin to chemically induced tumorigenesis. Carcinogenesis 2002;23:2103–9.

168. Zinser GM, Suckow M, Welsh J. Vitamin D receptor (VDR) ablation alters carcinogen-induced tumorigenesis in mammary gland, epidermis and lymphoid tissues. J Steroid Biochem Mol Biol 2005;97:153–64.

169. Mordan-McCombs S, Brown T, Wang WL, et al. Tumor progression in the LPB-Tag transgenic model of prostate cancer is altered by vitamin D receptor and serum testosterone status. J Steroid Biochem Mol Biol 2010;121:368–71.

170. Larriba MJ, Ordonez-Moran P, Chicote I, et al. Vitamin D receptor deficiency enhances Wnt/beta-catenin signaling and tumor burden in colon cancer. PLoS One 2011;6:e23524.

171. Zheng Y, Zhou H, Ooi LL, et al. Vitamin D deficiency promotes prostate cancer growth in bone. Prostate 2011;71:1012–21.

172. Garland CF, Garland FC. Do sunlight and vitamin D reduce the likelihood of colon cancer? Int J Epidemiol 1980;9:227–31.
173. Millen AE, Wactawski-Wende J, Pettinger M, et al. Predictors of serum 25-hydroxyvitamin D concentrations among postmenopausal women: the Women's Health Initiative Calcium plus Vitamin D clinical trial. Am J Clin Nutr 2010;91:1324–35.
174. Fedirko V, Bostick RM, Goodman M, et al. Blood 25-hydroxyvitamin D3 concentrations and incident sporadic colorectal adenoma risk: a pooled case-control study. Am J Epidemiol 2010;172:489–500.
175. Jenab M, Bueno-de-Mesquita HB, Ferrari P, et al. Association between prediagnostic circulating vitamin D concentration and risk of colorectal cancer in European populations: a nested case-control study. BMJ 2010;340:b5500. http://dx.doi.org/10.1136/bmj.b5500.
176. Lee JE, Li H, Chan AT, et al. Circulating levels of vitamin D and colon and rectal cancer: the Physicians' Health Study and a meta-analysis of prospective studies. Cancer Prev Res (Phila) 2011;4:735–43.
177. Wactawski-Wende J, Kotchen JM, Anderson GL, et al. Calcium plus vitamin D supplementation and the risk of colorectal cancer. N Engl J Med 2006;354:684–96.
178. Lappe JM, Travers-Gustafson D, Davies KM, et al. Vitamin D and calcium supplementation reduces cancer risk: results of a randomized trial. Am J Clin Nutr 2007;85:1586–91.
179. Ahearn TU, McCullough ML, Flanders WD, et al. A randomized clinical trial of the effects of supplemental calcium and vitamin D3 on markers of their metabolism in normal mucosa of colorectal adenoma patients. Cancer Res 2011;71:413–23.

Glucocorticoid-Induced Osteoporosis and Osteonecrosis

Robert S. Weinstein, MD

KEYWORDS

- Glucocorticoid-induced apoptosis • Osteoblasts • Osteocytes • Osteoclasts
- Bone vascularity • Bisphosphonates • Teriparatide • Denosumab

KEY POINTS

- Glucocorticoids are the most common cause of secondary osteoporosis and nontraumatic osteonecrosis.
- Adverse skeletal events are the most common glucocorticoid-related complications associated with successful litigation.
- Disparity between bone quantity and quality in glucocorticoid-induced osteoporosis (GIO) makes ultrasound or bone mineral density measurements inadequate for identifying patients at risk of fracture.
- Continuous treatment with 10 mg/d of prednisone for more than 90 days has a 7-fold increase in hip fractures and a 17-fold increase in vertebral fractures.
- The adverse effects of glucocorticoids on the skeleton are caused by direct actions on bone cells.
- Laboratory testing should include measurement of serum 25-hydroxyvitamin D, creatinine, and calcium (in addition to glucose, potassium, and lipids).
- The World Health Organization fracture prevention algorithm (FRAX) underestimates fracture risk in GIO.
- Bisphosphonates are first-line options for GIO and may also be useful in glucocorticoid-induced osteonecrosis.
- Teriparatide counteracts several fundamental aspects of the pathophysiology of GIO.
- Denosumab is useful in patients with renal insufficiency and stable serum calcium who are not candidates for bisphosphonates or teriparatide.
- Do not wait. Start antifracture treatment at the onset of a course of glucocorticoid therapy of more than 10 mg/d of prednisone expected to last more than 90 days.

Support: This material is based on work supported by a VA Merit Review Grant from the Office of Research and Development, Department of Veterans Affairs and the National Institutes of Health (P01-AG13918). The author has no potential conflicts of interest relevant to this article.
Division of Endocrinology and Metabolism, Center for Osteoporosis and Metabolic Bone Diseases, Department of Internal Medicine, and Central Arkansas Veterans Healthcare System at the University of Arkansas for Medical Sciences, 4301 West Markham Street, Slot 587, Little Rock, AR 72205-7199, USA
E-mail address: weinsteinroberts@uams.edu

Endocrinol Metab Clin N Am 41 (2012) 595–611
doi:10.1016/j.ecl.2012.04.004
0889-8529/12/$ – see front matter Published by Elsevier Inc.

INTRODUCTION

"A marked osteoporosis of the skeleton was found, it being easily possible to cut the vertebral bodies with a knife, the spongy part of the bone having largely disappeared." Cushing[1] described these adverse effects of long-term endogenous hypercortisolism on bone in his 1932 presentation to the Johns Hopkins Medical Society. Eighteen years later, only 1 year after the introduction of cortisone for the treatment of rheumatoid arthritis, clinicians became aware of the rapidly injurious skeletal effects of glucocorticoid administration.[2,3] At first, it was uncertain whether the hip fractures that had occurred were the result of falls caused by steroid myopathy or merely coincidental with cortisone therapy because vertebral fractures and radiographic osteoporosis had not yet been observed. However, within just a few more years, osteoporosis and fractures were clearly recognized as skeletal complications of treatment with cortisone, prednisolone, and prednisone.[4] Collapse of the femoral and humeral heads after high-dose therapy was described shortly thereafter.[5,6] Today, glucocorticoid administration is the most common cause of secondary osteoporosis and the leading cause of nontraumatic osteonecrosis. In patients receiving long-term therapy, glucocorticoids induce fractures in 30% to 50% and osteonecrosis in 9% to 40%.[7,8] Patients are seldom warned about these side effects and, as a result, adverse skeletal events are the most common glucocorticoid-related complications associated with successful litigation.[9]

GLUCOCORTICOID-INDUCED OSTEOPOROSIS
Risk Factors

Bone loss in glucocorticoid-induced osteoporosis (GIO) is biphasic, with a rapid reduction in bone mineral density (BMD) of 6% to 12% within the first year, followed by a slower annual loss of about 3% for as long as the glucocorticoids are administered.[10] However, the relative risk of fracture escalates by as much as 75% within the first 3 months after initiation of glucocorticoid therapy and this often occurs before a significant decline in BMD.[11] There is also a decrease in the risk of fractures within the first 3 months after the glucocorticoids are discontinued, before any improvement in BMD. The rapid onset and offset of the fracture risk suggest a qualitative defect in bone material properties not captured by bone densitometry.[11] Furthermore, more than one-third of postmenopausal women receiving long-term glucocorticoid therapy may have 1 or more asymptomatic vertebral fractures without abnormal results on calcaneal ultrasound or lumbar and hip BMD determinations.[12] Thus, the disparity between bone quantity and quality in GIO makes ultrasound or BMD measurements inadequate for identifying who is at risk of fractures.[13]

Several large case-controlled studies show clear and strong associations between glucocorticoid exposure and fracture.[11,14] An increase in vertebral and hip fractures occurs with as little as 2.5 to 7.5 mg/d of prednisolone (equivalent to 3.1–9.3 mg of prednisone). In a cohort study of patients aged 18 to 64 years receiving glucocorticoids for a variety of disorders, the combination of higher dose, longer duration, and continuous use had the greatest effect on the incidence of fractures.[14] Continuous treatment with 10 mg/d of prednisone for more than 90 days was associated with a 7-fold increase in hip fractures and a 17-fold increase in vertebral fractures.[14] At present, evidence suggests that the risk of fracture is small and intervention is not required with single-dose pack prescriptions, intermittent oral therapy with a cumulative exposure of less than 1 g per year, or replacement therapy for patients with hypopituitarism, adrenal insufficiency, or congenital adrenal hyperplasia, provided that the replacement doses are not excessive and the recommendations for increased dosage during periods of stress are not supraphysiologic or inappropriate (eg, as with mental stress as opposed to febrile or gastrointestinal illnesses).[7,15]

The risk of GIO is probably the same in men and women of all ethnicities.[16] Risk factors include advancing age, prolonged duration of treatment, increased daily dosage and cumulative dose (multiple courses of high-dose oral or intravenous therapy on a baseline of low doses also increase risk), low body mass index, prevalent fractures, frequent falls, underlying disease (especially organ transplants, inflammatory bowel disease and the accompanying malabsorption, rheumatoid arthritis, polymyalgia rheumatica, and chronic pulmonary disease), and polymorphisms in the glucocorticoid receptor (**Table 1**).[7,17–20] Another factor is the activity of the 11β-hydroxysteroid dehydrogenase (11β-HSD) system, a prereceptor modulator of corticosteroid action.[21] Two isoenzymes, 11β-HSD1 and 11β-HSD2, catalyze the interconversion of hormonally active glucocorticoids (such as cortisol or prednisolone) and inactive glucocorticoids (such as cortisone or prednisone). The 11β-HSD1 enzyme is an activator and the 11β-HSD2 enzyme is an inactivator. Increased fractures caused by glucocorticoid administration in the elderly may be attributed to the increase in 11β-HSD1 that occurs with aging.[21]

Table 1
Risk factors for GIO

Risk Factor	Explanation
Advancing age	Elderly patients receiving glucocorticoid therapy have a 26-fold higher risk of vertebral fractures than younger patients and a shorter interval between initiation of treatment and the occurrence of fracture[14]
Low body mass index	Significant risk factor for GIO and probably fractures[13]
Underlying disease	Rheumatoid arthritis, polymyalgia rheumatica, inflammatory bowel disease, chronic pulmonary disease, and transplantation are independent risk factors[7]
Family history of hip fracture, prevalent fractures, smoking, excessive alcohol consumption, frequent falls	All are independent risk factors for osteoporosis but have not been well studied in patients receiving glucocorticoids
Glucocorticoid receptor genotype	Individual glucocorticoid sensitivity may be regulated by polymorphisms in the glucocorticoid receptor gene[17]
11β-HSD isoenzymes	11β-HSD1 expression increases with aging and glucocorticoid administration and thereby enhances glucocorticoid activation[18]
Glucocorticoid dose (peak, current, or cumulative dose; duration of therapy; interval)	There may be no safe dose, although this is controversial. However, the risk of fracture escalates with increased doses and duration of therapy. Alternate day or inhalation therapy does not spare the skeleton[7,15]
Low BMD	Glucocorticoid-induced fractures occur independently of a decline in bone mass but patients with very low bone density may be at higher risk[7,13]

Abbreviation: 11β-HSD, 11β-hydroxysteroid dehydrogenase.

Natural and synthetic glucocorticoids differ in their vulnerability to 11β-HSD2, the inactivation enzyme. In dexamethasone, the 11-hydroxyl is already present as it is in prednisolone, but the fluorine atom at the 9α position of the B ring both extends the potency and occludes the 11β location. Dexamethasone causes more osteoporosis and osteonecrosis than prednisone, possibly because it is resistant to inactivation by 11β-HSD2.[8]

Pathogenesis

Histomorphometric studies in patients with GIO consistently show reduced numbers of osteoblasts on cancellous bone and diminished wall width, a measure of the work performed by these cells (**Box 1**, **Fig. 1**).[7,22,23] The decreased osteoblasts are caused by the direct effects of glucocorticoids decreasing the production of new osteoblast precursors and causing premature apoptosis of the mature, matrix-secreting osteoblasts. Inadequate numbers of osteoblasts and incomplete erosion cavity repair during bone remodeling are the main causes of the reduction in cancellous bone area, wall width, trabecular width, and bone formation rate typically found in GIO.[22] Increased osteocyte apoptosis also occurs and is associated with decreases in vascular endothelial growth factor (VEGF), skeletal angiogenesis, bone interstitial fluid, and bone strength.[24] Bone water represents at least 20% to 25% of the wet weight of bone and confers to bone much of its unique strength and resilience by reducing stress during dynamic loading. Tensile and compressive strength, modulus of elasticity, and hardness increase with decreasing bone water content but deformation and toughness, the energy absorbed before failure (ie, fracture), are greater for wet bone compared with dry bone. Both aging and glucocorticoid excess cause a reduction in bone blood flow and the volume of water present in the skeleton.[24]

Osteocytes and the lacunar-canalicular network are the strain-sensing system of bone and signal the need for remodeling to accommodate prevailing loads or repair damage. Transmission of fluid shear stresses to the lacunar-canalicular network is critical for the mechanosensing function of the osteocytes and the mechanical

---

Box 1
Fundamental histologic features of GIO

Cancellous bone

    Marked reduction in bone area with decreased trabecular width

    Diminished wall width

    Decreased osteoid area

    Decreased numbers of osteoblasts

    Increased prevalence of osteoblast and osteocyte apoptosis

    Normal or slightly increased numbers of osteoclasts

    Prolongation of the reversal phase

    Decreased rate of bone formation

    Decreased bone blood supply and interstitial fluid

Cortical bone

    Increased cortical porosity

    Increased prevalence of osteocyte apoptosis

    Decreased rate of bone formation

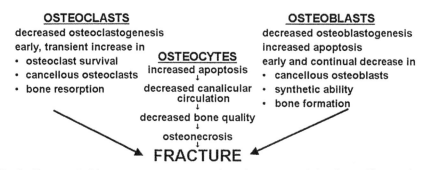

Fig. 1. Glucocorticoid excess causes osteoporosis and osteonecrosis by direct effects on bone cells.

adaptation of bone to mechanical forces. Thus, glucocorticoid-induced osteocyte apoptosis could account for the loss of bone strength that occurs before loss of BMD[25] and the resultant mismatch between bone quantity and quality in patients with GIO.[7,12,13,24]

Glucocorticoid excess also directly reduces osteoclast production but, in contrast with the increase in osteoblast apoptosis, the lifespan of osteoclasts is prolonged. Therefore, with long-term therapy, osteoclast numbers are usually maintained in the normal range, whereas osteoblasts and bone formation decrease.[22,26] These histologic features are distinct from those found in other forms of osteoporosis. Loss of gonadal function and secondary hyperparathyroidism are characterized by increased osteoclasts, osteoblasts, and bone formation rate. These different histologic features and the evidence that the skeletal effects of glucocorticoid excess override those caused by sex steroid deficiency, that fractures are similarly prevalent in amenorrheic and eumenorrheic women with Cushing syndrome, and that parathyroid hormone levels are not increased by exogenous glucocorticoids indicate that hypogonadism and secondary hyperparathyroidism are not part of the pathogenesis of GIO.[27–30]

The primary adverse effects of glucocorticoid excess on the skeleton are directly on the bone cells, as is evident from experiments in transgenic mice overexpressing 11β-HSD2, the enzyme that inactivates glucocorticoids in a prereceptor fashion.[23–26] Mice harboring the transgene in osteoblast and osteocytes are protected from prednisolone-induced apoptosis and decreased osteoblast number, osteoid production, and bone formation, but lost bone because the osteoclasts were still exposed to the prednisolone. However, bone strength was preserved in the transgenic animals in spite of the loss of bone, suggesting that osteocyte viability independently contributes to bone strength.[23] Using the same approach, overexpression of 11β-HSD2 in osteoclasts preserved bone but did not prevent the prednisolone-induced decrease in osteoblast number, osteoid production, and bone formation.[26]

Glucocorticoids reduce osteoblast differentiation by attenuating Akt (protein kinase B) phosphorylation and increasing activation of the redox-sensitive forkhead box subgroup O transcription factor family (FoxOs), which in turn inhibit wingless (Wnt)/β-catenin signaling, which is a critical pathway for the generation of osteoblasts.[31] Glucocorticoids also enhance the expression of Dickkopf-1, an antagonist of the Wnt pathway, and suppress bone morphogenetic proteins, factors required to induce osteoblast differentiation.[32] In addition, glucocorticoids increase production of peroxisome proliferator-activated receptor γ, a transcription factor that induces terminal adipocyte differentiation, while suppressing osteoblast differentiation, potentially contributing to increased marrow fat and reduced osteoblasts.[33]

In osteoblastic linage cells, glucocorticoids stimulate production of the receptor activator of NF-κB ligand (RANKL), which is essential for the generation and survival of osteoclasts, and reduce osteoblastic expression of osteoprotegerin (OPG), a decoy receptor for RANKL.[34] However, exogenous glucocorticoids may not alter RANKL or OPG mRNA levels in vivo.[26] Moreover, recent work indicates that RANKL produced by osteoblasts or their progenitors does not contribute to bone remodeling in mature animals and that osteocytes are the major RANKL-producing cells that control osteoclast formation.[35]

Patient Evaluation

Physicians who prescribe glucocorticoids should educate their patients about side effects and complications including osteoporosis and osteonecrosis, cataract and glaucoma, hypokalemia, hyperglycemia, hypertension, hyperlipidemia, weight gain, fluid retention, easy bruising, susceptibility to infection, impaired healing, myopathy, adrenal insufficiency, and the steroid withdrawal syndrome. Patients receiving long-term glucocorticoid therapy should carry a steroid therapy card or wear medication identification jewelry. A document signed by the patient acknowledging disclosure of the possible side effects should be placed in the patient's chart (**Boxes 2 and 3**).[7,36] Malpractice suits precipitated by failure to document disclosure of the skeletal complications to patients are common.[7,37] In a review of the Westlaw database from 1996 to 2008, avascular necrosis was reported as a complication of glucocorticoid therapy in 39% and osteoporosis and fractures in 12% of the litigation that went to court.[9] In spite of this, the bone complications are ignored by most specialists who prescribe glucocorticoids, possibly because of the physicians' greater concern for other coexisting disorders, their unfamiliarity with metabolic disorders of the skeleton, or lack of appreciation of the rapidity of the substantial increase in risk of fracture.[16]

Laboratory testing should include measurement of serum 25-hydroxyvitamin D (25OHD), creatinine, and calcium (in addition to glucose, potassium, and lipids). It is particularly important to check the 25OHD level before the administration of antiresorptive agents to avoid drug-induced hypocalcemia, especially because glucocorticoid use is independently associated with low serum 25OHD and the chances of severe vitamin D deficiency with levels less than 10 ng/mL in GIO are doubled.[38] The association of glucocorticoid use and vitamin D deficiency may be

---

Box 2
Evaluation of the patient about to receive glucocorticoids

Explain the rationale behind the use of glucocorticoids, expected benefits, and alternatives

Use the lowest possible dose and shortest possible course of treatment

Inform the patient of the side effects of glucocorticoid therapy

Document informed consent of the patient

Recommend a steroid identification card and medication identification jewelry

Measure:

    25-Hydroxyvitamin D

    Creatinine

    Calcium

    Glucose, potassium, and lipids

Obtain baseline height, vertebral morphologic assessment, and BMD

Box 3
Information for patients about to receive glucocorticoids

Under certain circumstances, serious medical problems must be treated with potent medications that are intended to improve the patient's condition but have the potential for severe side effects. Your doctor has decided that the risk of allowing your present illness to progress without glucocorticoid treatment outweighs the risk of the possible side effects. There are several similar glucocorticoid medications produced by different manufactures under many different names. The most common names are corticosteroids, cortisone, cortisol or hydrocortisone (Cortef), prednisone (Deltasone), prednisolone, methyl prednisolone (Medrol), and dexamethasone (Decadron or Dexasone). While receiving glucocorticoids, medication identification jewelry and carrying a card listing all your medications is recommended.

The following side effects are common and are seen in most individuals who receive these drugs for more than a few days:

1. Fluid retention and weight gain
2. Increased appetite
3. Fullness of the face
4. Easy bruising

Other less common side effects may occur after longer periods of drug administration:

1. Osteoporosis and fractures
2. Collapse of large joints such as the hip, shoulder, knee, or ankle
3. Loss of potassium
4. Increased blood glucose or loss of control of diabetes
5. Increased cholesterol and triglycerides
6. Glaucoma and cataracts
7. Delicate skin with impaired wound healing, stretch marks, discoloration, and acne
8. Increased susceptibility to infection, especially fungal infections
9. Fluid retention and congestive heart failure
10. Increased blood pressure
11. Muscle weakness
12. Indigestion and heartburn, abdominal pain, bloody or tarry stools
13. Insomnia
14. Increased sweating
15. Headache or dizziness
16. Memory problems, difficulty concentrating, depression, mood swings
17. Adrenal insufficiency and glucocorticoid withdrawal symptoms

This list is not all-inclusive. Patients receiving glucocorticoids should never adjust or stop the medication without consulting a physician. Your physician will discuss these side effects with you. By signing this document, you acknowledge that you have been informed of the reason for the use of glucocorticoid medication; the alternative treatments, if any; as well as the potential benefits and risks that are involved. You acknowledge that you have read the statements listed earlier and have been able to ask questions and express concerns, which have been satisfactorily responded to by your physician. You have been given a copy of this consent form.

Patient's signature _____ Witness _____

Physician's signature _____ Date _____

caused by glucocorticoid-induced enhancement of 24-hydroxylase transcription and increased inactivation of 25OHD, or may simply be a result of the underlying disease, nutritional status, and limited solar exposure of the patients.[38] Adequate calcium and vitamin D supplementation should be recommended.[7]

Bone turnover after long-term glucocorticoid therapy is low, so biochemical markers of bone metabolism are not usually helpful. However, if biomarkers have been already obtained and are increased, another problem besides GIO may be present. Prevalent fractures, vertebral morphologic assessment from digital images obtained by x-ray absorptiometry, spinal radiographs, or loss of height may help identify patients at risk of additional fractures. BMD measurements are inadequate for identifying which patients are particularly at risk, but BMD is useful in follow-up after intervention because the values should not decrease if the intervention was effective. The World Health Organization fracture prevention algorithm (FRAX) underestimates the risk of glucocorticoid-induced fractures because the current dose, cumulative dose, and duration of therapy are not entered into the calculation, the algorithm uses femoral neck density values but vertebral fractures are more common than hip fractures with glucocorticoid excess, and inclusion of the common risk factors for postmenopausal osteoporosis in the algorithm may not be applicable to GIO.[7]

Treatment

Bisphosphonates are considered first-line options for GIO at least in part because of the long experience with these drugs in postmenopausal osteoporosis, their ease of use, and low cost (**Table 2**).[7] Randomized, placebo-controlled trials have shown that alendronate, risedronate, and zoledronic acid are effective for this indication and reduce the risk of vertebral but not hip fractures.[41–43] Nitrogen-containing bisphosphonates induce apoptosis of osteoclasts and inhibit bone resorption,[44] but glucocorticoids antagonize this effect,[45] and this may account for the limited ability of these antiresorptive agents to protect BMD in GIO compared with other forms of osteoporosis.[38,46,47] In addition, alendronate decreases glucocorticoid-induced osteocyte apoptosis,[48] which may play a role in the preservation of bone strength.[25] The evidence for bisphosphonate treatment in GIO is not as strong as that for postmenopausal osteoporosis because the primary end point in the glucocorticoid treatment trials was BMD rather than fracture, and glucocorticoids induce a susceptibility to fracture independently of BMD. In addition, most studies were only 12 to 18 months in duration and insufficient numbers of patients were recruited to study hip fractures. Side effects and disadvantages of bisphosphonate therapy are given in **Table 2**.

An advantage of oral bisphosphonates is that they can be stopped if glucocorticoids are discontinued, but compliance with oral therapy is poor. Yearly infusions of zoledronic acid resolve this problem and provide rapid skeletal protection. If a patient presents for fracture protection and glucocorticoid administration has already been continuous with more than 10 mg/d of prednisone for longer than 90 days, there may not be time to wait for the delayed protective effects of oral bisphosphonates because of their average oral absorption of 0.7%, weekly or monthly administration, and lower molar potency compared with intravenous zoledronic acid.[49] For example, 63 mg of alendronate will be absorbed after 90 days of treatment with 70 mg/wk compared with 5 mg of zoledronic acid in 15 minutes, but the potency of alendronate is about 10-fold less than zoledronic acid. About 12% to 15% of patients with GIO who are receiving their first infusion of zoledronic acid experience an acute-phase reaction within 2 to 3 days and lasting less than 3 days.[43] The mild pyrexia, musculoskeletal pains, and flulike symptoms are effectively managed with acetaminophen or ibuprofen

Table 2
Treatment of GIO

Intervention	Advantages	Disadvantages
Alendronate (oral, 10 mg/d or 70 mg/wk), risedronate (5 mg/d or 35 mg/wk)	Osteoclast inhibition reduces bone loss. Alendronate also prevents glucocorticoid-induced osteocyte apoptosis. If glucocorticoids are discontinued, these drugs can be stopped	Antiresorptive agents do not directly address the decreased bone formation characteristic of glucocorticoid-induced bone disease. Additional problems include gastrointestinal side effects, rare uveitis, poor compliance with oral therapy, and the time required to obtain skeletal protection. Avoid in patients with a creatinine clearance less than 30 mL/min
Zoledronic acid (5 mg/y intravenously)	Osteoclast inhibition reduces bone loss. Increased compliance compared with oral treatment and rapid onset of skeletal effects. Gastrointestinal side effects are unlikely	Does not address the reduced bone formation caused by glucocorticoid excess. Avoid in patients with a creatinine clearance less than 30 mL/min
Teriparatide (20 μg/d subcutaneously)	Directly addresses the pathogenesis of GIO. Reduces vertebral fractures	Cost, daily injections are required, reduced response with high-dose glucocorticoids. Not studied in patients with increased parathyroid hormone levels. Adverse effects: mild hypercalcemia, headache, nausea, leg cramps, dizziness. Caution with preexisting nephrolithiasis. Check serum calcium at least once ≥16 h after injection and adjust oral calcium intake as needed[39]
Denosumab (60 mg subcutaneously every 6 mo)	Potent inhibitor of osteoclasts with ease of administration. Can be stopped if glucocorticoids are discontinued. Useful in renal insufficiency	Does not address the reduced bone formation caused by glucocorticoid excess. Not yet approved for GIO
Vertebroplasty, kyphoplasty	Commonly used to treat recent painful vertebral fractures	Beneficial effects similar to sham procedures. Dangers of cement leakage. Increased incidence of additional fractures in patients receiving glucocorticoids[40]

and seldom occur with subsequent infusions. Substantial BMD loss occurs in patients who discontinue bisphosphonates while receiving glucocorticoids, so the recommended duration of therapy is typically at least as long as the steroids are prescribed.[50] However, studies to determine the optimal duration of antifracture intervention have not been done. All the drugs used for the treatment of GIO require caution if the patient has childbearing potential.

Bisphosphonates are associated with osteonecrosis of the jaw, a disorder characterized by exposed maxillofacial bone for at least 8 weeks, typically diagnosed after a dental extraction or other invasive procedure, and associated with poor dental hygiene and infection with *Actinomyces*.[51] The disorder occurs mainly in patients with osteolytic breast cancer or multiple myeloma who receive frequent high-dose intravenous bisphosphonates in addition to chemotherapy. In patients with osteoporosis treated with bisphosphonates, the risk of osteonecrosis of the jaw is between 1 in 10,000 and 1 in 100,000 patient years.[51] Before prescribing bisphosphonates, the clinician should perform an oral examination and encourage patients to be seen by a dentist. Bisphosphonates may also be associated with atypical subtrochanteric or diaphyseal femoral fractures but, if so, the risk is about 2 per 10,000 patient years.[52] Glucocorticoid use has been reported in bisphosphonate-treated patients with osteonecrosis of the jaw and atypical femoral fractures, but evidence for a causal effect of the steroids is absent.

An alternative treatment of GIO is teriparatide, recombinant human parathyroid hormone (1–34). In an 18-month randomized, double-blind, controlled, head-to-head trial, teriparatide increased spinal BMD faster and to a greater extent than alendronate and also reduced vertebral fractures (0.6% vs 6.1%, P = .004).[53] Teriparatide represents a particularly rational approach to GIO by counteracting several fundamental aspects of its pathophysiology. The expected glucocorticoid-induced increase in osteoblast and osteocyte apoptosis and decrease in osteoblast number, bone formation, and bone strength are prevented by teriparatide. Decreased osteoblast apoptosis leads to an increase in bone formation and decreased osteocyte apoptosis is associated with preservation of bone strength.[54] Furthermore, teriparatide abrogates the negative impact of glucocorticoids on Akt activation and Wnt signaling. However, the anabolic effect of teriparatide is compromised by high-dose glucocorticoid therapy.[55] Dose and duration of glucocorticoid treatment, as well as host factors such as severity of the underlying illness, weight loss, concurrent medications, renal function, and low insulinlike growth factor I levels may contribute to the diminished efficacy of teriparatide in GIO compared with other forms of osteoporosis.[54] Disadvantages of teriparatide include the need for daily subcutaneous injections, refrigeration, cost, side effects (headache, nausea, dizziness, leg cramps), occasional mild hypercalcemia, and caution required in patients with nephrolithiasis or increased baseline levels of parathyroid hormone (see **Table 2**).[39]

Another potential treatment option is denosumab, a humanized monoclonal antibody to RANKL approved for the prevention of vertebral, nonvertebral, and hip fractures in women with postmenopausal osteoporosis, but not yet for GIO.[56] In a randomized, double-blind, placebo-controlled trial of denosumab in 61 patients with rheumatoid arthritis receiving less than 15 mg/d of prednisone and methotrexate, BMD of the spine and hip increased with denosumab to the same extent as in 88 patients receiving methotrexate and denosumab alone.[57] Furthermore, there was no difference in adverse effects compared with placebo and methotrexate. Denosumab may be considered for glucocorticoid-treated patients with renal insufficiency and stable serum calcium levels who are not candidates for bisphosphonates or teriparatide (see **Table 2**). The ease of administration as a subcutaneous injection every 6 months may increase compliance. In a murine model of glucocorticoid-induced bone disease treated with osteoprotegerin, a decoy receptor for RANKL representing a similar strategy in GIO as treatment with denosumab, bone strength and osteocyte viability were protected and associated with preservation of the osteocyte-lacunar-canalicular network.[58]

In patients with GIO, incapacitating adjacent vertebral fractures have been reported days after kyphoplasty, suggesting that caution should be exercised before recommending the procedure in these patients.[40]

GLUCOCORTICOID-INDUCED OSTEONECROSIS

Aseptic, avascular or ischemic necrosis, and bone infarctions are other terms for osteonecrosis. The most common joint involved is the hip and the most common cause of the disorder is trauma. Glucocorticoids are the second most common cause.[8] There are many other causes in adults including alcohol, sickle cell disease, ionizing radiation, Gaucher disease, Caisson disease or decompression sickness, and idiopathic causes. However, before concluding that any case of osteonecrosis is idiopathic, a thorough history for pain shots is essential. A pain shot is a general term for a glucocorticoid, narcotic, nonsteroidal antiinflammatory drug, or local anesthetic injection. If it was intra-articular or epidural, glucocorticoid and/or local anesthetic injections were likely. The patient may have received many of these injections but still deny the use of corticosteroids, cortisone, cortisol or hydrocortisone (Cortef), prednisone (Deltasone), prednisolone, methyl prednisolone (Medrol), or dexamethasone (Decadron or Dexasone).

Risk Factors

The incidence of glucocorticoid-induced osteonecrosis increases with higher doses and prolonged treatment, although it may occur with short-term exposure to high doses, by intra-articular injection, and without osteoporosis (**Box 4**). In the Westlaw database, oral doses as low as 290 mg of prednisone and courses as short as 6 days were thought to be responsible for osteonecrosis.[9] Many of these trials could have been avoided if informed consent had been documented.

Intra-articular glucocorticoids may be particularly dangerous because the injection may accelerate joint damage by alleviating pain, thus increasing weight bearing (a kind of Charcot arthropathy), in addition to the direct adverse effects of the steroids on bone. Osteonecrosis has been noted in just weeks to months after intra-articular injection of cumulative doses of 80 to 160 mg of methylprednisolone.[8]

Box 4
Risk factors for glucocorticoid-induced osteonecrosis

Risk factors

Dose and duration of therapy

Intra-articular administration

Polymorphisms in VEGF, GR, 11β-HSD2, COL2A1, PAI1, P-glycoprotein

Underlying disorders: renal insufficiency, transplantation, graft-versus-host disease, inflammatory bowel disease, human immunodeficiency virus (HIV), acute lymphoblastic leukemia

Dexamethasone causes greater skeletal complications than prednisone

Abbreviations: 11β-HSD2, 11β-hydroxysteroid dehydrogenase type2; COL2A1, collagen type II; PA1, plasminogen activator inhibitor 1; GR, glucocorticoid receptor.

Pathogenesis

Osteonecrosis has been postulated to be caused by fat embolism, vascular thrombosis, and fatigue fractures, but recent attention is focused on the role of osteocyte apoptosis.[7,8] Abundant apoptotic osteocytes and lining cells are found juxtaposed to the subchondral fracture crescent in femoral heads removed at surgery for glucocorticoid-induced osteonecrosis (**Fig. 2**).[59] Glucocorticoid-induced osteocyte apoptosis, a cumulative and irreparable defect, disrupts the mechanosensory function of the osteocyte-lacunar-canalicular system and thus starts the inexorable sequence of events leading to collapse of the joint.

Evaluation

Persistent hip or shoulder pain, especially with joint movement, tenderness, or reduced range of motion, warrants magnetic resonance imaging (MRI) because of the association of glucocorticoid therapy with osteonecrosis.[8] The pathognomonic, subchondral crescent sign seen on radiographic examination may not be present in the early stages of osteonecrosis and MRI can reveal extensive osteonecrosis before any change in the shape of the femoral head or appearance of a fracture crescent on radiographs.

Treatment

For advanced disease with obliteration of the acetabular articular space and osteophyte formation, total hip replacement is usually required. Osteonecrosis is the most common cause of total hip replacement in young adults, but problems with infection, osteolysis, dislocation, and revisions are worse with hip replacement for

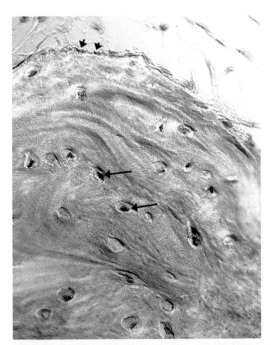

Fig. 2. Osteocyte apoptosis in glucocorticoid-induced osteonecrosis of the hip. Femoral head specimen taken from a patient with glucocorticoid-induced osteonecrosis during hip replacement. Apoptotic osteocytes (*arrows*) and lining cells (*arrowheads*) are stained brown by in situ end labeling (×200).

glucocorticoid-induced osteonecrosis than for osteoarthritis.[8,37] Because these replacements have about a 10-year lifespan, any delay in the need for surgery is welcome. For these reasons, recent evidence of the usefulness of bisphosphonates in the treatment of osteonecrosis is promising.

In a randomized, controlled, open-label trial, adults with osteonecrosis treated with alendronate had significant retardation of femoral head collapse and reduced need for total hip replacement compared with the control group over 24 months.[60] Sustained improvement in pain and ambulation was reported within months. In another study, a 10-year follow-up of patients with early to moderately advanced osteonecrosis treated with alendronate for only the first 3 years showed decreased use of analgesics, increased ability to function as desired, and improvement in standing and ambulation time within months that lasted up to 10 years.[61]

A recent report assessed the efficacy of treatment of early-stage osteonecrosis of the femoral head with core decompression and autologous implantation of bone marrow–derived and culture-expanded mesenchymal stem cells.[62] Five years after the procedure, 4% of the hips assigned to autologous implantation had deteriorated compared with 23% of the hips that received core decompression alone. However, this procedure is complicated and operator-dependent and may not be widely reproducible. Furthermore, even without surgical treatment, as many as 40% of small, medially located, early osteonecrotic lesions may not progress.[8]

AREAS OF UNCERTAINTY

Precise prediction of the risk of fracture is currently not possible in GIO and efforts to alert physicians prescribing glucocorticoids to their responsibilities to prevent bone complications have met with limited success. More data are needed to establish precise clinical thresholds for intervention and develop strategies to convey this information to physicians and patients. In addition, more research is required to ascertain the optimal duration of protective therapy, best treatment of premenopausal women, and efficacy of long-term use of teriparatide.[63]

SUMMARY

- Glucocorticoid administration is the most common cause of secondary osteoporosis and the leading cause of nontraumatic osteonecrosis.
- Patients are seldom warned about these side effects and, as a result, adverse skeletal events are the most common glucocorticoid-related complications associated with successful litigation.
- Disparity between bone quantity and quality in GIO makes ultrasound or BMD measurements inadequate for identifying patients at risk of glucocorticoid-induced fractures.
- Continuous treatment with 10 mg/d of prednisone for more than 90 days is associated with a 7-fold increase in hip fractures and a 17-fold increase in vertebral fractures.
- The adverse effects of glucocorticoids on the skeleton are primarily caused by direct actions on osteoblasts and osteoclasts, decreasing the production of both osteoblasts and osteoclasts, and increasing the apoptosis of osteoblasts while prolonging the lifespan of osteoclasts. Increased osteocyte apoptosis also occurs and is associated with decreases in VEGF, skeletal angiogenesis, bone interstitial fluid, and bone strength.
- Laboratory testing should include measurement of serum 25OHD, creatinine, and calcium (in addition to glucose, potassium, and lipids).

- The World Health Organization fracture prevention algorithm (FRAX) underestimates the risk of glucocorticoid-induced fractures.
- Bisphosphonates are considered first-line options for GIO and may also decrease pain, delay lesion expansion, and reduce the need for surgery in glucocorticoid-induced osteonecrosis.
- Teriparatide represents a particularly rational approach to GIO by counteracting several fundamental aspects of its pathophysiology.
- Denosumab may be considered for glucocorticoid-treated patients with renal insufficiency and stable serum calcium levels who are not candidates for bisphosphonates or teriparatide.
- Do not wait. Start antifracture treatment at the onset of a course of glucocorticoid therapy using more than 10 mg/d of prednisone and expected to last more than 90 days.

ACKNOWLEDGMENTS

The author thanks Drs Stavros C. Manolagas, Robert L. Jilka, Maria Almeida, and Charles A. O'Brien for their advice and helpful discussions, and Drs Stavros C. Manolagas, Robert L. Jilka, Maria Almeida, Fred H. Faas, and Irina Lendel for reviewing the manuscript.

REFERENCES

1. Cushing H. The basophil adenomas of the pituitary body and their clinical manifestations (pituitary basophilism). Bull Johns Hopkins Hosp 1932;50:137–95.
2. Boland EW, Headley NE. Management of rheumatoid arthritis with smaller (maintenance) doses of cortisone acetate. JAMA 1950;144:365–72.
3. Freyberg RH, Traeger CH, Patterson M, et al. Problems of prolonged cortisone treatment for rheumatoid arthritis. JAMA 1951;147:1538–43.
4. Bollet AJ, Black R, Bumin JJ. Major undesirable side-effects resulting from prednisolone and prednisone. JAMA 1955;157:459–63.
5. Heiman WG, Freiberger RH. Avascular necrosis of the femoral and humeral heads after high-dosage corticosteroid therapy. N Engl J Med 1960;263:672–5.
6. Pietrogrande V, Mastromarino R. Osteopathia da prolungato trattmento cortisonico. Ortop Tramatol 1957;25:791–810.
7. Weinstein RS. Clinical practice: glucocorticoid-induced bone disease. N Engl J Med 2011;365:62–70.
8. Weinstein RS. Glucocorticoid-induced osteonecrosis. Endocrine 2012;41(2): 183–90. DOI: 10.1007/s12020-011-9580-0.
9. Nash JJ, Nash AG, Leach ME, et al. Medical malpractice and corticosteroid use. Otolaryngol Head Neck Surg 2011;144:10–5.
10. LoCascio V, Bonucci E, Imbimbo B, et al. Bone loss in response to long-term glucocorticoid therapy. Bone Miner 1990;8:39–51.
11. van Staa TP, Laan RF, Barton IP, et al. Bone density threshold and other predictors of vertebral fracture in patients receiving oral glucocorticoid therapy. Arthritis Rheum 2003;48:3224–9.
12. Angeli A, Guglielmi G, Dovio A, et al. High prevalence of asymptomatic vertebral fractures in post-menopausal women receiving chronic glucocorticoid therapy: a cross-sectional outpatient study. Bone 2006;39:253–9.
13. Weinstein RS. Is long-term glucocorticoid therapy associated with a high prevalence of asymptomatic vertebral fractures in postmenopausal women? Nat Clin Pract Endocrinol Metab 2007;3:86–7.

14. Steinbuch M, Youket TE, Cohen S. Oral glucocorticoid use is associated with an increased risk of fracture. Osteoporos Int 2004;15:323–8.
15. de Vries F, Bracke M, Leufkens HG, et al. Fracture risk with intermittent high-dose oral glucocorticoid therapy. Arthritis Rheum 2007;56:208–14.
16. Curtis JR, Westfall AO, Allison JJ, et al. Longitudinal patterns in the prevention of osteoporosis in glucocorticoid-treated patients. Arthritis Rheum 2005;52:2485–94.
17. Thompson JM, Modin GW, Arnaud CD, et al. Not all postmenopausal women on chronic steroids and estrogen treatment are osteoporotic: predictors of bone mineral density. Calcif Tissue Int 1997;61:377–81.
18. Tatsuno I, Sugiyama T, Suzuki S, et al. Age dependence of early symptomatic vertebral fracture with high-dose glucocorticoid treatment for collagen vascular diseases. J Clin Endocrinol Metab 2009;94:1671–7.
19. van Staa TP, Leufkins H, Cooper C. Use of inhaled glucocorticoids and risk of fractures. J Bone Miner Res 2001;16:581–8.
20. Russcher H, Smit P, van den Akker ELT, et al. Two polymorphisms in the glucocorticoid receptor gene directly affect glucocorticoid-regulated gene expression. J Clin Endocrinol Metab 2005;90:5804–10.
21. Cooper MS, Rabbitt EH, Goddard PE, et al. Osteoblastic 11β-hydroxysteroid dehydrogenase type 1 activity increases with age and glucocorticoid exposure. J Bone Miner Res 2002;17:979–86.
22. Weinstein RS, Jilka RL, Parfitt AM, et al. Inhibition of osteoblastogenesis and promotion of apoptosis of osteoblasts and osteocytes by glucocorticoids: potential mechanisms of the deleterious effects on bone. J Clin Invest 1998;102:274–82.
23. O'Brien CA, Jia D, Plotkin LI, et al. Glucocorticoids act directly on osteoblasts and osteocytes to induce their apoptosis and reduce bone formation and strength. Endocrinol 2004;145:1835–41.
24. Weinstein RS, Wan C, Liu Q, et al. Endogenous glucocorticoids decrease vascularity and increase skeletal fragility in aged mice. Aging Cell 2010;9:147–61.
25. Seeman E. Bone quality-the material and structural basis of bone strength and fragility. N Engl J Med 2006;354:2250–61.
26. Jia D, O'Brien CA, Stewart SA, et al. Glucocorticoids act directly on osteoclasts to increase their lifespan and reduce bone density. Endocrinol 2006;147:5592–9.
27. Weinstein RS, Jia D, Powers CC, et al. The skeletal effects of glucocorticoid excess override those of orchidectomy in mice. Endocrinol 2004;145:1980–7.
28. Pearce G, Tabensky DA, Delmas PD, et al. Corticosteroid-induced bone loss in men. J Clin Endocrinol Metab 1998;83:801–6.
29. Tauchmanovà L, Pivonello R, Di Somma C, et al. Bone demineralization and vertebral fractures in endogenous cortisol excess: role of disease etiology and gonadal status. J Clin Endocrinol Metab 2006;91:1779–84.
30. Rubin MA, Bilezikian JP. The role of parathyroid hormone in the pathogenesis of glucocorticoid-induced osteoporosis: a reexamination of the evidence. J Clin Endocrinol Metab 2002;87:4033–41.
31. Almeida M, Han L, Ambrogini E, et al. Glucocorticoids and tumor necrosis factor (TNF) α increase oxidative stress and suppress WNT signaling in osteoblasts via mechanisms involving pkcβ/P66SHC/JNK and AKT/FOXO. J Biol Chem 2011; 286:44326–35.
32. Ohnaka K, Taniguchi H, Kawate H, et al. Glucocorticoid enhances the expression of dickkopf-1 in human osteoblasts: novel mechanism of glucocorticoid-induced osteoporosis. Biochem Biophys Res Commun 2004;318:259–64.
33. Lecka-Czernik B, Gubrij I, Moerman EJ, et al. Inhibition of Osf2/Cbfa1 expression and terminal differentiation by PPARγ2. J Cell Biochem 1999;74:357–71.

34. Hofbauer LC, Gori F, Riggs BL, et al. Stimulation of osteoprotegerin ligand and inhibition of osteoprotegerin production by glucocorticoids in human osteoblastic lineage cells: potential paracrine mechanisms of glucocorticoid-induced osteoporosis. Endocrinol 1999;140:4382–9.
35. Xiong J, Onal M, Jilka RJ, et al. Matrix-embedded cells control osteoclast formation. Nat Med 2011;17:1235–41.
36. Poetker DM, Smith TL. What rhinologists and allergists should know about the medico-legal implications of corticosteroid use: a review of the literature. Int Forum Allergy Rhinol 2012;2(2):95–103. DOI: 10.1002/alr.21016.
37. Mankin HF. Nontraumatic necrosis of bone (osteonecrosis). N Engl J Med 1992; 326:1473–9.
38. Skversky AL, Kumar J, Abramowitz MK, et al. Association of glucocorticoid use and low 25-hydroxyvitamin D levels: results from the National Health and Nutrition Examination Survey (NHANES): 2001-2006. J Clin Endocrinol Metab 2011;96: 3838–45.
39. Miller PD. Safety of parathyroid hormone for the treatment of osteoporosis. Curr Osteo Reports 2008;6:12–6.
40. Syed MI, Patel NA, Jan S, et al. Symptomatic refractures after vertebroplasty in patients with steroid-induced osteoporosis. Am J Neuroradiol 2006;27:1938–43.
41. Adachi JD, Saag KG, Delmas PD, et al. Two-year effects of alendronate on bone mineral density and vertebral fracture in patients receiving glucocorticoids: a randomized, double-blind, placebo-controlled extension trial. Arthritis Rheum 2001;44:202–11.
42. Reid DM, Hughes RA, Laan RF, et al. Efficacy and safety of daily risedronate in the treatment of corticosteroid-induced osteoporosis in men and women: a randomized trial. J Bone Miner Res 2000;15:1006–13.
43. Reid DM, Devogelaer J-P, Saag K, et al. Zoledronic acid and risedronate in the prevention and treatment of glucocorticoid-induced osteoporosis (HORIZON): a multicenter, double-blind, double-dummy, randomized controlled trial. Lancet 2009;373:1253–63.
44. Weinstein RS, Roberson PK, Manolagas SC, et al. Giant osteoclast formation aminobisphosphonate therapy. N Engl J Med 2009;360:53–62.
45. Weinstein RS, Chen JR, Powers CC, et al. Promotion of osteoclast survival and antagonism of bisphosphonate-induced osteoclast apoptosis by glucocorticoids. J Clin Invest 2002;109:1041–8.
46. Liberman UA, Weiss SR, Bröll J, et al. Effect of oral alendronate on bone mineral density and the incidence of fractures in postmenopausal osteoporosis. The alendronate phase III osteoporosis treatment study group. N Engl J Med 1995; 333:1437–43.
47. Orwoll E, Ettinger M, Weiss S, et al. Alendronate for the treatment of osteoporosis in men. N Engl J Med 2000;343:604–10.
48. Plotkin LI, Weinstein RS, Parfitt AM, et al. Prevention of osteocyte and osteoblast apoptosis by bisphosphonates and calcitonin. J Clin Invest 1999;104:1363–74.
49. Fleisch H. Bisphosphonates in bone disease: from the laboratory to the patient. 4th edition. San Diego (CA): Academic Press; 2000. p. 42.
50. Emkey R, Delmas PD, Goemaere S, et al. Changes in bone mineral density following discontinuation or continuation of alendronate therapy in glucocorticoid-treated patients: a retrospective, observational study. Arthritis Rheum 2003;48:1102–8.
51. Khosla S, Burr D, Cauley J, et al. Bisphosphonate-associated osteonecrosis of the jaw: report of a task force of the American society for bone and mineral research. J Bone Miner Res 2007;22:1479–91.

52. Black DM, Kelly MP, Genant HK, et al. Bisphosphonates and fractures of the subtrochanteric or diaphyseal femur. N Engl J Med 2010;362:1761–71.
53. Saag KG, Shane E, Boonen S, et al. Teriparatide or alendronate in glucocorticoid-induced osteoporosis. N Engl J Med 2007;357:2028–39.
54. Weinstein RS, Jilka RJ, Roberson PK, et al. Intermittent parathyroid hormone administration prevents glucocorticoid-induced osteoblast and osteocyte apoptosis, decreased bone formation, and reduced bone strength in mice. Endocrinol 2010; 151:2641–9.
55. Devogelaer JP, Adler RA, Recknor C, et al. Baseline glucocorticoid dose and bone mineral density response with teriparatide or alendronate therapy in patients with glucocorticoid-induced osteoporosis. J Rheumatol 2010;37:141–8.
56. Cummings SR, San Martin J, McClung MR, et al. Denosumab for prevention of fractures in postmenopausal women with osteoporosis. N Engl J Med 2009; 361:756–65.
57. Dore RK, Cohen SB, Lane NE, et al. Effects of denosumab on bone mineral density and bone turnover in patients with rheumatoid arthritis receiving concurrent glucocorticoids or bisphosphonates. Ann Rheum Dis 2010;69:872–5.
58. Weinstein RS, O'Brien CA, Zhao H, et al. Osteoprotegerin prevents glucocorticoid-induced osteocyte apoptosis in mice. Endocrinol 2011;152: 3323–31.
59. Weinstein RS, Nicholas RW, Manolagas SC. Apoptosis of osteocytes in glucocorticoid-induced osteonecrosis of the hip. J Clin Endocrinol Metab 2000; 85:2907–12.
60. Lai KA, Shen WJ, Yang CY, et al. The use of alendronate to prevent early collapse of the femoral head in patients with nontraumatic osteonecrosis. J Bone Joint Surg Am 2005;87:2155–9.
61. Agarwala S, Shah S, Joshi VR. The use of alendronate in the treatment of avascular necrosis of the femoral head: follow-up to eight years. J Bone Joint Surg Br 2009;91:1013–8.
62. Zhao D, Cui D, Wang B, et al. Treatment of early stage osteonecrosis of the femoral head with autologous implantation of bone marrow-deprived and cultures mesenchymal stem cells. Bone 2012;50:325–30.
63. Hansen KE, Wilson HA, Zapalowski C, et al. Uncertainties in the prevention and treatment of glucocorticoid-induced osteoporosis. J Bone Miner Res 2011; 26:1–8.

Unrecognized and Unappreciated Secondary Causes of Osteoporosis

Paul D. Miller, MD

KEYWORDS

- Bone • Cause • Secondary osteoporosis

KEY POINTS

- Renal tubular acidosis is a chronic form of metabolic acidosis that is caused by either the reduced capacity of the proximal tubule of the kidney to reabsorb the filtered bicarbonate load (proximal) or the reduced capacity of the distal renal tubule to maximally acidify the urine.[1–3]
- The bone is an reservoir for buffering hydrogen ions.
- The carbonate ion (from the splitting of calcium from calcium carbonate) buffers hydrogen ions.
- The focus for secondary causes of osteoporosis is separated into 5 systems: renal, hematological, gastrointestinal, endocrine and drugs associated with osteoporosis.
- There are many secondary causes of osteoporosis, including celiac disease, MGUS (monoclonal antibody of undetermined significance), impaired renal function, diabetes mellitus, and renal tubular acidosis.
- Through targeted laboratory tests, many secondary causes of osteoporosis can be identified.

INTRODUCTION

There are many secondary causes of osteoporosis.[4–6] However, before this article discusses specific secondary osteoporosis, it is important to define osteoporosis in the clinical sense.

The National Institutes of Health (NIH) consensus statement on how osteoporosis is defined is correct and scientific.[7] However, the NIH definition is not applicable in clinical practice, because bone quality, an important component of the definition and contributor to bone strength, cannot be measured in clinical practice at this time. After 1994, the World Health Organization (WHO) diagnostic criteria for postmenopausal osteoporosis was based on a bone mineral density (BMD) and a T score of −2.5 or lower,[8] but the diagnosis of osteoporosis could, and still can, be made after a low-trauma fragility fracture in women or men 50 years of age and older.[7] The classic fractures identified as being osteoporotic-type fractures are fractures of the hip and vertebrae, although

Colorado Center for Bone Research, 3190 South Wadsworth Boulevard, Lakewood, CO 80227, USA
E-mail address: millerccbr@aol.com

Endocrinol Metab Clin N Am 41 (2012) 613–628
http://dx.doi.org/10.1016/j.ecl.2012.05.005
0889-8529/12/$ – see front matter © 2012 Published by Elsevier Inc.

endo.theclinics.com

low-trauma fractures of the humerus, forearm, femur shaft, tibia, and/or fibula are also associated with a high risk for future fractures in untreated population studies. Even fragility fractures (or low dual-energy x-ray absorptiometry values) may be caused by metabolic bone diseases that are not osteoporosis (**Box 1**).[9,10]

Once a clinician is confident that a patient has osteoporosis, then the question is whether the diagnosis is postmenopausal osteoporosis, or osteoporosis of aging (the most common forms of osteoporosis) or some other form of osteoporosis. In men, the osteoporosis that develops in the elderly is usually related to hypogonadism.

Although estrogen deficiency is the most common cause of osteoporosis in postmenopausal women, there are many other conditions that may accompany estrogen deficiency and contribute to the impairment of bone strength in this population. Laboratory evaluation to detect any secondary mechanisms leading to derangements in bone metabolism in postmenopausal patients includes tests that may be ordered as a standard of care at the primary care level, and more in-depth tests that are considered in complex patients.[11–13] The basic primary, as opposed to secondary and more complex, laboratory assessment for causes of osteoporosis is listed in **Boxes 2** and **3**. This article also focuses on clinical issues related to targeted laboratory tests (see **Box 2**). Although 24-hour urine calcium and creatinine clearance are often considered to be a component of a basic evaluation for osteoporosis, this article classifies this important test as targeted because it is inconsistently performed and commonly misinterpreted at the primary care level. However, a 24-hour urine is strongly advised.

In this article, the focus for secondary causes of osteoporosis is separated into 5 systems: renal, hematological, gastrointestinal, endocrine, and drugs associated with osteoporosis.

RENAL-RELATED ASSOCIATIONS BETWEEN LOW BMD AND/OR FRACTURES, EXCLUDING PATIENTS ON DIALYSIS AND POSTTRANSPLANTATION BONE DISEASE
Hypercalciuria

The upper limit of normal for a 24-hour urine calcium has been identified as 4.0 mg/kg/d for women and 4.5 mg/kg/d for men.[14,15] The upper limit of the normal laboratory reference range was established in population studies showing that patients exceeding this level were often excreting more calcium than any specific reference range established by any particular study. There was also evidence that those who formed hypercalciuric calcium renal stone were at a higher risk for fractures and/or loss of BMD than is seen in hypercalciuric individuals who do not form stones.[16–21] Because of the difference in skeletal-related outcomes of hypercalciuric patients who form stones and those who do not form stones, it may be helpful to obtain a noncontrast computed tomography scan of the kidneys in some hypercalciuric patients with no history of a clinical renal

---

Box 1
Example of nonosteoporotic causes of low BMD or fractures

Osteomalacia

Genetic disorders (eg, osteogenesis imperfecta)

Renal bone disease

Bone marrow disorders (eg, multiple myeloma, mastocytosis, monoclonal gammopathy of undetermined significance [MGUS])

Paget disease, fibrous dysplasia

Metastatic cancer to bone

Box 2
Evaluation of secondary causes of osteoporosis: basic work-up

Careful history and physical examination

Basic laboratory tests:

Complete blood count

Biochemical profile (to include serum calcium, phosphorus, electrolytes, alkaline phosphatase, and creatinine)

Thyroid-stimulating hormone

25-Hydroxyvitamin D level

Serum protein electrophoresis

---

stone event; the finding of a silent radiographic stone may change clinical strategy toward consideration of intervention with a thiazide diuretic. What is the origin of high urinary calcium? Although it has been suggested that there are 3 possible sources of increased urinary calcium excretion (bone, renal, or gut),[22] it is difficult to discriminate among these sources in clinical practice. Although increased intact parathyroid hormone (PTH) or 1,25-dihydroxyvitamin D levels may suggest a renal leak or hyperabsorption from the gastrointestinal tract, clinical management may not differ as long as the clinician is certain that the patient does not have primary hyperparathyroidism as a cause of an increased PTH. Several normal serum calcium concentrations (rather than a single isolated normal value) may be necessary to exclude primary hyperparathyroidism. Restriction of calcium intake has been suggested in patients with gastrointestinal hyperabsorption as the mechanism for hypercalciuria.

Box 3
Evaluation of secondary causes of osteoporosis: comprehensive work-up

Serum parathyroid hormone

Bone-specific alkaline phosphatase (BSAP)

Serum immunoelectrophoresis and serum free light chains

Celiac disease testing

Biochemical bone turnover markers (BTM: c-telopeptide and propeptide type I collagen)

Serum free T^4 and fasting plasma cortisol

(May prefer 24-hour urinary free cortisol and midnight salivary cortisol)

1,25-Dihydroxyvitamin D

24-Hour urine for calcium, phosphorus, protein, and creatinine clearance

Small bowel biopsy (for celiac disease)

Serum prolactin

Serum insulinlike growth factor 1 (in anorexia, diabetes)

Fibroblastic growth factor 23[a]

Bone biopsy

[a] Chronic kidney disease (CKD), hypophosphatemia, osteomalacia, normal 25-hydroxyvitamin D and low 1,25-dihydroxyvitamin D, unexplained increase of BSAP, after tumor removal in oncogenic osteomalacia to monitor adequacy of tissue ablation.

However, without strong evidence that this dietary calcium restriction consistently reduces the risk of renal stone formation, there is the potential negative trade-off of reducing bone mass in others whose source of hypercalciuria is renal or bone. When should a clinician treat hypercalciuria? Should everyone identified with hypercalciuria be treated with agents, such as thiazide diuretics, that reduce urinary calcium excretion? In this author's opinion, no. Some patients may have low BMD and hypercalciuria without a causal relationship. Patients with hypercalciuria and no renal stones may never have a clinical event associated with their hypercalciuria and, in that regard, could be considered to have healthy hypercalciuria. Interventions to lower urinary calcium should treat those patients who have a negative clinical consequence, such as a renal stone or unexplained fracture, associated with the hypercalciuria.

Renal Tubular Acidosis

Renal tubular acidosis (RTA) is a chronic form of metabolic acidosis that is either caused by the reduced capacity of the proximal tubule of the kidney to reabsorb the filtered bicarbonate load (proximal), or the reduced capacity of the distal renal tubule to maximally acidify the urine.[1–3] The bone is a large reservoir for buffering hydrogen ions. The carbonate ion (from the splitting of calcium from calcium carbonate) buffers hydrogen ions. When this hydrogen ion load is greater than the normal daily acid load, the bone becomes the buffer. This may result in a spectrum of metabolic bone disorders from osteomalacia (with proximal RTA) to osteoporosis (with distal RTA), both of which can result in low BMD and/or fractures. However, in clinical practice, suspicion for RTA is best screened with serum electrolytes. The finding of an increased chloride (>110 mEq/L) and an low carbon dioxide (<18 meq/L) should lead to more sophisticated investigations into the possibility of an RTA, the most important of which is an arterial blood gas and a urine pH (best measured with a pH meter). An increased chloride and low serum CO_2 could also be caused by a respiratory alkalosis.[23]

Chronic Kidney Disease

The National Kidney Foundation classifies the severity of chronic kidney disease (CKD) from the glomerular filtration rate (GFR), as measured by 24-hour urine for creatinine clearance, or as estimated by the Cockcroft-Gault equation or, preferably, the Modification of Diet in Renal Disease (MDRD) equation (calculators are available at www.kidney.org/professionals/kdoqi/gfr_calculator.cfm):

- Stage 1: GFR 90 mL/min/1.73 m^2 or higher with urine abnormalities (hematuria, proteinuria)
- Stage 2: GFR 60 to 89 mL/min with urine abnormalities
- Stage 3: GFR 30 to 59 mL/min without urine abnormalities
- Stage 4: GFR 15 to 29 mL/min without urine abnormalities
- Stage 5: GFR lower than 15, or if the patient is on dialysis. (Another stage, called 5D, was added to the list to denote patients on dialysis, because the metabolic derangements in bone and systemic biology may differ between patients on dialysis and those not on dialysis.)[24]

This staging system is relevant to the discussion of bone fragility that follows.

The diagnosis of osteoporosis in these patients has no universally accepted criteria, except for agreement that the diagnosis of osteoporosis can be made in stage 1 to 3 CKD on the basis of the WHO BMD criteria or a fragility fracture, if there are no concomitant metabolic abnormalities that could suggest the presence of CKD–mineral and bone disorders (CKD-MBD).[25] CKD-MBD is a term used to encompass the systemic derangements in bone (mineralization, turnover, volume) that are linked to the systemic vascular calcification of severe CKD.

The diagnosis of osteoporosis in stage 4 to 5 and 5D CKD is best suggested by excluding other forms of renal osteodystrophy by quantitative histomorphometry or by attempting to classify the form of renal osteodystrophy by noninvasive means of assessing bone turnover, mineralization, and volume (CKD-MBD).[25] However, there are no clinical tools to make these distinctions between renal osteodystrophy and CKD-MBD in individual patients. Although many promising radiologic techniques that examine bone microarchitecture offer hope of being able to define turnover, mineralization, and volume noninvasively in severe CKD, they are investigational and unproven at this time in discriminating between renal osteodystrophy and osteoporosis.[26] As understanding of the relationships between turnover, mineralization, volume, and bone strength increase, these noninvasive imaging technologies may become the means to correlate turnover, mineralization, and volume with bone strength and open up a new way to classify skeletal strength. Because fracture risk is approximately doubled in patients even at stage 3 CKD compared with age-matched, body mass index (BMI)–matched, and BMD-matched persons without CKD, understanding the mechanisms that lead to the greater risk for fracture in these populations is important.[26] In the meantime, the clinician is left with quantitative bone histomorphometry (which requires biopsy) and biochemical markers of bone turnover to characterize the bone disease that may be responsible for low-trauma fractures in stage 5 CKD.[27,28] The clinician should use biochemical markers before bone biopsy to distinguish the form of renal osteodystrophy, because this distinction may prevent an unnecessary biopsy.

At the current time, the most useful of the biochemical profiling methods to discriminate among the major renal bone diseases in which an antiresorptive agent may not be desirable (adynamic bone disease) are bone-specific alkaline phosphatase and intact PTH. If a patient's bone-specific alkaline phosphatase level is increased, adynamic bone disease is highly unlikely. Assuming that other causes of this increased level (eg, Paget disease of bone, metastatic cancer) have already been excluded, the increased level could represent either osteomalacia or hyperparathyroid bone disease. However, a normal bone-specific alkaline phosphatase level does not exclude adynamic bone disease, whereas a low level is more often associated with low bone turnover. An increased PTH level does not exclude adynamic renal bone disease, but a low level (<150 pg/mL) suggests a low-bone-turnover state. A level 6 times or more greater than the upper limit of normal is more likely to be associated with high bone turnover. Thus, in clinical practice, patients with stage 4 or 5 CKD who have increased bone-specific alkaline phosphatase or very high (>6× the upper limit of the reference range) PTH values do not have adynamic bone disease.[27] Furthermore, once other causes of these aberrant biochemical abnormalities have been defined, then high-bone-turnover osteoporosis may be a consideration. In my opinion, if bone turnover markers suggest low bone turnover, bone biopsy is necessary before starting an antiresorptive agent.[5] The clinician should refer patients with suspected renal osteodystrophy or fracture with stage 4 to 5 CKD to a specialist dealing with such diseases because the other metabolic disturbances, such as an increased phosphate, low 25-hydroxyvitamin D and 1,25-dihydroxyvitamin D, and anemia, all need to be dealt with in such a complex disease.

HEMATOLOGICAL DISEASES

Monoclonal gammopathy of undetermined significance (MGUS) and multiple myeloma (MM) are 2 of the most common secondary causes of osteoporosis or fragility fractures.

MGUS is the most common plasma cell disorder; with an overall prevalence in the United States population of 3% in those 50 years of age and older, and nearly 7% of the population 80 years of age and older.[29] MGUS is defined as the detection of a monoclonal protein but with either no M protein, or a serum M protein value of 3 gm/dL or less, small amounts of light chains in the urine, and a proportion of plasma cells in the bone marrow of 10% or less in the absence of bone lesions, anemia, hypercalcemia, or renal failure related to the MGUS.[29] MGUS may be a precursor of more serious diseases, including MM, Waldenstrom macroglobulinemia, or primary amyloidosis. In the evaluation of patients, especially elderly patients with unexplained fractures, routine serum protein electrophoresis misses ~50% of patients with an M spike, and hence a more sensitive screening test using a combination of serum immunofixation and serum free light chains detects more than 95% of MM and/or MGUS.[30] The serum free κ/λ light chain ratio is a sensitive discriminator and also has prognostic value in helping to stratify risk for progression from MGUS to MM.[31] If there is doubt about the correct diagnosis or progression of disease, referral to an experienced hematologist/oncologist for bone marrow aspirations should be considered. It is important to know that, /although bone lytic lesions are rare in MGUS, they still have a higher risk for osteoporotic fragility fractures that may be either related to an increase in marrow-derived receptor activator of nuclear factor κ-B ligand or to a decrease in osteoblast activity caused by plasma cell production of an osteoblast inhibitor, Dickkopf-1.[32]

Mastocytosis

Mastocytosis as the mechanism for fragility fractures is a difficult disease to diagnose without bone marrow. Mastocytosis, if systemic, especially involving the skin, becomes an easier diagnosis if a skin biopsy shows the mast cells in the lesion. The proximity of the mast cell to bone remodeling surfaces and the production by this cell of a large number of chemical mediators and cytokines capable of modulating bone turnover (especially heparin) translates to skeletal involvement, ranging from severe osteolysis to significant osteosclerosis, with osteoporosis being the most frequently observed disorder.[33–38] Increased 24-hour urine excretion of N-methylhistamine may be valuable id there is suspicion of mastocytosis. However, the diagnosis requires a histologic confirmation.

GASTROINTESTINAL DISEASES
Celiac Disease

Celiac disease is a prevalent disorder and is one of the most common secondary causes of osteoporosis. The loss of small intestinal villa and accompanying pathophysiology leads to selective malabsorption of calcium (and iron) with a progressive negative calcium balance. Celiac disease laboratory detection is best accomplished by measuring serum antibodies to gluten, both the tissue transglutaminase (TT-IgA) antibody and the endomesial antibody (EmA). The sensitivity/specificity of these antibodies in patients with gastrointestinal symptoms is high: 87%/99% for TT-IgA and 87%/97% for EmA.[39] However, the sensitivity/specificity of these antibodies in asymptomatic celiac disease is less clear, because there have been few robust studies of small bowel biopsies, the gold standard for diagnosis, in asymptomatic patients. The sensitivity/specificity of the antibodies are correlated with the severity of the histologic findings; those with partial villous atrophy often have normal antibodies. From clinical experience, patients with osteoporosis who have no gastrointestinal symptoms and normal serum antibody levels should be considered for small bowel biopsies when there is a very low 24-hour urine calcium (<50 mg/d), unexplained secondary hyperparathyroidism, 25-hydroxyvitamin D deficiency, unexplained iron deficiency, or higher-than-expected bone turnover marker levels despite compliance with oral anti-resorptive therapy.

Crohn Disease and Other Inflammatory Bowel Diseases

In Crohn disease, the pathophysiology of osteoporosis is multifactorial, including the effect of inflammatory cytokines mediating disease activity (interleukin [IL]-6, IL-1, tumor necrosis factor α), intestinal malabsorption caused by disease activity or intestinal resection, the use of glucocorticoids, malnutrition, immobilization, and, often, a low BMI.[40,41] Ileum resection has been identified as the single most significant risk factor for osteoporosis.[42] Patients with Crohn disease are young, and the relationship between the host of factors potentially deleterious to the skeleton and increased risk for osteoporosis and fractures remains unclear. Because fat-soluble vitamins (including vitamin D) are absorbed in the terminal ileum where Crohn disease is most prevalent, these patients often have exceptionally low 24-hydroxyvitamin D serum levels.

Bariatric Surgery

Obesity is a serious public health issue that has reached pandemic proportions, and has been ranked the number 1 threat to American health by the Centers for Disease Control and Prevention since 2004. Results from the 2003 to 2005 National Health and Nutrition Examination Survey (NHANES) estimated that 33.8% of US adults were obese (BMI$\geq$30), and the prevalence of overweight and obesity combined (BMI$\geq$25) is 68% of the population.[43,44] Bariatric (weight loss) surgery is the only effective therapy for morbid obesity; it has been performed since the 1940s but has undergone a resurgence in the last 2 decades in response to the obesity pandemic and the need to address the myriad comorbidities for which obesity is directly responsible. Recent data indicate that the number of bariatric surgeries performed in the United States increased from 13,365 in 1998 to an estimated 200,000 in 2007.[45]

Bone loss caused by weight reduction is multifactorial and correlates strongly with the velocity at which the weight is lost. Decreased calcium, vitamin D, and protein intake during periods of caloric restriction result in decreased calcium absorption, a subsequent increase in PTH, and increased bone resorption. Proposed mechanisms include effects caused by increased levels of circulating cortisol, and decreased levels of circulating estrogen, insulinlike growth factor (IGF) 1, leptin, ghrelin, and glucagonlike peptide 2, particularly in patients who have undergone bariatric surgery.[45–51] Rapid weight loss of 45 kg to greater than 90 kg is common among patients who have had successful bariatric surgery. Combined with severely restricted oral intake, this decreased calcium absorption, and vitamin D deficiency, places these patients at high risk for rapid bone loss. Bone loss can affect more than 70% of patients who have undergone a malabsorptive procedure, and this may be associated with increased markers of bone resorption as soon as 8 weeks after bariatric surgery, regardless of whether the patient underwent a malabsorptive or restrictive bariatric procedure. In these patients, as soon as 12 months after undergoing gastric banding 48% may have a statistically significant bone mineral reduction of greater than 3%3. These patients require a higher vitamin D and calcium intake following surgery, and careful monitoring of the BMD and biochemical markers of bone turnover (at least annually). However, there are no data on whether these patients fracture more frequently. Bariatric surgery is also being performed in obese diabetics and has been shown to have a beneficial effect on glucose and insulin homeostasis, but this may also add to the complexity of the clinical picture of weight loss in diabetic patients who may have a predisposition to bone disease.

Osteoporosis Associated with Eating Disorders

Since the recognition of the importance of estrogen production and nutrition in the maintenance of skeletal health, clinical syndromes have been identified that include the development of bone mass loss and fractures in young women with the eating disorders anorexia nervosa and bulimia.[52,53]

The associations between eating disorders and skeletal fragility are systemic syndromes that involve psychological, nutritional, hypothalamic, ovarian, and bone-muscle-fat interrelationships.[54–60]

These patients often present to the osteoporosis clinic with low-trauma, nonvertebral fractures. They have low BMI, usually less than 17 kg/m², and have a unique biochemical profile including a low plasma estradiol without an increase of their follicle-stimulating hormone, consistent with the hypothalamic disorder that accompanies this syndrome. Other biochemical and hormonal abnormalities include increased cortisol, low IGF-1, and increased growth hormone. In this author's experience, quantitative bone histomorphometry shows low bone turnover, suggesting that the skeletal facility that may be seen even with normal BMD (eg, T scores) is a low-bone-turnover disease.

ENDOCRINE

Although many endocrine diseases may be associated with osteoporosis, the 3 most commonly seen in a primary care clinical practice are diabetes mellitus, primary hyperparathyroidism, and hyperthyroidism. Other less common endocrine associations with osteoporosis include Cushing disease and prolactinomas.

OSTEOPOROSIS ASSOCIATED WITH DIABETES MELLITUS

The deleterious effects of diabetes mellitus (DM) on the skeleton are multifactorial and both types 1 and 2 DM are associated with increased fracture risk.[61–65] Data from the Iowa Women's Health Study suggest that women with type 1 DM are 12 times more likely to sustain hip fractures than women without DM, and that women with type 2 DM have a 1.7-fold increased risk of sustaining hip fractures despite maintaining a normal bone mass.[65] Diabetes is associated with a reduction in BMD compared with age-matched and BMI-matched controls. However it is common to find an increased BMD in the obese. Low bone turnover is seen in patients with DM. The high prevalence of fractures in type 2 DM is likely to also be influenced by a greater risk of falls related to retinopathy-induced visual impairment, neuropathy-induced decreased balance, and sarcopenia.[61,62] The osteoporosis of DM is one of low bone turnover, with the main mechanism of bone loss being decreased bone formation. Insulin and amylin have an anabolic effect on bone, and their decrease in type 1 DM may lead to impaired bone formation, primarily because of a decrease in IGF-1 concentrations.[66] In vitro studies also show that sustained exposure to high glucose concentrations results in osteoblast dysfunction, and poor metabolic control has a clear negative impact on bone mass. In DM, there is increased bone marrow adiposity, which has also been linked with the osteoporosis of aging, glucocorticoid use, and immobility.[55,59] Several members of the nuclear hormone receptor family specifically control the critical adipogenic and osteogenic steps, and evidence has been mounting for an interdependence of adipogenesis and osteogenesis.[55,59,64] In the bone marrow microenvironment, the inverse relationship between adipogenic and osteogenic differentiation was shown to be mediated, at least in part, through crosstalk between pathways activated by steroid receptors (estrogen, thyroid, corticosteroid, and growth hormone receptors), the peroxisome proliferator activator receptors (PPARs), and other cytokine and paracrine factors. PPARs play a central role in initiating adipogenesis in bone marrow and other stromal-like cells in vitro and in vivo,[67] and their ligands (rosiglitazone and pioglitazone) play a prominent role in directing mesenchymal cell precursors toward adipocyte and away from osteoblast differentiation.[68] Other potential harmful metabolic abnormalities include accumulation of advanced glycosylation end products; acidosis; vitamin D deficiency, particularly in the obese diabetic, and renal impairment.

Primary Hyperparathyroidism and Osteoporosis

There is a gradient of skeletal health in primary hyperparathyroidism, from a clear link to fragility fractures in severe primary hyperparathyroidism to scant evidence for an increase in fracture risk in asymptomatic primary hyperparathyroidism.[69–71] There are conflicting studies relating the fracture risk in untreated primary hyperparathyroidism or the benefit/lack of benefit of parathyroid surgery on the modification of risk.[72,73] Given the complexity of skeletal effects of chronic exposure to increased PTH levels, the uncertain relationship between BMD and fracture risk with primary hyperparathyroidism, discordant findings on fracture risk at different skeletal sites before and after surgery, and limitations of study design, severity of disease, and patient selection in many reports, further study is indicated.[74,75] The NIH has held 3 separate consensus conferences on when surgery should be considered in asymptomatic primary hyperparathyroidism.[76] There is a role for medical monitoring of these patients whose average blood calcium is less than 11.0 mg/dL; who are not forming kidney stones; who are not fracturing or losing BMD because of the primary hyperparathyroidism (and not because of other causes of bone loss such as estrogen deficiency)[77]; and who do not have unexplained, sustained increases of bone-specific alkaline phosphatase. Although there may be a forme fruste of normocalcemic primary hyperparathyroidism, whose serum calcium concentration repeatedly remains within the laboratory-defined normal reference range despite an increased PTH, and in which causes of secondary hyperparathyroidism have been excluded, surgery in this type of patient should only be considered after consultation with a parathyroid expert.[78]

One other important point concerning the diagnosis of primary hyperparathyroidism is that, although the combination of an increased serum calcium and PTH is most often caused by primary hyperparathyroidism, another parathyroid condition in which no parathyroid adenoma or hyperplasia is found is familial hypercalcemia hypocalciuria (FHH).[79] The diagnosis is established by the calculation of the ratio of the clearance of calcium to the clearance of creatinine (<0.01), and now with genetic testing of the inactivating calcium-sensing receptor gene mutation. This differential is important because parathyroid surgery is not indicated in most cases of FHH.

DRUGS ASSOCIATED WITH LOW BMD AND/OR FRACTURES

Box 4 provides a list of medications that can be associated with the loss of BMD and/or an increased risk of fractures.[80] This list is not complete, and this article focuses on a few of the more commonly encountered drugs that are seen in clinical practice: Depo-Provera, aromatase inhibitors, and protein pump inhibitors (PPIs).

Depo-Provera

Depo-Provera (medroxyprogesterone) is the most widely used contraceptive worldwide. Because of its wide use in younger women and the documentation that administration of Depo-Provera may be associated with a loss of BMD, the US Food and

---

Box 4
Drugs associated with low BMD or fractures[a]

Glucocorticoids

Unfractionated heparin

Aromatase inhibitors

Gonadotrophin-releasing hormone agonists

Medroxyprogesterone

Excessive thyroid replacement

Thiazolidinediones

PPIs

Selective serotonin reuptake inhibitors

Antiseizure medications

Calcineurin inhibitors (eg, cyclosporine)

[a] This list is not complete.

Drug Administration has attached a black-box warning to its label, which has been controversial because of the lack of reliable evidence of any negative short-term or long-term outcomes.[81–84] In longitudinal observations, the loss of BMD with use of depomedroxyprogesterone acetate rapidly returns to baseline after discontinuation.[85] Because the risk of fracture is small (if any), and the benefit of affordable and widely available parenteral contraception is great, the use of medroxyprogesterone acetate should not be limited by its effect on the skeleton, although the association with loss of BMD should be discussed with the patient.

Aromatase Inhibitors

The aromatase inhibitors are highly effective at reducing the reoccurrence of breast cancer. Aromatase inhibitors are now regarded as front-line adjuvant therapy in women with estrogen receptor–positive breast cancer.[86] They reduce endogenous estrogen production by 80% to 90% by blocking the peripheral conversion of androgens to estrogen, and have largely replaced the selective estrogen receptor modulator, tamoxifen, as the preferred treatment option for postmenopausal women. The existing biomarker data indicate that all 3 aromatase inhibitors increase bone turnover, although some studies indicate a proportionately greater effect of exemestane on formation than resorption. Increased rates of bone loss have also been reported; for example, in the ATAC (Arimidex, Tamoxifen, Alone or in Combination) trial, median rates of bone loss at the spine and hip were 4.1% and 3.9%, respectively, over 2 years.[87,88] Data on fractures are confounded by prior or concomitant use of tamoxifen, which is not associated with bone loss of fractures. In the ATAC study, there was a greater risk for fractures after 5 years in subjects on this aromatase inhibitor.[87] Prevention of bone loss associated with aromatase inhibitor therapy has been shown with intravenous zoledronic acid, 4 mg every 6 months, oral risedronate 35 mg once weekly, and denosumab 60 mg subcutaneously every 6 months, although data on fracture reduction are lacking.[89–93] Management decisions on whether or not to intervene with antiresorptive agents for aromatase inhibitors are lacking but should follow those decisions for management of postmenopausal osteoporosis: monitoring BMD and bone turnover markers at intervals dictated by individual patient considerations.

PPIs

PPIs have received a great deal of attention since the initial claims from database retrospective analysis suggesting that a small increase in the risk of hip fractures is associated with long-term use of PPIs.[94–97] Because of their widespread use (7 registered PPIs available and more than US$14 billion annual sales), a common question from patients and physicians alike is related to their effects on bone. Data support an acid-suppressive association.

Data support an association between acid-suppressive medication, duration of use, and increased fracture risk. The limitations of observational studies (particularly the effects of potential but unmeasured confounding factors), have to be recognized. Furthermore, a mechanism of action whereby PPIs might be associated with an increased fracture risk is not known, with theories ranging from effects on gastrointestinal acid production and calcium absorption to effects on bone cell activity or BMD. It is reasonable to maintain PPIs in patients who need them, advise optimum calcium and vitamin D intake, and focus on other means to reduce their fracture risk, including reducing the risk for falls.

SUMMARY

There are many secondary causes of osteoporosis, besides those mentioned earlier, that also need to be recognized; for example, human immunodeficiency virus and the drugs used to treat the disease; stroke and immobilization; chronic heart, liver, and lung disease; and autoimmune diseases. As patients who present with osteoporosis are studied, many unrecognized causes begin to appear. Albert Einstein once stated that "Everything should be made as simple as possible but not simpler." This is also true of the many findings of secondary contributors to low BMD or fractures in these patients; in this sense, osteoporosis becomes a kaleidoscope of general medicine. Keep looking and keep finding.

REFERENCES

1. Krieger NS, Frick KK, Bushinsky DA. Mechanism of acid-induced bone resorption. Curr Opin Nephrol Hypertens 2004;13(4):423–36.
2. Lemann J Jr, Bushinsky DA, Hamm LL. Bone buffering of acid and base in humans. Am J Physiol Renal Physiol 2003;285(5):F811–32 Review.
3. Grieff M, Bushinsky DA. Diuretics and disorders of calcium homeostasis. Semin Nephrol 2011;31(6):535–41 Review.
4. Painter SE, Kleerekoper M, Camacho PM. Secondary osteoporosis: a review of the recent evidence. Endocr Pract 2006;12:436–45.
5. Miazgowski T, Kleerekoper M, Felsenberg D, et al. Secondary osteoporosis: endocrine and metabolic causes of bone mass deterioration. J Osteoporos 2012;2012:907214.
6. Bogoch ER, Elliot-Gibson V, Wang RY, et al. Secondary causes of osteoporosis in fracture patients. J Orthop Trauma 2012. [Epub ahead of print].
7. Osteoporosis prevention, diagnosis and therapy. NIH Consens Statement 2000; 17(1):1–45 Review.
8. Assessment of fracture risk and its application to screening for postmenopausal osteoporosis. Report of a WHO Study Group. World Health Organ Tech Rep Ser 1994;843:1–129.
9. Miller PD, Bonnick SL, Rosen CJ. Consensus of an international panel on the clinical utility of bone mass measurements in the detection of low bone mass in the adult population. Calcif Tissue Int 1996;58:207–14.

10. Miller PD, Zapalowski C, Kulak CA, et al. Bone densitometry: the best way to detect osteoporosis and to monitor therapy. J Clin Endocrinol Metab 1999;84:1867–71.

11. Adler RA. Laboratory testing for secondary osteoporosis evaluation. Clin Biochem 2012. [Epub ahead of print].

12. Tannenbaum C, Clark J, Schwartzman K, et al. Yield of laboratory testing to identify secondary contributors to osteoporosis in otherwise healthy women. J Clin Endocrinol Metab 2003;87:4431–7.

13. Lewiecki EM, Bilezikian JP, Khosla S, et al. Osteoporosis update from the 2010 Santa Fe Bone Symposium. J Clin Densitom 2011;14(1):1–21.

14. Worcester EM, Coe FL. Clinical practice. Calcium kidney stones. N Engl J Med 2010;363(10):954–63.

15. Consensus conference. Prevention and treatment of kidney stones. J Am Med Assoc 1988;260(7):977–81.

16. Asplin JR, Bauer KA, Kinder J, et al. Bone mineral density and urine calcium excretion among subjects with and without nephrolithiasis. Kidney Int 2003; 63(2):662–9.

17. Pietschmann F, Breslau NA, Pak CYC. Reduced vertebral bone density in hypercalciuric nephrolithiasis. J Bone Miner Res 1992;7:1383–8.

18. Jaeger P, Lippuner K, Casez JP, et al. Low bone mass in idiopathic renal stone formers: magnitude and significance. J Bone Miner Res 1994;9(10):1525–32.

19. Giannini S, Nobile M, Sartori L, et al. Bone density and skeletal metabolism are altered in idiopathic hypercalciuria. Clin Nephrol 1998;50(2):94–100.

20. Da Silva AMM, Dos Reis LM, Pereira RC, et al. Bone involvement in idiopathic hypercalciuria. Clin Nephrol 2002;57(3):183–91.

21. Tasca A, Cacciola A, Ferrarese P, et al. Bone alterations in patients with idiopathic hypercalciuria and calcium nephrolithiasis. Urology 2002;59(6):865–9.

22. Pak CY, Kaplan R, Bone H, et al. A simple test for the diagnosis of absorptive, resorptive and renal hypercalciurias. N Engl J Med 1975;292(10):497–500.

23. Bushinsky DA. Acidosis and bone. Miner Electrolyte Metab 1994;20(1–2):40–52 Review.

24. National Kidney Foundation. K/DOQI clinical practice guidelines for chronic kidney disease: evaluation, classification, and stratification. Am J Kidney Dis 2002;39:S1–266.

25. Kidney Disease: Improving Global Outcomes (KDIGO) CKD–MBD Work Group. KDIGO clinical practice guideline for the diagnosis, evaluation, prevention, and treatment of chronic kidney disease–mineral and bone disorder (CKD–MBD). Kidney Int 2009;76(Suppl 113):S1–130.

26. Jamal S, West S, Miller PD. Fracture risk assessment in patients with chronic kidney disease. Osteoporos Int 2012;23(4):1191–8.

27. Miller PD. Fragility fractures in chronic kidney disease: an opinion-based approach. Cleve Clin J Med 2009;76:715–23.

28. Miller PD. The kidney and bisphosphonates. Bone 2011;49(1):77–81.

29. Bida JP, Kyle RA, Therneau TM, et al. Disease associations with monoclonal gammopathy of undetermined significance: a population-based study of 17,398 patients. Mayo Clin Proc 2009;84(8):685–93.

30. Jagannath S. Value of serum free light chain testing for the diagnosis and monitoring of monoclonal gammopathies in hematology. Clin Lymphoma Myeloma 2007;7(8):518–23.

31. Varettoni M, Corso A, Cocito F, et al. Changing pattern of presentation of monoclonal gammopathy of undetermined significance: a single-center experience with 1,400 patients. Medicine (Baltimore) 2010;89(4):211–6.

32. Tian E, Zhan F, Walker R, et al. The role of the Wnt-signaling antagonist DKK1 in the development of osteolytic lesions in multiple myeloma. N Engl J Med 2003; 349(26):2483–94.

33. Barete S, Assous N, de Gennes C, et al. Systemic mastocytosis and bone involvement in a cohort of 75 patients. Ann Rheum Dis 2010;69:1838–41.

34. Valent P, Akin C, Escribano L, et al. Standards and standardization in mastocytosis: consensus statements on diagnostics, treatment recommendations and response criteria. Eur J Clin Invest 2007;37:435–53.

35. Lidor C, Frisch B, Gazit D, et al. Osteoporosis as the sole presentation of bone marrow mastocytosis. J Bone Miner Res 1990;5:871–6.

36. De Gennes C, Kuntz D, de Vernejoul MC. Bone mastocytosis: a report of nine cases with a bone histomorphometric study. Clin Orthop Relat Res 1992;279:281–91.

37. Brumsen C, Papapoulos SE, Lentjes EG, et al. A potential role for the mast cell in the pathogenesis of idiopathic osteoporosis in men. Bone 1990;31:556–61.

38. Oranje AP, Mulder PG, Heide R, et al. Urinary N-methyl histamine as an indicator of bone marrow involvement in mastocytosis. Clin Exp Dermatol 2002;27:502–6.

39. van der Windt DA, Jellema P, Mulder CJ, et al. Diagnostic testing for celiac disease among patients with abdominal symptoms: a systematic review. JAMA 2010;303(17):1738–46.

40. Moschen AR, Kaser A, Enrich B, et al. The RANKL/OPG system is activated in inflammatory bowel disease and relates to the state of bone loss. Gut 2005;54: 479–87.

41. Compston J. Osteoporosis in inflammatory bowel disease. Gut 2003;52:63–4.

42. van Hogezand RA, Banffer D, Zwinderman AH, et al. Ileum resection is the most predictive factor for osteoporosis in patients with Crohn's disease. Osteoporos Int 2006;17:535–42.

43. Flegal KM, Carroll MD, Ogden CL, et al. Prevalence and trends in obesity among US adults, 1999-2008. JAMA 2010;303(3):235–41.

44. Sturm R. Increases in morbid obesity in the USA: 2000-2005. Public Health 2007; 121(7):492–6.

45. Mechanick JI, Kushner RF, Sugerman HJ, et al. American Association of Clinical Endocrinologists, The Obesity Society, and American Society for Metabolic & Bariatric Surgery Medical guidelines for clinical practice for the perioperative nutritional, metabolic, and nonsurgical support of the bariatric surgery patient. Endocr Pract 2008;14(Suppl 1):1–83.

46. Shapses SA, Cifuentes M. Body weight/composition and weight change: effects on bone health. In: Holick MF, Dawson-Hughes B, editors. Nutrition and bone health. New Jersey: Humana Press; 2004. p. 549–73.

47. Shapses SA, Riedt CS. Bone, body weight, and weight reduction: what are the concerns? J Nutr 2006;136:1453–6.

48. Coates PS, Fernstrom JD, Fernstrom MH, et al. Gastric bypass surgery for morbid obesity leads to an increase in bone turnover and a decrease in bone mass. J Clin Endocrinol Metab 2004;89(3):1061–5.

49. Pugnale N, Giusti V, Suter M, et al. Bone metabolism and risk of secondary hyperparathyroidism 12 months after gastric banding in obese pre menopausal women. Int J Obes Relat Metab Disord 2003;27(1):110–6.

50. Haria DM, Sibonga JD, Taylor HC. Hypocalcemia, hypovitaminosis D osteopathy, osteopenia, and secondary hyperparathyroidism 32 years after jejunoileal bypass. Endocr Pract 2005;11:335–40.

51. Bal BS, Finelli FC, Shope TR, et al. Nutritional deficiencies after bariatric surgery. Nat Rev Endocrinol 2012. http://dx.doi.org/10.1038/nrendo.2012.48.

52. Lindsay R. Prevention and treatment of osteoporosis with ovarian hormones. Ann Chir Gynaecol 1988;77(5–6):219–23.
53. Walker MD, Novotny R, Bilezikian JP, et al. Race and diet interactions in the acquisition, maintenance, and loss of bone. J Nutr 2008;138:1256S–60S.
54. Biller BM, Caughlin JF, Sake V, et al. Osteopenia in women with hypothalamic amenorrhea: a prospective study. Obstet Gynecol 1991;78:996–1001.
55. Rosen CJ, Kiblanski A. Bone, fat, and body composition: evolving concepts in the pathogenesis of osteoporosis. Am J Med 2009;122(5):409–14.
56. Fazeli PK, Bredella MA, Freedman L, et al. Marrow fat and preadipocyte factor-1 levels decrease with recovery in women with anorexia nervosa. J Bone Miner Res 2012. http://dx.doi.org/10.1002/jbmr.1640.
57. Bredella MA, Fazeli PK, Freedman LM, et al. Young women with cold-activated brown adipose tissue have higher bone mineral density and lower pref-1 than women without brown adipose tissue: a study in women with anorexia nervosa, women recovered from anorexia nervosa, and normal-weight women. J Clin Endocrinol Metab 2012;97(4):E584–90.
58. Divasta AD, Feldman HA, Giancaterino C, et al. The effect of gonadal and adrenal steroid therapy on skeletal health in adolescents and young women with anorexia nervosa. Metabolism 2012;61(7):1010–20.
59. Rosen C, Karsenty G, MacDougald O. Foreword: interactions between bone and adipose tissue and metabolism. Bone 2012;50(2):429.
60. Kawai M, Rosen CJ. Bone: adiposity and bone accrual-still an established paradigm? Nat Rev Endocrinol 2010;6(2):63–4.
61. Hofbauer LC, Brueck CC, Singh SK, et al. Osteoporosis in patients with diabetes mellitus. J Bone Miner Res 2007;22:1317–28.
62. Inzerillo AM, Epstein S. Osteoporosis and diabetes mellitus. Rev Endocr Metab Disord 2004;5:261–8.
63. de Liefde II, van der Klift M, de Laet CE, et al. Bone mineral density and fracture risk in type-2 diabetes mellitus: the Rotterdam Study. Osteoporos Int 2005;16: 1713–20.
64. de Paula FJ, Horowitz MC, Rosen CJ. Novel insights into the relationship between diabetes and osteoporosis. Diabetes Metab Res Rev 2010;26(8):622–30. http://dx.doi.org/10.1002/dmrr.1135.
65. Nicodemus KK, Folsom AR, Iowa Women's Health Study. Type 1 and type 2 diabetes and incident hip fractures in postmenopausal women. Diabetes Care 2001; 24:1192–7.
66. Rosen CJ, Motyl KJ. No bones about it: insulin modulates skeletal remodeling. Cell 2010;142(2):198–200.
67. Kawai M, Rosen CJ. PPARγ: a circadian transcription factor in adipogenesis and osteogenesis. Nat Rev Endocrinol 2011;6(11):629–36.
68. Rosen CJ. Revisiting the rosiglitazone story-lessons learned. N Engl J Med 2010; 363(9):803–6.
69. Bilezikian JP. Bone strength in primary hyperparathyroidism. Osteoporos Int 2003;14(Suppl 5):113–7.
70. Silverberg SJ, Shane E, de la CL, et al. Skeletal disease in primary hyperparathyroidism. J Bone Miner Res 1989;4(3):283–91.
71. Khosla S, Melton LJ III, Wermers RA, et al. Primary hyperparathyroidism and the risk of fracture: a population-based study. J Bone Miner Res 1999;14(10):1700–7.
72. Silverberg SJ, Shane E, Jacobs TP, et al. A 10-year prospective study of primary hyperparathyroidism with or without parathyroid surgery. N Engl J Med 1999;341: 1249–55.

73. Rubin MR, Bilezikian JP, McMahon DJ, et al. The natural history of primary hyperparathyroidism with or without parathyroid surgery after 15-years. J Clin Endocrinol Metab 2008;93(9):3462–70.
74. Silverberg SJ, Lewiecki EM, Mosekilde L, et al. Presentation of asymptomatic primary hyperparathyroidism: proceedings of the third international workshop. J Clin Endocrinol Metab 2009;94(2):351–65.
75. Lewiecki EM. Management of skeletal health in asymptomatic primary hyperparathyroidism. J Clin Densitom 2010;13(4):324–34.
76. Bilezikian JP, Potts JT Jr, Fuleihan GE, et al. Summary statement from a workshop on asymptomatic primary hyperparathyroidism: a perspective for the 21st century. J Bone Miner Res 2002;17:N2–11.
77. Miller PD, Bilezikian JP. Bone densitometry in asymptomatic primary hyperparathyroidism. J Bone Miner Res 2002;17(Suppl 2):N98–102.
78. Bilezikian JP, Silverberg SJ. Normocalcemic primary hyperparathyroidism. Arq Bras Endocrinol Metabol 2010;54(2):106–9.
79. Eldeiry LS, Ruan DT, Brown EM, et al. Primary hyperparathyroidism and FHH: relationships and clinical implications. Endocr Pract 2012;9:1–19.
80. Pitts CJ, Kearns AE. Update on medications with adverse skeletal effects. Mayo Clin Proc 2011;86(4):338–43.
81. Kaunitz AM, Grimes DA. Removing the black-box warning for depot medroxyprogesterone acetate. Contraception 2011;84(3):212–3.
82. ACOG Committee Opinion No. 415: depot medroxyprogesterone acetate and bone effects. Obstet Gynecol 2008;112(3):727–30.
83. Meier C, Brauchli YB, Jick SS, et al. Use of depot medroxyprogesterone acetate and fracture risk. J Clin Endocrinol Metab 2010;95(11):4909–16.
84. Renner RM, Edelman AB, Kaunitz AM. Depot medroxyprogesterone acetate contraceptive injections and skeletal health. Womens Health (Lond Engl) 2010; 6(3):339–42.
85. Kaunitz AM, Miller PD, Rice VM, et al. Bone mineral density in women aged 25-35 years receiving depot medroxyprogesterone acetate: recovery following discontinuation. Contraception 2006;74(2):90–9.
86. McCloskey E. Effects of third-generation aromatase inhibitors on bone. Eur J Cancer 2006;42:1044–51.
87. Eastell R, Hannon RA, Cuzick J, et al. Effect of an aromatase inhibitor on BMD and bone turnover markers: 2-year results of the Anastrozole, Tamoxifen, Alone or in Combination (ATAC) trial. J Bone Miner Res 2006;21:1215–23.
88. Perez EA, Josse RG, Pritchard KI, et al. Effect of letrozole versus placebo on bone mineral density in women with primary breast cancer completing 5 or more years of adjuvant tamoxifen: a comparison study to NCIC CTG MA.17. J Clin Oncol 2006;24:3629–35.
89. Brufsky A, Harker WG, Beck JT, et al. Zoledronic acid inhibits adjuvant letrozole-induced bone loss in postmenopausal women with early breast cancer. J Clin Oncol 2007;25:829–36.
90. Markopoulos C, Tzoracoleftherakis E, Polychronis A, et al. Management of anastrozole-induced bone loss in breast cancer patients with oral risedronate: results from the ARBI prospective clinical trial. Breast Cancer Res 2010;12:R24.
91. Hines SL, Sloan JA, Atherton PJ, et al. Zoledronic acid for treatment of osteopenia and osteoporosis in women with primary breast cancer undergoing adjuvant aromatase inhibitor therapy. Breast 2010;19:92–6.
92. Van Poznak C, Hannon RA, Mackey JR, et al. Prevention of aromatase inhibitor-induced bone loss using risedronate: the SABRE trial. J Clin Oncol 2010;28:967–75.

93. Ellis GK, Bone HG, Chlebowski R, et al. Effect of denosumab on bone mineral density in women receiving adjuvant aromatase inhibitors for non-metastatic breast cancer: subgroup analyses of a phase 3 study. Breast Cancer Res Treat 2009;118:81–7.

94. Grisso JA, Kelsey JL, O'Brien LA, et al. Risk factors for hip fracture in men. Hip Fracture Study Group. Am J Epidemiol 1997;145:786–93.

95. Vestergaard P, Rejnmark L, Mosekilde L. Proton pump inhibitors, histamine H2 receptor antagonists, and other antacid medications and the risk of fracture. Calcif Tissue Int 2006;19:76–83.

96. Yu EW, Blackwell T, Ensrud KE, et al. Acid suppressive medications and risk of bone loss and fracture in older adults. Calcif Tissue Int 2008;83:251–9.

97. Yang YX, Lewis JD, Epstein S, et al. Long-term proton pump inhibitor therapy and risk of hip fracture. JAMA 2006;296:2947–53.

Male Osteoporosis

Matthew T. Drake, MD, PhD*, Sundeep Khosla, MD

KEYWORDS

- Osteoporosis • Men • Fracture • Epidemiology • DXA • QCT • Sex steroids

KEY POINTS

- Osteoporosis is a major health threat in aging men, with hip fractures associated with the greatest morbidity and mortality.
- Trabecular bone loss in men begins in early adulthood, while cortical bone loss occurs from midlife onwards.
- Declining bioavailable estradiol levels are closely associated with age-associated bone loss in men.

INTRODUCTION

Osteoporosis is defined as an asymptomatic bone disease marked by low bone mass and skeletal microarchitectural deterioration resulting in increased fracture risk.[1] Although osteoporosis has been widely recognized by medical professionals and the public as a significant health issue in aging women, it is now also increasingly viewed as a major health threat to the aging male population in terms of morbidity, mortality, and health care resource expenditure.

MALE FRACTURE EPIDEMIOLOGY

Despite not undergoing a menopausal transition as women do, men sustain bone loss of approximately 0.5% to 1.0% per year beginning by the sixth decade.[2] Current estimates are that approximately 20% of Americans with osteopenia or osteoporosis are men and that 1 in 8 men aged older than 50 years will incur an osteoporotic-type fracture during his lifetime, with roughly 30% of hip fractures occurring in men.[3] Fractures at both the hip and vertebrae have been shown to increase morbidity and mortality in men,[4,5] with hip fractures in men associated with an approximately 2- to 3-fold increased mortality risk relative to women.[6]

Department of Medicine, Division of Endocrinology, College of Medicine, Mayo Clinic, 200 First Street Southwest, Rochester, MN 55905, USA
* Corresponding author. Endocrine Research Unit, Guggenheim 7-11, Mayo Clinic, 200 First Street Southwest, Rochester, MN 55905.
E-mail address: drake.matthew@mayo.edu

Endocrinol Metab Clin N Am 41 (2012) 629–641
doi:10.1016/j.ecl.2012.05.001
0889-8529/12/$ – see front matter © 2012 Elsevier Inc. All rights reserved.

Fracture incidence in men has 2 peaks: one around adolescence and a second sustained peak that occurs at advanced age. Before 50 years of age, men experience more fractures than women, which is likely primarily caused by increased rates of high-energy trauma, such as athletic and work-place related injuries, in younger men relative to women.[7] Men subsequently experience an exponential increase in fractures beginning after about 75 years of age, although the absolute fracture incidence in older men remains less than in age-matched women.

Using data from the year 2000, it has been estimated that approximately 9.0 million new osteoporotic fractures occur yearly, and that roughly 39% of these occur in men.[5] In the General Practice Research Database in the United Kingdom followed from 1988 to 1998, 103,052 men among the 5 million adults followed sustained a fracture over 10.4 million person-years of follow-up.[7] In men, aging was associated with an increased risk for fracture of the vertebrae, femur, forearm, humerus, clavicle, scapula, pelvis, and ribs; thus, these fracture types were considered more likely to be associated with osteoporosis. Similar to these findings, other studies of aged men have also shown increased rates of nonvertebral fractures of the proximal femur, humerus, and forearm.[8,9] Taken together, these findings suggest that osteoporotic fractures in men primarily involve the hip, vertebrae, humerus, and forearm, although fractures at other sites, including the ribs, pelvis, and clavicle, are also associated with male aging.

Hip Fractures

In men, hip fractures are associated with the greatest morbidity and mortality. Although current evidence suggests that hip fracture rates in Western populations seem to have stabilized over the past 2 decades, hip fracture rates may be increasing in other parts of the world, including Asia.[10] Indeed, current estimates are that the number of men worldwide with hip fractures will be between 1.8 and 6.8 million by 2050.[3,11] Although absolute incidence rates vary geographically, overall incidence rates worldwide have been found to increase exponentially beginning at roughly 75 years of age.[12] Mortality is substantially higher in men compared with women following hip fracture. Men are nearly twice as likely to die during their immediate postfracture hospitalization,[13] and roughly one-third of men die within the first year following fracture.[14,15] Morbidity is also increased in men compared with women following hip fracture; nearly half of men require skilled institutionalized care following hip fracture,[16] and men are far less likely when compared with women to return to full independence at 1 year following hip fracture.[17] Further, although it is well documented that both men and women continue to be undertreated for their osteoporosis following hip fracture,[18] men seem to be disproportionally more likely to be undertreated.[19]

Vertebral Fractures

Like hip fractures, vertebral fracture incidence in men increases with age. As shown in the European Prospective Osteoporosis Study of 3174 men (mean age 63.1 years) who had spinal radiographs performed at a mean of 3.8 years following a baseline film, the age-standardized incidence of morphometric fractures was 5.7 per 1000 person-years, a rate slightly lower than the 10.7 per 1000 person-years determined in women.[20] As expected, the incidence in both sexes increased markedly with progressive age. Similar trends have been demonstrated in numerous other studies performed both in the United States and Europe,[21–24] with small differences in incidence/prevalence rates between the studies likely reflecting subject inclusion criteria, study methodologies, and geographic variation. Importantly, vertebral fractures increase the likelihood of subsequent fractures in both sexes,[25,26] have been shown to be a positive predictor of age-adjusted mortality in men,[26] and are associated with multiple indices of poorer life quality.[27]

Although fracture data in men at sites other than the spine and hip are more limited, there is now good evidence that low-trauma fractures of the upper arm (forearm and humerus) and ankle are associated with an increased risk for future fractures in men.[28]

PREVALENCE OF LOW BONE MASS IN MEN

As defined by the World Health Organization, osteopenia is a bone mineral density (BMD) measured by dual-energy x-ray absorptiometry (DXA) between 1.0 and 2.5 standard deviations (SD) less than the young adult (aged 20–29 years) normative reference mean, with osteoporosis defined as a BMD value of less than 2.5 SD less than the mean value. Using femoral BMD data from the Third National Health and Nutrition Survey and a BMD normative reference range derived from non-Hispanic whites, Looker and colleagues[29] found that substantial numbers of men had low bone mass. Using a male reference range, 3% to 6% of men had osteoporosis and 28% to 47% had osteopenia. Using a female reference mean, 1% to 4% of men had osteoporosis, whereas 15% to 33% were osteopenic. By comparison, Melton and colleagues[30] used a population-based sample of Rochester, Minnesota men to determine a prevalence estimate of 19% for osteoporosis in men aged 50 years and older when using a male reference range but only 3% when using a female reference range. There remains some debate as to whether sex-specific reference ranges may be more appropriate than a single female-based reference range for describing low bone mass in men,[31,32] although it is clear that the use of a male-specific database identifies more men as having diminished bone mass (osteopenia and osteoporosis). Estimates of low bone mass from DXA data in men other than non-Hispanic whites are more limited but suggest that non-Hispanic white men have the highest prevalence of osteopenia/osteoporosis, followed by Mexican-American men and non-Hispanic black men,[29] which are results that are consistent with the hip fracture incidence among men of different ethnic backgrounds.[33]

RISK FACTORS FOR BONE LOSS IN MEN

Because of the combination of an improved male longevity, the significant morbidity associated with fractures in aged men, and the broad availability of pharmacologic agents that documented efficacy for reducing fracture risk, it is increasingly important to identify men at an increased fracture risk for low BMD-associated fractures. There are many reasons why male bone loss occurs, which can broadly be grouped into primary (age-associated and idiopathic) and secondary (all other) causes (**Box 1**). In individual men, bone loss may result from a single cause or be caused by a combination of multiple factors. A more thorough review of risk factors associated with bone loss is men is beyond the scope of this review but has been reviewed recently.[34]

CAUSE OF MALE BONE LOSS

Although DXA is the best-established clinical method for assessing bone loss, DXA only allows for assessment of areal BMD and, therefore, lacks the ability to distinguish between cortical and trabecular bone components. Recent advances in bone imaging, however, have allowed for significant enhancement in our understanding of age-associated bone loss. Chief among these advances has been the application of quantitative computed tomography (QCT) to both central and peripheral skeletal sites, which is technology that allows for true assessments of volumetric BMD

Box 1
Primary and secondary causes of male osteoporosis

Primary Osteoporosis

    Age-related osteoporosis

    Idiopathic osteoporosis

Secondary Osteoporosis

    Alcoholism

    Chronic obstructive pulmonary disease

    Glucocorticoid excess (exogenous or endogenous)

    Gastrointestinal disorders

        Malabsorption syndromes

        Inflammatory bowel disease, celiac sprue

        Primary biliary cirrhosis

        Postgastrectomy

    Hypercalciuria

    Hyperthyroidism

    Hyperparathyroidism

    Hypogonadism

        Idiopathic

        Androgen deprivation therapy for prostate cancer

    Lifestyle choices

        Cigarette smoking

        Sedentary lifestyle

    Medication/drug related

        Anticonvulsants

        Chemotherapeutics

        Glucocorticoids

        Thyroid hormone

    Neuromuscular disorders

    Posttransplant osteoporosis

    Systemic illnesses

        Mastocytosis

        Monoclonal gammopathy

            Multiple myeloma

            Monoclonal gammopathy of undetermined significance

        Other malignancies

        Rheumatoid arthritis

Data from Khosla S, Amin S, Orwoll E. Osteoporosis in men. Endocr Rev 2008;29(4):441–64.

(vBMD) and bone microstructural changes either cross-sectional or longitudinal. Accordingly, Riggs and colleagues[35] recently assessed bone geometry and vBMD by QCT at the lumbar spine and femoral neck and peripheral QCT at the distal radius and tibia in a population-based sample of 323 men aged 20 to 97 years from Rochester, Minnesota. As seen in **Fig. 1**, a substantial (approximately 46%) nearly linear loss of lumbar spine (comprised primarily of trabecular bone) vBMD occurred across the adult male lifespan. In contrast, cortical vBMD as assessed at the radius remained essentially stable until approximately the sixth decade in men, thereafter decreasing nearly linearly by approximately 18%.

In addition to changes in vBMD, changes in bone geometry also occur with aging. As again demonstrated by Riggs and colleagues,[35] aging in men was associated with increases in bone cross-sectional area at the femoral neck caused by progressive periosteal apposition with concomitant increases in endocortical resorption, ultimately resulting in a slight decline in cortical area and thickness. Importantly, however, this net outward cortical displacement increases resistance to bending stresses, thereby providing a partial biomechanical adaptation to limit the overall loss of bone strength caused by the decreases in cortical area and thickness.[36]

Additional studies from the Osteoporotic Fractures in Men cohort examining changes in vBMD and bone dimensions at the femoral neck and shaft by QCT in a cohort of 3358 men aged 65 to 100 years demonstrated that at the femoral neck, trabecular vBMD was 22.1% lower in men aged more than 85 years compared with men aged 65 to 69 years but that cortical vBMD was similar between the two groups.[37] Confirming the results described by Riggs and colleagues,[36] increased endocortical resorption and periosteal apposition with resultant cortical thinning but outward cortical displacement was also observed at the femoral neck in the older versus younger men. At the femoral shaft by comparison, both the cross-sectional and medullary areas were increased (9% and 22% respectively) in the older versus younger men, with percent shaft cortical bone and shaft cortical vBMD both 4% lower in the older men.

Together, these studies demonstrate that although trabecular bone loss in men (and, indeed, in women) begins in early adulthood, cortical bone loss only seems to begin with midlife. Further, although an increase in periosteal apposition leads to an

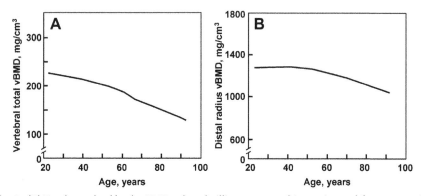

Fig. 1. (A) Total vertebral body vBMD values (milligrams per cubic centimeter) from a population sample (n = 323) of men in Rochester, Minnesota aged 20 to 97 years. (B) Cortical vBMD values at the distal radius in the same male cohort. (*Adapted from* Riggs BL, Melton Iii LJ 3rd, Robb RA, et al. Population-based study of age and sex differences in bone volumetric density, size, geometry, and structure at different skeletal sites. J Bone Miner Res 2004;19(12):1945–54; with permission from the American Society of Bone and Mineral Research.)

increase in bone cross-sectional area with aging, a simultaneous increase in endocortical resorption ultimately results in the overall decline in cortical area.

MALE BONE MICROSTRUCTURAL CHANGES WITH AGING

The more recent development of high-resolution peripheral QCT (HRpQCT), which can be used to image peripheral skeletal sites (wrist and tibia) at much higher resolutions than standard QCT, has allowed for an even more accurate noninvasive assessment of bone microstructure. In a population-based cross-sectional study of 278 men in Rochester, Minnesota aged 21 to 97 years highly characteristic of the United States white population, Khosla and colleagues[38] used HRpQCT to examine bone microstructure at the ultradistal radius. Relative to young aged-matched women aged 20 to 29 years, men had markedly greater bone volume (BV)/tissue volume (TV) and trabecular thickness (26% and 28% respectively) but little difference in trabecular number or separation. Although cross-sectional decreases in trabecular BV/TV were approximately 26% in both sexes between 20 to 90 years of age, the structural basis for these declines was fundamentally different. Women lost trabeculae and increased trabecular separation over the lifespan, whereas men primarily sustained trabecular thinning without trabecular loss. Importantly, these data are in accordance with previous histomorphometric studies of cadaveric transiliac bone biopsies obtained over approximately the same age range of 20 to 90 years, suggesting that the changes determined by HRpQCT may be similar at other skeletal sites. If so, this may partially explain the reduced fracture incidence seen in men compared with women with aging because decreases in trabecular number are anticipated to have a greater impact on bone strength relative to decreases in trabecular thickness.[39]

THE ROLE OF SEX STEROIDS IN MALE OSTEOPOROSIS

Although the role of declining sex steroid levels in bone loss is best recognized in women, marked changes in sex steroid levels also occur over the male lifespan. Unlike women in whom menopausal-associated ovarian failure is the primary cause, declining sex-steroid levels in men are principally caused by a greater than twofold age-associated increase in sex hormone binding globulin (SHBG) levels.[40] This SHBG increase limits the biologically available (free [1%–3%] and albumin-associated [35%–55%]) sex steroids, leading to declines in bioavailable testosterone (T) and estrogen (E) levels of 64% and 47%, respectively, over the male lifespan.[40]

Although T is the predominant male sex steroid, both cross-sectional[41–46] and longitudinal[47] evidence indicates that levels of bioavailable estradiol (E2) rather than T are better correlated with male BMD. In support of this, a longitudinal study that evaluated sex steroid levels in a younger male cohort (aged 22–39 years, an age range in the final stages of skeletal maturation) versus an older male cohort (aged 60–90 years, an age range in which age-related bone loss occurs) over a 4-year interval found that although distal forearm BMD (primarily reflecting cortical bone compartment changes) in the younger cohort increased approximately 0.42% to 0.43% per year, distal forearm BMD in the older men declined by 0.49% to 0.66% per year.[47] Importantly, the increased BMD in younger men and the decreased BMD in older men were more closely associated with bioavailable E2 levels than with T levels. Further, in older men, there seemed to be a threshold bioavailable E2 level of approximately 40 pM (11 pg/mL), which was less than the bone loss rates seemed to increase. Further vBMD analyses showed that this bioavailable E2 threshold correlated better with cortical than trabecular sites.[48] Above this threshold, however, there was no firm relationship seen between bone loss rates and bioavailable E2 levels. Additional work has supported this threshold effect for bioavailable and total E2,[49] although the absolute threshold determined by other investigators has varied slightly depending on whether E2 levels were determined by immunoassay (approximately 20–25 pg/mL) or mass spectroscopy (16 pg/mL).[50,51]

Although correlative, the previous findings provide no direct evidence of a causal role for E in male bone health with aging. To directly assess the role of sex steroids (E and T) on skeletal health in aging men, Falahati-Nini and colleagues[52] undertook a direct interventional study in which they suppressed endogenous T and E production (by treatment with both a gonadotropin-releasing hormone agonist and an aromatase inhibitor) while simultaneously providing physiologic replacement levels of E and T by topical patch placement. Following the determination of the baseline bone turnover markers while on the previous endogenous suppression/physiologic replacement regime, patients were randomized into 1 of 4 groups: group A (-T, -E) discontinued both patches, group B (-T, +E) continued only the E patch, group C (+T, -E) continued only the T patch, and group D (+T, +E) continued both patches. Accordingly, the study design permitted the determination of bone metabolism changes caused by either E or T because endogenous sex steroid production was suppressed throughout the study.

As seen in **Fig. 2**, the complete absence of both T and E (group A) resulted in significant increases in bone resorption, which was completely prevented by treatment with both T and E (group D). Treatment with E alone was almost completely able to prevent the increase in bone resorption (group B), whereas T alone had only modest effects (group C). Comparatively, the significant decline in serum bone formation markers (osteocalcin and amino-terminal propeptide of type I collagen [P1NP]) that occurred with a deficiency of both T and E (group A) was completely prevented by the supplementation of both T and E (group D); treatment with either E or T alone lead to only slight decreases in osteocalcin levels, whereas P1NP levels were maintained with E (group B) but not T (group C) treatment. Together, these results are consistent with a dominant role for E as the major sex steroid regulating skeletal health in aged men.

With male aging, levels of bioavailable T decline even more precipitously than those of bioavailable E. Despite this decrease, however, the extent to which the diminution of bioavailable T levels impacts bone loss associated with male aging is less clear when compared with the role of declining bioavailable E levels. As shown, T imparts modest effects on bone resorption and also affects bone formation (see **Fig. 2**). As recently demonstrated, increased femoral neck BMD occurred in aged men who received low-dose T replacement for 2 years[53] despite the absence of BMD increases at any other site examined (lumbar spine, total hip, or distal radius). Whether the effect of T on femoral neck BMD in this study was direct or rather the result of T aromatization to E, however, is unclear. Current evidence suggests that T also likely plays a role in cortical appositional bone growth, although this has been most convincingly demonstrated in rodent studies[54] and the extent to which T has this function with aging in men is less clear.

Finally, it has been suggested that T may play a more indirect role in male skeletal health with aging by allowing for relative maintenance of balance and muscle strength in men compared with women.[51] As such, the slightly lower fracture incidence in aged men relative to age-matched women may be partially reflective of the increased frequency of falling that occurs with aging in women relative to men,[55,56] with fractures after falls occurring 2.2-fold higher in women than men.[57]

OTHER POTENTIAL CAUSES OF MALE BONE LOSS

A variety of other factors have been postulated to play a role in age-associated male bone loss. These factors include an age-associated increase in parathyroid hormone

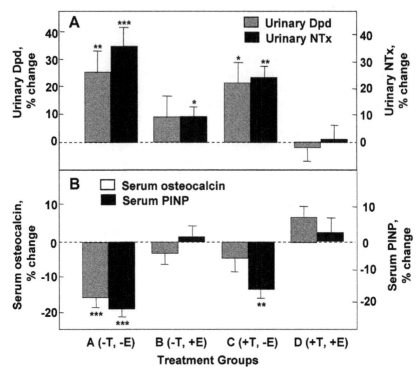

Fig. 2. Percent changes in markers of (A) bone resorption (urinary deoxypyridinoline [Dpd] and N-telopeptide of type I collagen [NTX]) and (B) bone formation (serum osteocalcin and N-terminal extension peptide of type I collagen [P1NP]) in elderly men (mean age, 68 years) pharmacologically made acutely hypogonadal and subsequently treated with either an aromatase inhibitor (group A), E alone (group B), T alone (group C), or both E and T (group D). Significance for change from baseline: asterisk, $P<.05$; double asterisk, $P<.01$; triple asterisk, $P<.001$. (*Adapted from* Falahati-Nini A, Riggs BL, Atkinson EJ, et al. Relative contributions of testosterone and estrogen in regulating bone resorption and formation in normal elderly men. J Clin Invest 2000;106(12):1553–60; with permission from the American Society for Clinical Investigation.)

levels,[58] decreases in growth hormone and circulating bioavailable insulinlike growth factor levels,[59] and inherent changes or loss of stem or osteoprogenitor cells.[60] Additionally, nutrition also seems to be critical for optimal skeletal health because the failure to maintain an adequate intake of vitamin D, calcium, or protein has shown to lead to worsened bone health in men.[12]

CARE FOR MALE PATIENTS WITH BONE LOSS

Reducing the substantial fracture risk that occurs with bone loss in men is now more widely recognized as an important goal of optimal patient care. Despite this recognition, however, most studies using pharmacologic interventions have been performed in women; further, the comparatively fewer studies in men have typically assessed BMD changes as a surrogate for fracture risk. Nonetheless, current evidence suggests that the most commonly prescribed therapies (nitrogen-containing bisphosphonates and teriparatide) are as efficacious in men as they are in women.

Bisphosphonates

Alendronate,[61] risedronate,[62] ibandronate,[63] and zoledronate[64] have all been shown to increase BMD and reduce biochemical markers of bone turnover in men with low bone mass, with alendronate, risedronate, and zoledronate having received Food and Drug Administration (FDA) approval for the treatment of osteoporosis in men. Importantly, BMD changes with bisphosphonate therapy seem to be equivalent in men with low free T levels as in men with normal levels,[61] perhaps indicating why bisphosphonate therapy is effective in limiting bone loss in men receiving androgen deprivation therapy for prostate cancer. Bisphosphonates have also been shown to be effective for limiting bone loss in men receiving corticosteroid therapy[65] or in the setting of acute immobilization.[66]

Teriparatide

Once daily recombinant parathyroid hormone 1–34 increases BMD in men with low bone mass and seems to reduce the risk for vertebral fractures.[67] As with bisphosphonates, results seem to be similar in magnitude to those seen in women, and teriparatide has received FDA approval for the treatment of osteoporosis in men.

Denosumab

The receptor activator of nuclear factor kappa-B (RANK) ligand inhibitor was initially approved for the treatment of osteoporosis in women and was more recently FDA-approved for the treatment of men with nonmetastatic prostate cancer with osteopenia and a high risk of fracture receiving androgen-deprivation therapy.

A more complete review of additional potential pharmacologic agents for the management of male bone loss is beyond the scope of this review. Accordingly, the reader is referred to a recently published meta-analysis of the comparative effectiveness of currently available pharmacologic agents for reducing fracture risk in men.[68]

ADDITIONAL SUPPORTIVE CARE

In addition to pharmacologic interventions, ensuring that men with low bone mass receive appropriate supportive care is essential for limiting fracture risk. Such care includes confirming that patients have adequate vitamin D and calcium intake both before and while maintained on therapy. In older community-dwelling men aged 65 years and older, moderate reductions in bone loss at the hip and spine and reduced nonvertebral fracture incidence were seen in patients receiving dietary vitamin D and calcium supplementation for 3 years compared with patients who received placebo.[69] Notably, recommendations from the Institute of Medicine on dietary intakes of calcium and vitamin D have been recently published, with skeletal-related outcomes as the primary end point for most included studies.[70,71]

Finally, defining appropriate generalized exercise prescriptions in patients at increased fracture risk remains an important part of the care plan for most patients because increases in physical performance are expected to increase muscle mass and tone, thereby reduce frailty and decreasing fall risk. To date, however, studies that have attempted to examine this approach to exercise in at-risk patients have not used standardized methods. Because of the significant heterogeneity among studies that examined the role of exercise in fracture reduction, a recent review concluded that currently available data do not allow for proper quantitative assessment of the risk associated with exercise in at-risk patients.[34]

SUMMARY

Although much work over the preceding 2 decades has enlightened our understanding of male bone loss, significant challenges to providing optimal care to our male patients persist. Osteoporosis in men remains an underrecognized clinical problem that will continue to grow in importance with the aging of the population. Despite significant advances in our understanding of the epidemiology, risk factors, causes, and therapeutic approaches to male osteoporosis, much work awaits if we are to limit future morbidity and mortality associated with bone loss in men.

REFERENCES

1. Consensus development conference: diagnosis, prophylaxis, and treatment of osteoporosis. Am J Med 1993;94(6):646–50.
2. Melton LJ 3rd, Khosla S, Achenbach SJ, et al. Effects of body size and skeletal site on the estimated prevalence of osteoporosis in women and men. Osteoporos Int 2000;11(11):977–83.
3. Cooper C, Campion G, Melton LJ 3rd. Hip fractures in the elderly: a world-wide projection. Osteoporos Int 1992;2(6):285–9.
4. Johnell O, Kanis JA. An estimate of the worldwide prevalence, mortality and disability associated with hip fracture. Osteoporos Int 2004;15(11):897–902.
5. Johnell O, Kanis JA. An estimate of the worldwide prevalence and disability associated with osteoporotic fractures. Osteoporos Int 2006;17(12):1726–33.
6. Center JR, Nguyen TV, Schneider D, et al. Mortality after all major types of osteoporotic fracture in men and women: an observational study. Lancet 1999;353(9156):878–82.
7. van Staa TP, Dennison EM, Leufkens HG, et al. Epidemiology of fractures in England and Wales. Bone 2001;29(6):517–22.
8. Schuit SC, van der Klift M, Weel AE, et al. Fracture incidence and association with bone mineral density in elderly men and women: the Rotterdam study. Bone 2004;34(1):195–202.
9. Jonsson BY, Siggeirsdottir K, Mogensen B, et al. Fracture rate in a population-based sample of men in Reykjavik. Acta Orthop Scand 2004;75(2):195–200.
10. Cooper C, Cole ZA, Holroyd CR, et al. Secular trends in the incidence of hip and other osteoporotic fractures. Osteoporos Int 2011;22(5):1277–88.
11. Gullberg B, Johnell O, Kanis JA. World-wide projections for hip fracture. Osteoporos Int 1997;7(5):407–13.
12. Khosla S, Amin S, Orwoll E. Osteoporosis in men. Endocr Rev 2008;29(4):441–64.
13. Diamond TH, Thornley SW, Sekel R, et al. Hip fracture in elderly men: prognostic factors and outcomes. Med J Aust 1997;167(8):412–5.
14. Kiebzak GM, Beinart GA, Perser K, et al. Undertreatment of osteoporosis in men with hip fracture. Arch Intern Med 2002;162(19):2217–22.
15. Bass E, French DD, Bradham DD, et al. Risk-adjusted mortality rates of elderly veterans with hip fractures. Ann Epidemiol 2007;17(7):514–9.
16. Poor G, Atkinson EJ, O'Fallon WM, et al. Determinants of reduced survival following hip fractures in men. Clin Orthop Relat Res 1995;(319):260–5.
17. Schurch MA, Rizzoli R, Mermillod B, et al. A prospective study on socioeconomic aspects of fracture of the proximal femur. J Bone Miner Res 1996;11(12):1935–42.
18. Curtis JR, McClure LA, Delzell E, et al. Population-based fracture risk assessment and osteoporosis treatment disparities by race and gender. J Gen Intern Med 2009;24(8):956–62.

19. Shibli-Rahhal A, Vaughan-Sarrazin MS, Richardson K, et al. Testing and treatment for osteoporosis following hip fracture in an integrated U.S. healthcare delivery system. Osteoporos Int 2011;22(12):2973–80.

20. Incidence of vertebral fracture in Europe: results from the European Prospective Osteoporosis Study (EPOS). J Bone Miner Res 2002;17(4):716–24.

21. O'Neill TW, Felsenberg D, Varlow J, et al. The prevalence of vertebral deformity in European men and women: the European Vertebral Osteoporosis Study. J Bone Miner Res 1996;11(7):1010–8.

22. Davies KM, Stegman MR, Heaney RP, et al. Prevalence and severity of vertebral fracture: the Saunders County Bone Quality Study. Osteoporos Int 1996;6(2):160–5.

23. Santavirta S, Konttinen YT, Heliovaara M, et al. Determinants of osteoporotic thoracic vertebral fracture. Screening of 57,000 Finnish women and men. Acta Orthop Scand 1992;63(2):198–202.

24. Szulc P, Munoz F, Marchand F, et al. Semiquantitative evaluation of prevalent vertebral deformities in men and their relationship with osteoporosis: the MINOS study. Osteoporos Int 2001;12(4):302–10.

25. Melton LJ 3rd, Atkinson EJ, Cooper C, et al. Vertebral fractures predict subsequent fractures. Osteoporos Int 1999;10(3):214–21.

26. Hasserius R, Karlsson MK, Nilsson BE, et al. Prevalent vertebral deformities predict increased mortality and increased fracture rate in both men and women: a 10-year population-based study of 598 individuals from the Swedish cohort in the European Vertebral Osteoporosis Study. Osteoporos Int 2003;14(1):61–8.

27. Burger H, Van Daele PL, Grashuis K, et al. Vertebral deformities and functional impairment in men and women. J Bone Miner Res 1997;12(1):152–7.

28. Center JR, Bliuc D, Nguyen TV, et al. Risk of subsequent fracture after low-trauma fracture in men and women. JAMA 2007;297(4):387–94.

29. Looker AC, Orwoll ES, Johnston CC Jr, et al. Prevalence of low femoral bone density in older U.S. adults from NHANES III. J Bone Miner Res 1997;12(11):1761–8.

30. Melton LJ 3rd, Atkinson EJ, O'Connor MK, et al. Bone density and fracture risk in men. J Bone Miner Res 1998;13(12):1915–23.

31. Khosla S. Update in male osteoporosis. J Clin Endocrinol Metab 2010;95(1):3–10.

32. Kanis JA, Bianchi G, Bilezikian JP, et al. Towards a diagnostic and therapeutic consensus in male osteoporosis. Osteoporos Int 2011;22(11):2789–98.

33. Silverman SL, Madison RE. Decreased incidence of hip fracture in Hispanics, Asians, and blacks: California hospital discharge data. Am J Public Health 1988;78(11):1482–3.

34. Drake MT, Murad MH, Mauck KF, et al. Risk factors for low bone mass-related fractures in men: a systematic review and meta-analysis. J Clin Endocrinol Metab 2012;97(6):1861–70.

35. Riggs BL, Melton Iii LJ 3rd, Robb RA, et al. Population-based study of age and sex differences in bone volumetric density, size, geometry, and structure at different skeletal sites. J Bone Miner Res 2004;19(12):1945–54.

36. Turner CH. Bone strength: current concepts. Ann N Y Acad Sci 2006;1068:429–46.

37. Marshall LM, Lang TF, Lambert LC, et al. Dimensions and volumetric BMD of the proximal femur and their relation to age among older U.S. men. J Bone Miner Res 2006;21(8):1197–206.

38. Khosla S, Riggs BL, Atkinson EJ, et al. Effects of sex and age on bone microstructure at the ultradistal radius: a population-based noninvasive in vivo assessment. J Bone Miner Res 2006;21(1):124–31.

39. Silva MJ, Gibson LJ. Modeling the mechanical behavior of vertebral trabecular bone: effects of age-related changes in microstructure. Bone 1997;21(2):191–9.

40. Khosla S, Melton LJ 3rd, Atkinson EJ, et al. Relationship of serum sex steroid levels and bone turnover markers with bone mineral density in men and women: a key role for bioavailable estrogen. J Clin Endocrinol Metab 1998;83(7):2266–74.

41. Slemenda CW, Longcope C, Zhou L, et al. Sex steroids and bone mass in older men. Positive associations with serum estrogens and negative associations with androgens. J Clin Invest 1997;100(7):1755–9.

42. Greendale GA, Edelstein S, Barrett-Connor E. Endogenous sex steroids and bone mineral density in older women and men: the Rancho Bernardo Study. J Bone Miner Res 1997;12(11):1833–43.

43. Center JR, Nguyen TV, Sambrook PN, et al. Hormonal and biochemical parameters in the determination of osteoporosis in elderly men. J Clin Endocrinol Metab 1999;84(10):3626–35.

44. van den Beld AW, de Jong FH, Grobbee DE, et al. Measures of bioavailable serum testosterone and estradiol and their relationships with muscle strength, bone density, and body composition in elderly men. J Clin Endocrinol Metab 2000;85(9):3276–82.

45. Amin S, Zhang Y, Sawin CT, et al. Association of hypogonadism and estradiol levels with bone mineral density in elderly men from the Framingham study. Ann Intern Med 2000;133(12):951–63.

46. Szulc P, Munoz F, Claustrat B, et al. Bioavailable estradiol may be an important determinant of osteoporosis in men: the MINOS study. J Clin Endocrinol Metab 2001;86(1):192–9.

47. Khosla S, Melton LJ 3rd, Atkinson EJ, et al. Relationship of serum sex steroid levels to longitudinal changes in bone density in young versus elderly men. J Clin Endocrinol Metab 2001;86(8):3555–61.

48. Khosla S, Riggs BL, Robb RA, et al. Relationship of volumetric bone density and structural parameters at different skeletal sites to sex steroid levels in women. J Clin Endocrinol Metab 2005;90(9):5096–103.

49. Gennari L, Merlotti D, Martini G, et al. Longitudinal association between sex hormone levels, bone loss, and bone turnover in elderly men. J Clin Endocrinol Metab 2003;88(11):5327–33.

50. Mellstrom D, Vandenput L, Mallmin H, et al. Older men with low serum estradiol and high serum SHBG have an increased risk of fractures. J Bone Miner Res 2008;23(10):1552–60.

51. Khosla S, Melton LJ 3rd, Riggs BL. The unitary model for estrogen deficiency and the pathogenesis of osteoporosis: is a revision needed? J Bone Miner Res 2011; 26(3):441–51.

52. Falahati-Nini A, Riggs BL, Atkinson EJ, et al. Relative contributions of testosterone and estrogen in regulating bone resorption and formation in normal elderly men. J Clin Invest 2000;106(12):1553–60.

53. Nair KS, Rizza RA, O'Brien P, et al. DHEA in elderly women and DHEA or testosterone in elderly men. N Engl J Med 2006;355(16):1647–59.

54. Wakley GK, Schutte HD Jr, Hannon KS, et al. Androgen treatment prevents loss of cancellous bone in the orchidectomized rat. J Bone Miner Res 1991;6(4): 325–30.

55. Sattin RW, Lambert Huber DA, DeVito CA, et al. The incidence of fall injury events among the elderly in a defined population. Am J Epidemiol 1990;131(6):1028–37.

56. Paspati I, Galanos A, Lyritis GP. Hip fracture epidemiology in Greece during 1977-1992. Calcif Tissue Int 1998;62(6):542–7.

57. Stevens JA, Sogolow ED. Gender differences for non-fatal unintentional fall related injuries among older adults. Inj Prev 2005;11(2):115–9.
58. Kennel KA, Riggs BL, Achenbach SJ, et al. Role of parathyroid hormone in mediating age-related changes in bone resorption in men. Osteoporos Int 2003;14(8): 631–6.
59. Boonen S, Mohan S, Dequeker J, et al. Down-regulation of the serum stimulatory components of the insulin-like growth factor (IGF) system (IGF-I, IGF-II, IGF binding protein [BP]-3, and IGFBP-5) in age-related (type II) femoral neck osteoporosis. J Bone Miner Res 1999;14(12):2150–8.
60. Undale AH, Westendorf JJ, Yaszemski MJ, et al. Mesenchymal stem cells for bone repair and metabolic bone diseases. Mayo Clin Proc 2009;84(10):893–902.
61. Orwoll E, Ettinger M, Weiss S, et al. Alendronate for the treatment of osteoporosis in men. N Engl J Med 2000;343(9):604–10.
62. Ringe JD, Faber H, Farahmand P, et al. Efficacy of risedronate in men with primary and secondary osteoporosis: results of a 1-year study. Rheumatol Int 2006;26(5):427–31.
63. Orwoll ES, Binkley NC, Lewiecki EM, et al. Efficacy and safety of monthly ibandronate in men with low bone density. Bone 2010;46(4):970–6.
64. Orwoll ES, Miller PD, Adachi JD, et al. Efficacy and safety of a once-yearly i.v. infusion of zoledronic acid 5 mg versus a once-weekly 70-mg oral alendronate in the treatment of male osteoporosis: a randomized, multicenter, double-blind, active-controlled study. J Bone Miner Res 2010;25(10):2239–50.
65. Sambrook PN, Roux C, Devogelaer JP, et al. Bisphosphonates and glucocorticoid osteoporosis in men: results of a randomized controlled trial comparing zoledronic acid with risedronate. Bone 2012;50(1):289–95.
66. Bauman WA, Wecht JM, Kirshblum S, et al. Effect of pamidronate administration on bone in patients with acute spinal cord injury. J Rehabil Res Dev 2005;42(3): 305–13.
67. Girotra M, Rubin MR, Bilezikian JP. The use of parathyroid hormone in the treatment of osteoporosis. Rev Endocr Metab Disord 2006;7(1–2):113–21.
68. Murad MH, Drake MT, Mullan RJ, et al. Comparative effectiveness of drug treatments to prevent fragility fractures: a systematic review and network meta-analysis. J Clin Endocrinol Metab 2012, Mar 30. [Epub ahead of print].
69. Dawson-Hughes B, Harris SS, Krall EA, et al. Effect of calcium and vitamin D supplementation on bone density in men and women 65 years of age or older. N Engl J Med 1997;337(10):670–6.
70. Ross AC, Manson JE, Abrams SA, et al. The 2011 report on dietary reference intakes for calcium and vitamin D from the Institute of Medicine: what clinicians need to know. J Clin Endocrinol Metab 2011;96(1):53–8.
71. Rosen CJ, Gallagher JC. The 2011 IOM report on vitamin D and calcium requirements for North America: clinical implications for providers treating patients with low bone mineral density. J Clin Densitom 2011;14(2):79–84.

Combination Anabolic and Antiresorptive Therapy for Osteoporosis

Natalie E. Cusano, MD, John P. Bilezikian, MD*

KEYWORDS

- Combination therapy • PTH(1–34) • Teriparatide • PTH(1–84) • Antiresorptive
- Bisphosphonate

KEY POINTS

- Osteoanabolic agents directly stimulate bone formation to improve both bone mass and skeletal microarchitecture, properties not shared by antiresorptive agents.
- Despite many attempts to show an advantage of simultaneous combination therapy with osteoanabolic and antiresorptive drugs, most studies have shown that monotherapy with the full-length molecule of parathyroid hormone, PTH(1–84), or its fully active, but truncated amino-terminal fragment, PTH(1–34), is as good, if not better than, combination therapy.
- Treatment with an antiresorptive following PTH(1–34) or PTH(1–84) therapy is necessary to maintain increases in bone mass.

INTRODUCTION

The full-length molecule of parathyroid hormone, PTH(1–84), and its fully active, fore-shortened variant, PTH(1–34) (teriparatide), represent the only available osteoanabolic treatments for osteoporosis at this time. Osteoanabolic agents are an attractive therapeutic option for postmenopausal women and for men with osteoporosis because of their direct stimulation of bone formation, an action that is not shared by any antiresorptive agent. PTH increases bone mineral density (BMD) at the lumbar spine, primarily a cancellous site, with more modest increases in the hip region, a site that is an admixture of cancellous and cortical bone. The early effect of PTH is an initial rapid increase in bone formation markers, subsequently followed by an increase in bone resorption markers. The pharmacokinetics of this effect suggest that PTH can

Disclosures: Dr Bilezikian is a consultant for Eli Lilly, NPS Pharmaceuticals, Merck, Warner-Chilcott, GSK, Novartis, and Amgen, and receives research support from NPS Pharmaceuticals and GSK. Dr Cusano has no conflicts of interest to report.
Division of Endocrinology, Department of Medicine, College of Physicians and Surgeons, Columbia University, 630 West 168th Street, PH 8W-864, New York, NY 10032, USA
* Corresponding author.
E-mail address: jpb2@columbia.edu

Endocrinol Metab Clin N Am 41 (2012) 643–654
doi:10.1016/j.ecl.2012.04.005
0889-8529/12/$ – see front matter © 2012 Elsevier Inc. All rights reserved.

initially stimulate processes associated with bone formation before bone resorption is stimulated. Bone biopsies from subjects treated with PTH(1–34) have confirmed that bone formation occurs first on quiescent surfaces in a manner that suggests a modeling mechanism.[1] The modeling process is a characteristic of the growing skeleton and is not usually seen in the mature human skeleton. The adult human skeleton typically demonstrates bone remodeling, a process by which mature bone is replaced by more resilient, young bone. Continued therapy with PTH does lead to a stimulation of bone remodeling, but in this setting bone formation exceeds bone resorption so that bone accrual is favored, even when remodeling is stimulated by PTH. It is estimated that 70% of the ultimate anabolic effect is due to remodeling.

The concept of the anabolic window describes the period of time when PTH directly stimulates bone formation before stimulation of bone remodeling, but it also includes, to a lesser extent, the period of time during remodeling when bone formation is favored over bone resorption (**Fig. 1**).[2] These actions of PTH on skeletal dynamics are limited. Over a 2-year treatment period, the increased rate of bone turnover is mitigated, with levels falling toward baseline. The 18- to 24-month approval period of PTH(1–84) and PTH(1–34) is consistent with these modeling and remodeling dynamics. PTH(1–34) is approved worldwide, including in Europe and the United States, for the treatment of advanced osteoporosis in men and postmenopausal women at high risk for fracture, as well as for the treatment of glucocorticoid-induced osteoporosis. PTH(1–84) is approved in Europe and elsewhere, but not in the United States, for the treatment of postmenopausal osteoporosis.

The anabolic actions of PTH are confirmed further by detailed skeletal microstructure studies of Dempster and colleagues.[3] Their study evaluated paired iliac crest bone biopsy specimens from both men and women with osteoporosis before and after treatment with PTH(1–34) 400 IU daily (approximately equivalent to 25 μg daily). By histomorphometry, cortical width was maintained in men and significantly increased in women (632 ± 95 μm at baseline to 951 ± 130 μm posttreatment, $P<.001$). There was no increase in cortical porosity. There was a significant increase in the width of

PTH as an anabolic agent for bone: A kinetic model

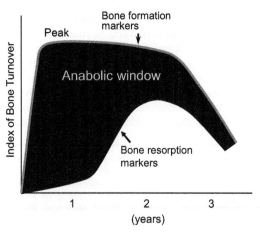

Fig. 1. The anabolic window. The graph demonstrates the concept that bone formation is first stimulated by PTH(1–34) or PTH(1–84), followed by an increase in bone resorption. (*From* Cusano NE, Costa AG, Silva BC, et al. Therapy of osteoporosis in men with teriparatide. J Osteoporos 2011;2011:463675; with permission.)

bone packets on the endocortical surface in both men and women, associated with a significant decrease in the eroded perimeter. Microcomputed tomography of the bone biopsy specimens confirmed these findings, and in addition demonstrated an increase in trabecular connectivity, to as much as 253% (**Fig. 2**). Graeff and colleagues[3] evaluated high-resolution computed tomography imaging data from a subset of participants in the European Study of Forsteo (EUROFORS) treated with PTH(1–34) 20 µg daily for 12 months. In treatment-naïve patients, there were significant increases in apparent trabecular number (+12.9% ± 22% from baseline to 12 months; P<.05) and trabecular thickness (+8.4% ± 7% from baseline to 12 months; P<.001), accompanied by reductions in trabecular separation (−10.5% ± 18%; P not significant).

Given that osteoanabolic therapy uniquely helps to restore deteriorated skeletal microstructure that forms the structural basis for osteoporosis, it may be expected that this approach would be routinely used as first-line treatment for osteoporosis. However, anabolic therapy is restricted in time and to subjects who are at high risk for fracture. It is thus used in a very small number of patients with osteoporosis. The study population that led to approval of PTH(1–34) had advanced osteoporosis. The trial was shortened to an average of only 21 months in women and 11 months in men, because of the discovery of rat osteosarcoma in toxicity studies (see later discussion). These explanations are the obvious ones for why the drug is limited in use with a black-box warning in the United States. Other limitations to more widespread use include that it has to be given by daily subcutaneous injection, a route and frequency of administration that are not ideal. The drugs are also very expensive. Another point is that the antiresorptive agents such as alendronate,[4] risedronate,[5] and zoledronic acid[6] have also been shown to be efficacious in severely osteoporotic individuals, and their use is associated with greater convenience and less expense. The only head-to-head comparison between PTH(1–34) and an antiresorptive dealt with

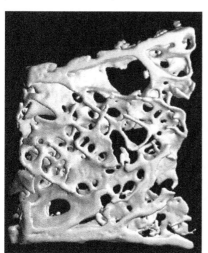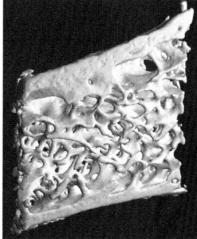

Fig. 2. Improved trabecular connectivity after PTH(1–34) therapy. Paired biopsies from a 64-year-old woman. The sample on the left was taken before treatment and the one on the right was taken from the contralateral side after treatment. In this patient, cortical thickness increased from 0.32 mm to 0.42 mm, and connectivity density increased from 2.9/mm³ to 4.6/mm³. (*Reproduced from* Dempster DW, Cosman F, Kurland ES, et al. Effects of daily treatment with parathyroid hormone on bone microarchitecture and turnover in patients with osteoporosis: a paired biopsy study. J Bone Miner Res 2001;16:1850; with permission of the American Society for Bone and Mineral Research.)

a special group of individuals who had glucocorticoid-induced osteoporosis. In that study by Saag and colleagues,[7,8] PTH(1–34) was superior to alendronate in protecting against vertebral fractures over a 3-year period.

The points covered in this review address questions regarding sequential and combination therapy with osteoanabolic and antiresorptive drugs. Most patients who receive PTH(1–34) or PTH(1–84) have previously received an antiresorptive drug; is there an influence of previous antiresorptive treatment on subsequent therapy with PTH? In patients who have been treated with antiresorptive therapy, is it better to add the osteoanabolic agent or it is better to switch from the antiresorptive to the osteoanabolic alone? Can one use simultaneous de novo osteoanabolic and antiresorptive agents in a manner that will expand the anabolic window? Finally, because PTH(1–34) and PTH(1–84) are approved only for up to 2 years, is it necessary to follow this treatment course with antiresorptive therapy? These questions are addressed in this article.

OSTEOANABOLIC THERAPY FOLLOWING ANTIRESORPTIVE THERAPY ("SWITCHING")

Kurland and colleagues[9] have shown that the level of baseline bone turnover in subjects not previously treated with any antiresorptive therapy affects the subsequent response to PTH(1–34): the lower the level of turnover, the more sluggish the initial densitometric response to PTH(1–34). In support of this idea, Ettinger and colleagues[10] showed that in women following an average of 29 months of raloxifene or alendronate treatment, densitometric gains with PTH(1–34) following raloxifene were rapid, but following alendronate were delayed. Of note, median baseline levels of bone turnover marker levels in subjects previously treated with alendronate were lower than those previously treated with raloxifene by approximately 50%. It appeared that alendronate, by virtue of its more potent antiresorptive effects, interfered with the rapid effects of PTH(1–34) to stimulate bone formation. Providing additional support for this idea is the Open-label Study to Determine How Prior Therapy with Alendronate or Risedronate in Postmenopausal Women with Osteoporosis Influences the Clinical Effectiveness of Teriparatide (OPTAMISE) by Miller and colleagues,[11] in which patients previously treated with either risedronate or alendronate for at least 24 months were then switched to PTH(1–34). Median baseline levels of bone turnover markers in individuals first treated with risedronate were higher than those first treated with alendronate. The individuals first treated with risedronate responded more exuberantly to PTH(1–34) with more rapid increases in BMD. The results are consistent with the smaller effect of risedronate on bone turnover, thus permitting a more rapid response to PTH(1–34).

In a secondary analysis of the EUROFORS study, Boonen and colleagues[12] studied the effects of 2 years of PTH(1–34) treatment on BMD and bone formation markers in postmenopausal women previously treated with at least 1 year of antiresorptive therapy: alendronate, risedronate, etidronate, and nonbisphosphonate antiresorptives. Bone formation markers increased significantly in all groups after 1 month of PTH(1–34) treatment, although subjects previously treated with alendronate had significantly lower baseline values. BMD responses were similar in all previous antiresorptive groups, but previous etidronate users showed a greater increase at the lumbar spine. These results are consistent with the OPTAMISE trial results. In addition, the EUROFORS study demonstrated that duration of previous antiresorptive therapy and time between stopping previous therapy and starting PTH(1–34) did not affect the BMD response at any skeletal site.

As demonstrated in these studies, within a short period of time any delay due to previous antiresorptive therapy, if present, is overcome in terms of patient response to therapy.[13–15] If there is a delay in subsequent responsiveness to PTH after antiresorptive therapy, it appears to be surmounted within approximately 6 months.

OSTEOANABOLIC THERAPY FOLLOWING ONGOING ANTIRESORPTIVE THERAPY ("ADDING")

In postmenopausal women with a history of antecedent estrogen therapy, Lindsay and colleagues[16] and Lane and colleagues[17] showed rapid and sustained increases in lumbar spine BMD with PTH(1–34) in glucocorticoid-induced osteoporosis. The magnitude of the changes was similar to that when using PTH alone. When Cosman and colleagues[18] used alendronate as the antecedent antiresorptive, the addition of PTH(1–34) was also associated with prompt increases in BMD. The same BMD gains were seen whether PTH(1–34) was used in a 3-month cyclical fashion or continuously with a backdrop of continuous alendronate administration.

FURTHER EXAMINATION OF THE QUESTION: SWITCHING VERSUS ADDING

In a protocol that focused on regimens of switching versus adding, as well as antiresorptive potency per se, the study of Cosman and colleagues[15] is noteworthy. Subjects previously treated with either raloxifene or alendronate for at least 18 months were then administered PTH(1–34) and antiresorptive together (add regimen) or PTH(1–34) alone (switch regimen, antiresorptive discontinued) for the next 18 months. While bone turnover markers increased more in the switch group (from either alendronate or raloxifene to PTH(1–34)), the densitometric gains were greatest when PTH(1–34) was added to the antiresorptive drug. The results seem counterintuitive at first, but the data show that the anabolic window (the difference between increases in bone formation over bone resorption) was greater with the add regimen (**Fig. 3**).[19] The study had too few subjects to determine whether the greater gains in BMD with the add regimen might have been associated with better fracture results. In addition, raloxifene was associated with greater changes in bone turnover markers and bone density at the lumbar spine than was alendronate, consistent with the findings of Ettinger and colleagues.[10] This latter point demonstrates again that the more potent the antiresorptive agent (ie, alendronate), the greater its

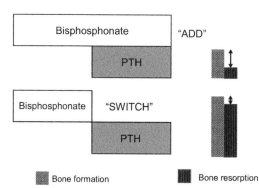

Fig. 3. The anabolic window (the difference between increases in bone formation over bone resorption) in the *add* regimen (PTH(1–34) added to alendronate or raloxifene) versus the *switch* regimen (antiresorptive discontinued prior to PTH(1–34)). (*Data from* Cosman F, Wermers RA, Recknor C, et al. Effects of teriparatide in postmenopausal women with osteoporosis on prior alendronate or raloxifene: differences between stopping and continuing the antiresorptive agent. J Clin Endocrinol Metab 2009;94:3772–80.)

lasting effect on bone turnover in comparison with a less potent antiresorptive (ie, raloxifene).

SIMULTANEOUS USE OF OSTEOANABOLIC AND ANTIRESORPTIVE THERAPY

The idea of using osteoanabolic and antiresorptive therapy together in subjects who have not previously been treated is attractive, based on the different mechanisms of action of these therapeutic classes. If bone resorption is inhibited by an antiresorptive while bone formation is stimulated by an osteoanabolic agent, combination therapy might give better results than therapy with either agent alone. Implicit in this postulate is that the anabolic window is expanded. Despite the intuitive appeal of this reasoning, important data to the contrary have been provided by Black and colleagues[20] and Finkelstein and colleagues.[21] These 2 groups independently conducted trials using a form of PTH alone, alendronate alone, or the combination of PTH and alendronate.

The Parathyroid Hormone and Alendronate for Osteoporosis (PaTH) study conducted by Black and colleagues[20] investigated the combination of alendronate and PTH(1–84) in 238 postmenopausal women who were randomly allocated to 1 of 3 daily treatment groups: alendronate 10 mg (60 women), PTH(1–84) 100 µg (119 women), or both agents combined (59 women). After 12 months, there were no differences ($P = .84$) between the PTH(1–84) alone (+6.3%) or combination groups (+6.1%) in lumbar spine BMD by dual-energy x-ray absorptiometry (DXA), whereas both PTH(1–84) alone or in combination showed greater increases than the alendronate group, although not statistically significant (+4.6%: $P = .15$ combination vs alendronate). All 3 groups showed equivalent increases at the femoral neck site of the hip. The study also monitored changes by quantitative computed tomography (QCT). Increases in vertebral trabecular BMD in the women treated with PTH(1–84) alone were approximately 2-fold greater than those in the combination or alendronate groups (25.5% PTH(1–84) vs 12.9% combination vs 10.5% alendronate; $P = .01$ between the PTH(1–84) and combination groups). Bone turnover markers in the combination group were similar to those seen in the group treated with alendronate alone, with a rapid decrease in markers of both formation and resorption. The superiority of PTH(1–84) therapy over combination therapy with the trabecular site analysis by QCT could be explained by the observation that the bone turnover markers in the combination-therapy group mirrored the alendronate-only arm, with rapid and sustained reductions. The PTH(1-84)-only arm showed the expected increase in bone turnover markers. Thus, the osteoanabolic potential of PTH(1–84) on trabecular bone was impaired by the simultaneous use of alendronate (**Fig. 4**).

Finkelstein and colleagues[21] used a similar experimental paradigm, but used PTH(1–34) instead of PTH(1–84) and men instead of women. Osteoporotic men (n = 83) were randomized to receive daily alendronate 10 mg (28 men), PTH(1–34) 40 µg (27 men), or the combination of both drugs (28 men). Alendronate was given for 30 months, with PTH(1–34) started at month 6 and continued for 24 months. The amount of daily PTH(1–34) was twice the 20 µg dose approved by the Food and Drug Administration. After 30 months, BMD at the lumbar spine by DXA increased to a greater extent in men treated with PTH(1–34) alone than in the other groups (18.1% PTH(1–34) vs 14.8% combination vs 7.9% alendronate; $P<.001$ for the 3-way comparison). Femoral neck BMD also increased to a greater extent in the group treated with PTH(1–34) alone (9.7% PTH(1–34) vs 6.2% combination vs 3.2% alendronate; $P = .001$). Increases in vertebral trabecular BMD by QCT were markedly higher with PTH(1–34) alone (48% PTH(1–34) vs 17% combination vs 3% alendronate; $P<.001$). Bone turnover markers in the combination group were again similar to those

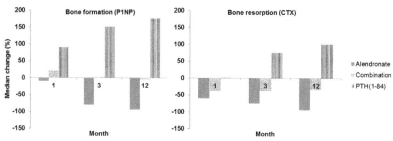

Fig. 4. Changes in markers of bone turnover in the different treatment groups in the Parathyroid Hormone and Alendronate for Osteoporosis (PaTH) study. Bone turnover markers in the combination-therapy group paralleled the alendronate-only arm. PTH, parathyroid hormone; ALN, alendronate; P1NP, N-propeptide of type I Collagen; CTX, C-terminal telopeptide of type I collagen. (*Data from* Black DM, Greenspan SL, Ensrud KE, et al. The effects of parathyroid hormone and alendronate alone or in combination in postmenopausal osteoporosis. N Engl J Med 2003;349:1207–15.)

seen in the group treated with alendronate alone, namely a rapid decrease in markers of both formation and resorption.[22] The study results are similar to those of the PaTH trial, suggesting that the impaired response to combination therapy, in contrast to PTH alone, might be due to the dominating effects of alendronate on bone remodeling dynamics when both drugs are used simultaneously.

The results of these 2 combination-therapy studies led to the concept that an antiresorptive agent that does not impair the anabolic actions of PTH to increase bone formation while mitigating its effects on bone resorption may lead to results that favor a combination-therapy approach. To this end, Deal and colleagues[23] explored the effects of raloxifene, an antiresorptive agent less potent than bisphosphonates, in combination with PTH(1–34) in a pilot, 6-month study of postmenopausal women. Bone formation markers increased to the same extent in the PTH(1–34) and combination groups. As hypothesized, when raloxifene was used in combination with PTH(1–34), bone resorption markers were significantly lower than in the PTH(1–34)-only group. The combination of PTH(1–34) and raloxifene had greater densitometric effects than did monotherapy with PTH(1–34), although the results were only statistically significant at the total hip. In the presence of raloxifene, PTH(1–34) appears to stimulate bone formation, unimpeded, but its ability to stimulate bone resorption is reduced. This pilot study needs to be followed by a longer-term study that more definitely establishes this concept.

Yet another approach has been taken by Cosman and colleagues,[24] whereby a single dose of zoledronic acid was given along with a course of daily PTH(1–34). This approach to combination therapy is based on animal studies of Gasser and colleagues[25] in which a single dose of bisphosphonate led to greater improvements in BMD in rats treated with concurrent PTH(1–34) than in rats treated with chronic bisphosphonate therapy. Cosman and colleagues[24] found that the combination of a single dose of zoledronic acid with daily PTH(1–34) in postmenopausal women was associated with a rapid reduction in bone turnover markers, but only transiently. This observation is different from the findings of the combination approaches summarized above, when daily use of bisphosphonate and PTH was associated with a sustained reduction in bone turnover markers. With the combination of zoledronic acid and PTH(1–34), BMD increased after 6 months at the spine and hip to a greater degree than either drug alone. However, the major differences after 6 months were much less apparent at the end of the 12-month study. At the lumbar spine, combination therapy was not greater than PTH(1–34) alone (7.3% vs 7.3%; *P* not significant); at the hip, the combination-therapy arm was not better than zoledronic acid alone (2.3% vs 2.2%; *P* not significant). However, if one looked at both sites, lumbar spine and hip, as composite end points, only combination therapy provided improvement in BMD that was greater than either zoledronic acid or PTH(1–34) alone.

ANTIRESORPTIVES AFTER OSTEOANABOLIC THERAPY

Kurland and colleagues[26] were the first to show that when PTH(1–34) is not followed by an antiresorptive agent, lumbar spine bone density falls precipitously. These investigators followed 21 men from their initial study[10] for up to 2 years after discontinuation of PTH(1–34), 12 of whom opted for immediate treatment with a bisphosponate following PTH(1–34). In the men who began bisphosphonate therapy immediately, there were continued gains of 5.1% at the lumbar spine, compared with a decline of 3.9% in the men not receiving bisphosphonate therapy. Within 1 year of completing PTH(1–34), 6 of the 9 men who had initially chosen no follow-up treatment decided to begin bisphosphonates. At 2 years of post-PTH follow-up, lumbar spine BMD improved by 2.6% in the delayed group, representing a BMD 0.8% below the post-PTH values. In the men who immediately started bisphosphonate therapy and continued treatment for the entire 2-year post-PTH period, there were gains of 8.9% at the lumbar spine above their post-PTH values.

This study was followed by the second phase of the PaTH study[27] in which a controlled, randomized, blinded, prospective study was designed to address the question as to whether antiresorptive therapy is necessary after PTH is discontinued. Postmenopausal women who had received PTH(1–84) for 12 months were randomly assigned to an additional 12 months of therapy with alendronate 10 mg daily or placebo. In subjects who received alendronate, there was a further 4.9% gain in lumbar spine BMD, whereas those who received placebo experienced a significant decline of 1.7%. By QCT analysis, the net increase over 24 months in trabecular spine BMD was 31% among those treated with alendronate after PTH(1–84), compared with 14% in the placebo group, with the placebo group experiencing an approximate 10% decline in trabecular BMD after discontinuation of PTH. There were similar, dramatic differences in hip BMD when those who followed PTH with alendronate were compared with those who were treated with placebo after PTH (13% vs 5%). The results of this study establish the importance of following PTH(1–84) or PTH(1–34) therapy with an antiresorptive to maintain or improve BMD.

Cosman and colleagues[28] studied postmenopausal women treated with concurrent PTH(1–34) and raloxifene for 12 months, followed by raloxifene alone for 12 months. Continued raloxifene only partially maintained PTH-induced BMD gains at the spine and hip. BMD declined by 0.7% to 2.9% (*P* not significant) at all sites except the femoral neck, where BMD increased modestly (+1.3%; *P* = .04). As a result of these data, the standard of care is now to follow the 2-year period of PTH therapy with an antiresorptive, preferably a bisphosphonate.

There are only observational data to provide guidance as to the question of fracture protection after discontinuation of PTH therapy. In a 30-month observational cohort following the pivotal Fracture Prevention Trial (FPT) of PTH(1–34),[29] subjects were given the option of bisphosphonate therapy or not taking any further medications after PTH(1–34).[30] A majority (60%) were treated with antiresorptive therapy at some time after PTH discontinuation, with greater use in the former placebo group. As noted from the PaTH trial, gains in BMD were maintained in those who elected to begin antiresorptive therapy immediately after PTH(1–34). There were progressive reductions in BMD noted throughout the 30-month observational period in subjects who elected not to follow PTH(1–34) with any therapy. In a group that began antiresorptive therapy 6 months after PTH(1–34) discontinuation, major reductions in BMD were seen during these first 6 months, but no further reductions were observed after antiresorptive therapy was instituted.[31] Despite these densitometric data, vertebral fracture risk was reduced by more than 40% in individuals previously treated with PTH(1–34) (with or without subsequent bisphosphonate therapy) compared with the former placebo group that persisted for as long as 18 months after PTH(1–34) discontinuation. In a logistic regression model, bisphosphonate use for 12 months or longer added little to overall risk reduction of new vertebral fractures in this posttreatment period. Nonvertebral fragility fractures 30 months after treatment discontinuation were reported by proportionately fewer women previously treated with PTH (followed with or without a bisphosphonate) compared with those treated with placebo (with or without a bisphosphonate; $P<.03$). However, the data for those who did or did not follow PTH(1–34) treatment with an antiresorptive were not separately analyzed. One may expect a residual but transient protection against fracture after PTH treatment without subsequent antiresorptive therapy, which would wane over time. Additional studies are needed to address fracture outcomes specifically. However, the results of the PaTH study and other trials establish the importance of treatment with an antiresorptive following PTH(1–34) or PTH(1–84) therapy to maintain increases in bone mass.

SAFETY

PTH therapy is well tolerated for the recommended 2-year treatment period. Clinical trials have shown a very small risk of hypercalcemia at the approved 20-µg dose.[29,32] Hypercalcemia is even less likely to occur if calcium supplementation is reduced to 500 mg/d with the initiation of PTH(1–34). PTH(1–34) does not appear to significantly increase urinary calcium excretion.[32,33] Other possible side effects of therapy include nausea, vomiting, dizziness, headache, and increased serum uric acid concentrations, but none of these other adverse events have been problematic clinically.[29]

In animal toxicity studies, male and female rats treated with PTH(1–34) or PTH(1–84) at doses 3 to 58 times the equivalent human dose for 75 years of equivalent human time develop osteosarcoma.[34] The results are consistent with exposure of an anabolic agent to an animal with persistence of growth plates throughout life and limited bone-remodeling capability. The uncontrolled, exuberant effects of PTH in rats are not seen in the human skeleton. In human subjects, the remodeling system eventually takes over after exposure to PTH(1–34) or PTH(1–84), limiting the extent to which PTH can stimulate bone formation in an uncontrolled manner. Clinical experience with PTH(1–34) now extends to more than 9 years. The number of reported cases of osteosarcoma in human subjects treated with PTH(1–34) does not exceed the level that one would expect on the basis of the epidemiology of osteosarcoma in the adult human population.[35,36] The data thus far do not support an epidemiologic or causal relationship between PTH and osteosarcoma in human subjects, although continued vigilance is necessary.

SUMMARY

With the availability of antiresorptives and osteoanabolic therapy for the treatment of osteoporosis, it is still unclear as to how and whether combination or sequential therapeutic approaches can be used in a manner that is advantageous over monotherapy. Despite many attempts to show an advantage of simultaneous combination therapy, most studies have shown that monotherapy with PTH(1–34) or PTH(1–84) is as good, if not better than, combination therapy with osteoanabolic and antiresorptive drugs.

Nevertheless, the importance of following PTH(1–34) or PTH(1–84) therapy with an antiresorptive agent to maintain increases in bone mass is clear.

REFERENCES

1. Lindsay R, Cosman F, Zhou H, et al. A novel tetracycline labeling schedule for longitudinal evaluation of the short-term effects of anabolic therapy with a single iliac crest bone biopsy: early actions of teriparatide. J Bone Miner Res 2006;21: 366–73.
2. Bilezikian JP. Combination anabolic and antiresorptive therapy for osteoporosis: opening the anabolic window. Curr Osteoporos Rep 2008;6:24–30.
3. Graeff C, Timm W, Nickelsen TN, et al. Monitoring teriparatide-associated changes in vertebral microstructure by high-resolution CT in vivo: results from the EUROFORS study. J Bone Miner Res 2007;22:1426–33.
4. Liberman UA, Weiss SR, Broll J, et al. Effect of oral alendronate on bone mineral density and the incidence of fractures in postmenopausal osteoporosis. The Alendronate Phase III Osteoporosis Treatment Study Group. N Engl J Med 1995;333:1437–43.
5. Harris ST, Watts NB, Genant HK, et al. Effects of risedronate treatment on vertebral and nonvertebral fractures in women with postmenopausal osteoporosis: a randomized controlled trial. Vertebral Efficacy With Risedronate Therapy (VERT) Study Group. JAMA 1999;282:1344–52.
6. Black DM, Delmas PD, Eastell R, et al. Once-yearly zoledronic acid for treatment of postmenopausal osteoporosis. N Engl J Med 2007;356:1809–22.
7. Saag KG, Zanchetta JR, Devogelaer JP, et al. Effects of teriparatide versus alendronate for treating glucocorticoid-induced osteoporosis: thirty-six-month results of a randomized, double-blind, controlled trial. Arthritis Rheum 2009;60: 3346–55.
8. Saag KG, Shane E, Boonen S, et al. Teriparatide or alendronate in glucocorticoid-induced osteoporosis. N Engl J Med 2007;357:2028–39.
9. Kurland ES, Cosman F, McMahon DJ, et al. Parathyroid hormone as a therapy for idiopathic osteoporosis in men: effects on bone mineral density and bone markers. J Clin Endocrinol Metab 2000;85:3069–76.
10. Ettinger B, San Martin J, Crans G, et al. Differential effects of teriparatide on BMD after treatment with raloxifene or alendronate. J Bone Miner Res 2004;19: 745–51.
11. Miller PD, Delmas PD, Lindsay R, et al. Early responsiveness of women with osteoporosis to teriparatide after therapy with alendronate or risedronate. J Clin Endocrinol Metab 2008;93:3785–93.
12. Boonen S, Marin F, Obermayer-Pietsch B, et al. Effects of previous antiresorptive therapy on the bone mineral density response to two years of teriparatide treatment in postmenopausal women with osteoporosis. J Clin Endocrinol Metab 2008;93: 852–60.
13. Boonen S, Milisen K, Gielen E, et al. Sequential therapy in the treatment of osteoporosis. Curr Med Res Opin 2011;27:1149–55.
14. Cusano NE, Bilezikian JP. Combination antiresorptive and osteoanabolic therapy for osteoporosis: we are not there yet. Curr Med Res Opin 2011;27:1705–7.
15. Cosman F, Wermers RA, Recknor C, et al. Effects of teriparatide in postmenopausal women with osteoporosis on prior alendronate or raloxifene: differences between stopping and continuing the antiresorptive agent. J Clin Endocrinol Metab 2009;94:3772–80.

16. Lindsay R, Nieves J, Formica C, et al. Randomised controlled study of effect of parathyroid hormone on vertebral-bone mass and fracture incidence among postmenopausal women on oestrogen with osteoporosis. Lancet 1997;350:550–5.
17. Lane NE, Sanchez S, Modin GW, et al. Parathyroid hormone treatment can reverse corticosteroid-induced osteoporosis. Results of a randomized controlled clinical trial. J Clin Invest 1998;102:1627–33.
18. Cosman F, Nieves J, Zion M, et al. Daily and cyclic parathyroid hormone in women receiving alendronate. N Engl J Med 2005;353:566–75.
19. Cusano NE, Bilezikian JP. Teriparatide: variations on the theme of a 2-year therapeutic course. IBMS Bone Key 2010;7:84–7.
20. Black DM, Greenspan SL, Ensrud KE, et al. The effects of parathyroid hormone and alendronate alone or in combination in postmenopausal osteoporosis. N Engl J Med 2003;349:1207–15.
21. Finkelstein JS, Hayes A, Hunzelman JL, et al. The effects of parathyroid hormone, alendronate, or both in men with osteoporosis. N Engl J Med 2003;349:1216–26.
22. Finkelstein JS, Leder BZ, Burnett SM, et al. Effects of teriparatide, alendronate, or both on bone turnover in osteoporotic men. J Clin Endocrinol Metab 2006;91:2882–7.
23. Deal C, Omizo M, Schwartz EN, et al. Combination teriparatide and raloxifene therapy for postmenopausal osteoporosis: results from a 6-month double-blind placebo-controlled trial. J Bone Miner Res 2005;20:1905–11.
24. Cosman F, Eriksen EF, Recknor C, et al. Effects of intravenous zoledronic acid plus subcutaneous teriparatide [rhPTH(1-34)] in postmenopausal osteoporosis. J Bone Miner Res 2011;26:503–11.
25. Gasser JA, Ingold P, Venturiere-Rebmann A, et al. Chronic subcutaneous, but not single intravenous, dosing of rats with bisphosphonates results in reduced bone anabolic response to PTH. In: American Society for Bone and Mineral Research 28th Annual Meeting. Philadelphia, September 15–19, 2006: F386; SA386.
26. Kurland ES, Heller SL, Diamond B, et al. The importance of bisphosphonate therapy in maintaining bone mass in men after therapy with teriparatide [human parathyroid hormone(1-34)]. Osteoporos Int 2004;15:992–7.
27. Black DM, Bilezikian JP, Ensrud KE, et al. One year of alendronate after one year of parathyroid hormone (1-84) for osteoporosis. N Engl J Med 2005;353:555–65.
28. Cosman F, Nieves JW, Zion M, et al. Effect of prior and ongoing raloxifene therapy on response to PTH and maintenance of BMD after PTH therapy. Osteoporos Int 2008;19:529–35.
29. Neer RM, Arnaud CD, Zanchetta JR, et al. Effect of parathyroid hormone (1-34) on fractures and bone mineral density in postmenopausal women with osteoporosis. N Engl J Med 2001;344:1434–41.
30. Lindsay R, Scheele WH, Neer R, et al. Sustained vertebral fracture risk reduction after withdrawal of teriparatide in postmenopausal women with osteoporosis. Arch Intern Med 2004;164:2024–30.
31. Prince R, Sipos A, Hossain A, et al. Sustained nonvertebral fragility fracture risk reduction after discontinuation of teriparatide treatment. J Bone Miner Res 2005;20:1507–13.
32. Orwoll ES, Scheele WH, Paul S, et al. The effect of teriparatide [human parathyroid hormone (1-34)] therapy on bone density in men with osteoporosis. J Bone Miner Res 2003;18:9–17.
33. Kaufman JM, Orwoll E, Goemaere S, et al. Teriparatide effects on vertebral fractures and bone mineral density in men with osteoporosis: treatment and discontinuation of therapy. Osteoporos Int 2005;16:510–6.

34. Vahle JL, Sato M, Long GG, et al. Skeletal changes in rats given daily subcutaneous injections of recombinant human parathyroid hormone (1-34) for 2 years and relevance to human safety. Toxicol Pathol 2002;30:312–21.

35. Harper KD, Krege JH, Marcus R, et al. Comments on Initial experience with teriparatide in the United States. Curr Med Res Opin 2006;22:1927.

36. Harper KD, Krege JH, Marcus R, et al. Osteosarcoma and teriparatide? J Bone Miner Res 2007;22:334.

Future Directions in Osteoporosis Therapeutics

Henry Bone, MD

KEYWORDS

• Osteoporosis • Osteocytes • Antiresorptives • Anabolic agents

In the coming years we can expect to see a transition from the twentieth-century medications that have had such a great impact on osteoporosis treatment to newer medications and new ways of using the old drugs, perhaps with more systematic sequential or coordinated therapies.

OLDER ANTIRESORPTIVES

Bisphosphonates

Bisphosphonates have played a very important role in establishing efficacious treatment of osteoporosis for a wide range of patients. Alendronate is generic in most countries at the time of writing, and other bisphosphonates will be soon. Thus there are widely available, relatively inexpensive medications requiring weekly or monthly, oral or parenteral administration, with reasonably good, well-established efficacy and limited toxicity. Some controversies have arisen over safety and tolerability, especially regarding the rare problems of osteonecrosis of the jaw[1] and atypical femoral fractures.[2] These concerns may become lesser or greater impediments to the use of these medications as more experienced is gained. Provided concerns about toxicity and tolerability do not increase, the cost-effectiveness of generic bisphosphonates will keep them in an important role for the foreseeable future, as constraining the cost of medications assumes ever greater priority. These medications may turn out to be important in coordinated therapeutic regimens[3,4] as well as for continued use in monotherapy.

Calcitonin

Salmon calcitonin was initially introduced as a subcutaneously injected medication, but considerations including cost, convenience, and tolerability led to the introduction of the more popular nasal alternative. At present, several oral formulations of salmon calcitonin are being developed and a recent report indicates an improved effect on bone mineral density.[5] The main concern about calcitonin for the clinical treatment of osteoporosis has been that the efficacy is relatively modest. However, the

Section of Endocrinology and Metabolism, Michigan Bone and Mineral Clinic, St. John Hospital and Medical Center, 22201 Moross Road, Detroit, Michigan 48236, USA
E-mail address: hgbone.md@att.net

Endocrinol Metab Clin N Am 41 (2012) 655–661
doi:10.1016/j.ecl.2012.05.003
0889-8529/12/$ – see front matter © 2012 Published by Elsevier Inc.

exceptional safety record of calcitonin may make it a therapeutic option for some individuals with moderate fracture risk, particularly if the newer preparations result in even modest improvements in efficacy. A recent meta-analysis found a convincing reduction in acute pain after vertebral compression fractures,[6] and the use of calcitonin for this purpose is likely to continue.

HORMONE THERAPY IN THE PREVENTION AND MANAGEMENT OF OSTEOPOROSIS

The most important factor in the pathogenesis of postmenopausal osteoporosis is the absence of adequate levels of estrogen for the control of bone remodeling. In comparative clinical trials, estrogen has been shown to be comparable with oral bisphosphonate treatment in controlling bone turnover and increasing bone density.[7,8] The antifracture efficacy reported from the Women's Health Initiative places estrogen on a par with efficacious antiresorptive agents.[9] Estrogen can of course mitigate or eliminate most of the symptoms encountered by postmenopausal women, such as vasomotor flushing, vaginal atrophy, and so forth.[10] This fact makes hormone products particularly attractive in the early postmenopausal years, and this has led to emphasis on the role of estrogen in the prevention of osteoporosis. Hormone therapy became controversial as a result of the Women's Health Initiative. The issues or controversies with estrogen therapy are related to the effects on other organs besides bone, and this has been extensively discussed.[10] Noteworthy is that for women initiating hormone therapy in the usual period before age 60 years there was an overall favorable effect on all-cause mortality.[11] The results were particularly favorable in the case of women who had undergone hysterectomy and therefore took estrogens without medroxyprogesterone.[12] However, in women older than 70 years, and especially those taking combination conjugated equine estrogen plus medroxyprogesterone acetate, there were a sufficient number of unfavorable events to outweigh the benefits when women of all ages were combined in the originally published analysis.[9] As the subsequent analyses have been published and follow-up analyses are reported, it is increasingly clear that for substantial number of earlier postmenopausal women estrogen is a reasonable intermediate-term option for prevention or treatment of postmenopausal bone loss.[10,13] The use in established osteoporosis has not been as extensively explored, but the available results are favorable.[14,15] The fact that estrogen reduces pro-osteolytic signaling to osteoclasts, directly blocking bone resorption, may contribute to its utility in conjunction with anabolic agents, such as parathyroid hormone derivatives.[16,17]

NEWER ANTIRESORPTIVES
RANK Ligand Blockade

Control of accelerated bone resorption continues to be a mainstay of antiosteoporotic treatment. Denosumab is a recently introduced monoclonal antibody that blocks the effect of RANK ligand on the osteoclast lineage.[18] This extremely potent antiresorptive agent has produced a sustained progressive effect on bone density with what appears to be less attenuation of the rate of gain after the first few years than has been seen with other potent antiresorptive drugs.[19] This finding suggests that the remodeling transient and maturation of bone mineral may not be the only important factors driving the increase in bone density. In clinical trials, the antifracture efficacy during the blinded 3-year initial observation period was highly significant and comparable with the better results achieved with other antiresorptive medications.[20] However, clinical data on patients with degrees of immunosuppression attributable to steroid exposure, transplantation, and so forth remain to be obtained.

Safety information regarding denosumab is generally reassuring thus far, but unfortunately the product information lists several "adverse reactions" that were not significantly different in rate between the active treatment group and placebo controls. This has resulted in considerable concern on the part of many patients. Overall adverse events were quite well balanced versus the placebo control in the randomized trials, with some apparent specific differences. Mortality was nonsignificantly lower in the active treatment group.[20] The crossover extension study has not demonstrated any worsening trends to date,[19] and imbalances in certain adverse-event categories reported in years 1 to 3 do not appear to be reproduced in those individuals crossed over from placebo to active treatment. Osteonecrosis of the jaw, however, has been reported in a small number of cases.[19] As dosed, denosumab has the interesting pharmacodynamic property of allowing some release of bone remodeling from control at about the end of the 6-month dosing interval after an injection. This property may lend itself to some form of coordinated or cyclic treatment paradigm, but this has yet to be elucidated (see the article by Bilezikian elsewhere in this issue).

Cathepsin K Inhibition

The osteoclast resorbs bone under the ruffled border by extrusion of acid into the confined space, thereby dissolving bone mineral, and by means of cathepsin K, a proteolytic enzyme that is active at low pH. It is this enzyme that is principally responsible for digestion of bone matrix. Several pharmaceutical companies have attempted to produce cathepsin K inhibitors as therapeutics for osteoporosis. Some of these have been unsuccessful because of toxicity or tolerability issues.[21] The bulk of the available clinical data comes from odanacatib.[22,23] This mechanism appears to blunt bone resorption with very little effect on bone formation. It is thought that the rate of bone formation is responsive to signaling by matrix proteins that are liberated by osteoclasts as well as molecules that are directly produced by the osteoclasts themselves. Numerous candidates have been nominated as important signaling molecules, but at the time of writing it is not clear which are the most important or how these substances may interact with signal osteoblasts. In any case, this class, uniquely among clinically developed antiresorptives, appears to decrease bone resorption with little or no sustained decrease in bone formation.[24] It should be noted that because widely used bone resorption markers are actual products of cathepsin K action, the degree to which bone resorption is actually suppressed could be overestimated by measurement of N-telopeptide or C-telopeptide. Extension of the phase II study of odanacatib has demonstrated a progressive increase in bone-density measurements.[25] The finding that bone formation can be maintained despite decreased bone resorption may make this mechanism especially suitable for use in conjunction with one or more anabolic agents.

ANABOLIC AGENTS
Teriparatide and Parathyroid Hormone

Teriparatide is the 1–34 N-terminal fragment of parathyroid hormone. Teriparatide has been extensively used and is widely registered for the treatment of osteoporosis, and parathyroid hormone(1–84) is available in several countries for the same indication. As discussed by Leder and Uihlein elsewhere in this issue, parathyroid hormone acts directly on osteoblasts to stimulate bone formation. There is a secondary stimulation of bone resorption, but by appropriate timing of the systemic exposure to increased parathyroid hormone (PTH) levels, the anabolic effect can be emphasized. By contrast, sustained elevation of parathyroid hormone such as seen in primary or secondary hyperparathyroidism can have a predominantly catabolic effect on bone.

Attempts have been made to emulate the effect of teriparatide with PTH secreta-gogues, but this has not worked out very well so far, perhaps because of overly pro-longed PTH exposure with insufficient recovery between doses.[26] Such medications may be important in the future if extremely short "spikes" of PTH can be induced, but improved pharmacokinetics and pharmacodynamics will be required if this approach is to be successful. Analogues of parathyroid hormone and PTH-related protein, acting on the common receptor may prove to be important anabolic agents if they can be shown to have improved therapeutic profiles or reduced adverse effects.

Sclerostin Blockade

As reviewed by Leder and Uihlein elsewhere in this issue, sclerostin is an endogenous regulator of Wnt signaling, produced by cells of the osteoblast/osteocyte lineage. Sclerostin suppresses bone formation and increases bone resorption. A new strategy for the enhancement of bone formation is the inhibition of sclerostin signaling, specif-ically with a monoclonal antibody. Conceivably, a small molecule might also be used if one could be successfully designed. Clinical trials are under way with an antisclerostin antibody, but the trial results are not yet in the public domain. Whether consolidation therapy will be required after sclerostin blockade remains to be seen.

COORDINATED THERAPY

Coordinated therapy, the systematic concurrent or sequential use of 2 or more drugs, has been discussed for many years and is reviewed by Bilezikian elsewhere in this issue. The original paradigm was introduced by Harold Frost many years ago.[27] The nearest practical illustration was follow-up treatment with alendronate after parathyroid hormone in the extension of the phase II parathyroid hormone study[4] and in the PATH trial.[3] The paradigm of the anabolic stimulatory drug followed by the antiresorptive agent is consistent with Frost's early suggestions and may well turn out to be one that will endure, in part because of the inherent biological logic and also because from a pharma-coeconomic standpoint, the anabolic agents, which are thus far relatively expensive, are more appealing if they can be used for a limited period of time. Thus they could accel-erate an increase in bone density, to be followed by consolidation with generally less expensive agents afterward. It is difficult to imagine more potent antiresorptive drugs than those that are currently available. For this reason, it seems unlikely that newer anti-resorptive drugs will produce substantially greater gains in bone density or antifracture effect than are achieved with the potent bisphosphonates and denosumab. It also seems likely that there may be practical limitations to the use of potent anabolic agents, whether using the parathyroid hormone mechanism or Wnt signaling, or other mechanisms. Therefore, it seems almost inevitable that some form of therapeutic coordination will be necessary to optimize long-term results in patients with osteoporosis.

Stumbling blocks or impediments to the achievement of ideal coordinated treat-ment regimens include regulatory restrictions on the simultaneous use of 2 investiga-tional drugs. The challenges are increased when agents that might be particularly useful in coordination with each other are not sponsored by the same company. This situation adds complexity to the coordination of development programs, and is another reason why such regimens are more likely to be investigated late in the life cycle of at least one of the drugs. Furthermore, reimbursement pressure from govern-ments and other insurers may be an impediment to the development of new drugs for addressing osteoporosis, as well as for other indications. Another important consider-ation as we go forward is the perhaps disproportionate concern on the part of patients about possible adverse effects that have been so widely publicized. Addressing concerns about long-term safety and cost-effectiveness will make long-term trial extensions increasingly important, but will add to the cost of development.

FUTURE TARGETS

It is increasingly clear that osteocytes have a central role in the regulation of bone-cell activity and ultimately the biomechanical properties of bone.[28] Many of the functions of Frost's hypothetical mechanostat[29] are evidently performed by osteocytes. A better understanding of the relationship between current and investigational agents and osteocyte function may lead to important insights into the regulation of bone strength and perhaps ultimately to specific therapeutic agents. More specific modulation of osteocyte function by novel agents may eventually lead to optimized bone mass. Insights into the specific contributions of bone structural elements to the important biomechanical properties of intact bones may also lead to new therapies and a better understanding of old ones. For instance, the biomechanical contribution of bone diameter suggests that a focus on periosteal bone apposition may prove fruitful.[30,31]

One of the great current challenges in the treatment of osteoporosis is actual implementation of the useful treatments that are already available. The extent to which new medications and treatment paradigms address this implementation challenge will be an important determinant of their success.

REFERENCES

1. Khosla S, Burr D, Cauley J, et al. Bisphosphonate-associated osteonecrosis of the jaw: report of a task force of the American Society for Bone and Mineral Research. J Bone Miner Res 2007;22(10):1479–91.
2. Shane E, Burr D, Ebeling PR, et al. Atypical subtrochanteric and diaphyseal femoral fractures: report of a task force of the American Society for Bone and Mineral Research. J Bone Miner Res 2010;25(11):2267–94.
3. Rittmaster RS, Bolognese M, Ettinger MP, et al. Enhancement of bone mass in osteoporotic women with parathyroid hormone followed by alendronate. J Clin Endocrinol Metab 2000;85(6):2129–34.
4. Black DM, Bilezikian JP, Ensrud KE, et al. One year of alendronate after one year of parathyroid hormone (1-84) for osteoporosis. N Engl J Med 2005;353(6):555–65.
5. Binkley N, Bolognese M, Sidorowicz-Bialynicka A, et al. A phase 3 trial of the efficacy and safety or oral recombinant calcitonin: the ORACAL trial. J Bone Miner Res 2012. DOI: 10.1002/jbmr.1602.
6. Knopp-Sihota JA, Newburn-Cook CV, Homik J, et al. Calcitonin for treating acute and chronic pain of recent and remote osteoporotic vertebral compression fractures: a systematic review and meta-analysis. Osteoporos Int 2012;23(1):17–38.
7. Bone HG, Greenspan SL, McKeever C, et al. Alendronate and estrogen effects in postmenopausal women with low bone mineral density. Alendronate/Estrogen Study Group. J Clin Endocrinol Metab 2000;85(2):720–6.
8. Greenspan SL, Resnick NM, Parker RA. Combination therapy with hormone replacement and alendronate for prevention of bone loss in elderly women: a randomized controlled trial. JAMA 2003;289(19):2525–33.
9. Rossouw JE, Anderson GL, Prentice RL, et al. Risks and benefits of estrogen plus progestin in healthy postmenopausal women: principal results from the Women's Health Initiative randomized controlled trial. JAMA 2002;88(3):321–33.
10. North American Menopause Society. The 2012 hormone therapy position statement of: the North American Menopause Society. Menopause 2012;19(3): 257–71.

11. Rossouw JE, Prentice RL, Manson JE, et al. Postmenopausal hormone therapy and risk of cardiovascular disease by age and years since menopause. JAMA 2007;297(13):1465–77.

12. Anderson GL, Limacher M, Assaf AR, et al. Effects of conjugated equine estrogen in postmenopausal women with hysterectomy: the Women's Health Initiative randomized controlled trial. JAMA 2004;291(14):1701–12.

13. Stevenson JC. A woman's journey through the reproductive, transitional and post-menopausal periods of life: impact on cardiovascular and musculo-skeletal risk and the role of estrogen replacement. Maturitas 2011;70(2):197–205.

14. Lindsay R, Hart DM, Aitken JM, et al. Long-term prevention of postmenopausal osteoporosis by oestrogen. Evidence for an increased bone mass after delayed onset of oestrogen treatment. Lancet 1976;1(7968):1038–41.

15. Lufkin EG, Wahner HW, O'Fallon WM, et al. Treatment of postmenopausal osteo-porosis with transdermal estrogen. Ann Intern Med 1992;117(1):1–9.

16. Lane NE, Sanchez S, Modin GW, et al. Parathyroid hormone treatment can reverse corticosteroid-induced osteoporosis. Results of a randomized controlled clinical trial. J Clin Invest 1998;102(8):1627–33.

17. Lindsay R, Nieves J, Formica C, et al. Randomised controlled study of effect of para-thyroid hormone on vertebral-bone mass and fracture incidence among postmen-opausal women on oestrogen with osteoporosis. Lancet 1997;350(9077):550–5.

18. Stolina M, Kostenuik PJ, Dougall WC, et al. RANKL inhibition: from mice to men (and women). Adv Exp Med Biol 2007;602:143–50.

19. Papapoulos S, Chapurlat R, Libanati C, et al. Five years of denosumab exposure in women with postmenopausal osteoporosis: results from the first two years of the FREEDOM extension. J Bone Miner Res 2012. [Epub ahead of print]. DOI: 10.1002/jbmr.1479.

20. Cummings SR, San Martin J, McClung MR, et al. FREEDOM Trial. Denosumab for prevention of fractures in postmenopausal women with osteoporosis [Erratum in: N Engl J Med. 2009 Nov 5;361(19):1914]. N Engl J Med 2009;361(8):756–65.

21. Rünger TM, Adami S, Benhamou CL, et al. Morphea-like skin reactions in patients treated with the cathepsin K inhibitor balicatib. J Am Acad Dermatol 2012;66(3): e89–96.

22. Bone HG, McClung MR, Roux C, et al. Odanacatib, a cathepsin-K inhibitor for osteoporosis: a two-year study in postmenopausal women with low bone density. J Bone Miner Res 2010;25(5):937–47.

23. Eisman JA, Bone HG, Hosking DJ, et al. Odanacatib in the treatment of postmen-opausal women with low bone mineral density: three-year continued therapy and resolution of effect. J Bone Miner Res 2011;26(2):242–51. DOI: 10.1002/jbmr.212.

24. Costa AG, Cusano NE, Silva BC, et al. Cathepsin K: its skeletal actions and role as a therapeutic target in osteoporosis. Nat Rev Rheumatol 2011;7(8):447–56. DOI: 10.1038/nrrheum.2011.77.

25. Binkley N, Bone H, Gilchrist N, et al. Treatment with the cathepsin K inhibitor oda-nacatib in postmenopausal women with low BMD: 5 year results of a phase 2 trial. Presented at the American Society of Bone & Mineral Research Meeting. San Diego, September 16-20, 2011.

26. Fitzpatrick LA, Dabrowski CE, Cicconetti G, et al. The effects of ronacaleret, a calcium-sensing receptor antagonist, on bone mineral density and biochemical markers of bone turnover in postmenopausal women with low bone mineral density. J Clin Endocrinol Metab 2011;96(8):2441–9.

27. Frost HM. Treatment of osteoporosis by manipulation of coherent bone cell pop-ulations. Clin Orthop Relat Res 1979;(143):227–44.

28. Bonewald LF. The amazing osteocyte. J Bone Miner Res 2011;26(2):229–38. DOI: 10.1002/jbmr.320.
29. Frost HM. The mechanostat: a proposed pathogenic mechanism of osteoporosis and the bone mass effects of mechanical and nonmechanical agents. Bone Miner 1987;2(2):73–85.
30. Davison KS, Siminoski K, Adachi JD, et al. Bone strength: the whole is greater than the sum of its parts. Semin Arthritis Rheum 2006;36(1):22–31.
31. Turner CH. Biomechanics of bone: determinants of skeletal fragility and bone quality. Osteoporos Int 2002;13(2):97–104.

Index

Note: Page numbers of article titles are in **boldface** type.

Endocrinol Metab Clin N Am 41 (2012) 663–678
http://dx.doi.org/10.1016/S0889-8529(12)00086-2
0889-8529/12/$ – see front matter © 2012 Elsevier Inc. All rights reserved.

endo.theclinics.com

Moving?

Make sure your subscription moves with you!

To notify us of your new address, find your **Clinics Account Number** (located on your mailing label above your name), and contact customer service at:

Email: journalscustomerservice-usa@elsevier.com

800-654-2452 (subscribers in the U.S. & Canada)
314-447-8871 (subscribers outside of the U.S. & Canada)

Fax number: 314-447-8029

Elsevier Health Sciences Division
Subscription Customer Service
3251 Riverport Lane
Maryland Heights, MO 63043

*To ensure uninterrupted delivery of your subscription, please notify us at least 4 weeks in advance of move.

Printed and bound by CPI Group (UK) Ltd, Croydon, CR0 4YY

03/10/2024

01040459-0002